W0043047

Acquired Immunodeficiency Syndrome

Current Issues and Scientific Studies

Acquired Immunodeficiency Syndrome

Current Issues and Scientific Studies

EDITED BY

PASCAL JAMES IMPERATO, M.D.

The Medical Society of the State of New York
Lake Success, New York

PLENUM MEDICAL BOOK COMPANY
NEW YORK AND LONDON

Library of Congress Cataloging in Publication Data

Acquired Immunodeficiency Syndrome: current issues and scientific studies /
edited by Pascal James Imperato.
    p.   cm.
A collection of articles originally appearing in the New York State journal of
medicine.
Includes bibliographies and index.

ISBN-13: 978-1-4612-8092-7   e-ISBN-13: 978-1-4613-0807-2
DOI: 10.1007/978-1-4613-0807-2

1. AIDS (Disease) I. Imperato, Pascal James. II. New York State journal of
medicine.
[DNLM: 1. Acquired Immunodeficiency Syndrome—collected works. WD 308
A186545]
RC607.A26A3414   1989
616.97′92—dc19
DNLM/DLC   88-13378
for Library of Congress   CIP

This volume consists of reprints of articles from the
New York State Journal of Medicine, issues of May 1987,
February 1988, and May 1988, supplemented with a new introduction.

© 1989 Medical Society of the State of New York

Softcover reprint of the hardcover 1st edition 1989

Plenum Medical Book Company is an imprint of Plenum Publishing Corporation
233 Spring Street, New York, N.Y. 10013

All rights reserved

No part of this book may be reproduced, stored in a retrieval system, or transmitted
in any form or by any means, electronic, mechanical, photocopying, microfilming,
recording, or otherwise, without written permission from the Publisher

Printed on acid-free paper

Foreword

When Pascal James Imperato, MD, assumed the editorship of the *New York State Journal of Medicine* in 1986, the acquired immunodeficiency syndrome (AIDS) epidemic in the United States was already six years old. During the time of his editorship, two thematic issues of the *Journal* have been devoted to AIDS. In addition, a large number of original communications have been regularly published on the subject. This volume brings together important articles published on AIDS in the *Journal* during 1987 and 1988.

In the early years of the epidemic the Medical Society of the State of New York (MSSNY) was aware that it had a responsibility to both the profession and the public to add its efforts to those already mobilized in the attempt to understand and control this tragic disease. Early on, the MSSNY thought that its efforts would be best spent on public education. However, as both state and federal legislatures followed ages of precedent in the belief that all problems can be solved by passing laws, the MSSNY felt that there was an urgency for educating legislators. Apparently it was not alone in this belief, for the MSSNY received an invitation from New York's Senator Daniel Patrick Moynihan to present a symposium on AIDS to him and his Washington, DC, staff. The senator invited all the New York State congressmen and their aides to attend the symposium. This first effort of the MSSNY took place in the spring of 1987 and was very well received by those who attended.

As a consequence of this experience the MSSNY leadership appointed a task force on AIDS in the summer of 1987 and charged it to work with all divisions of the MSSNY, chiefly the Division of Scientific and Educational Activities and the Division of Communications, and to coordinate all AIDS-related activities of the MSSNY. Administration, legal counsel, and the Division of Governmental Affairs were soon included in the task force. The Committee on Preventive Medicine, a committee in the Division of Scientific and Educational Activities, had been far ahead of everyone else in the MSSNY in its knowledge of the AIDS epidemic and in its thinking as to the part MSSNY should play. The task force has been expertly guided by this committee and its gifted chairman, Duncan W. Clark, MD, in all of its activities.

Soon after its formation, the task force recommended to the MSSNY council, with subsequent council approval, a series of positions which resulted in the adoption of a Position Paper on AIDS. This included detailed statements on the following subjects:

- Prevention and control of human immunodeficiency virus (HIV) infection
- The role of the physician in HIV surveillance
- Drug abuse and HIV infection
- The physician's duty to treat

- Exclusion by the New York State Department of Health of qualified laboratories from HIV testing
- Protection of health care workers
- Responsibilities of physicians and other health care workers
- Public education
- AIDS confidentiality

The Symposium on AIDS in Washington, DC, had been so successful that the MSSNY, under the auspices of the task force and the Division of Governmental Affairs, held two informational symposia for state senators and assemblymen and their staffs in Albany, New York. These were presented in February 1988 and March 1989. This effort has convinced the MSSNY that it has given legislators a better understanding of the overall AIDS problem. This, hopefully, will lead to cooperative efforts at helpful legislation.

Recent efforts taken by the MSSNY at the behest of the task force and the Committee on Preventive Medicine, chaired by Dr Duncan W. Clark, have included a request that the New York State Department of Health make available to county health departments helpful information contained in its Health Data Base, with due regard for existing statutes on confidentiality and discrimination. The MSSNY also called on the American Medical Association to adopt the position that "states should apply the same public health measures to contain the HIV epidemic as are used to control the spread of other communicable and sexually transmissible diseases" and also to take the position that "physicians are permitted to test patients for the presence of HIV infections in the same manner as they currently test for other infections and conditions."

A further effort at public education on AIDS is presently being planned as a joint project of MSSNY and its Auxiliary. This will be a statewide effort to educate parents, school board members, teachers, and students. David M. Benford, MD, and Mrs Marie Rizzutto, presidents of MSSNY and the Auxiliary, respectively, are spearheading this with the task force.

In assembling this large collection of papers on AIDS Dr Imperato has taken on a prodigious task. It is hoped that this book will demonstrate the need for continued, careful, and extensive research into the methods of spread of AIDS in all groups and the importance of both professional and public education in this area. The latter should begin in the early years of elementary school with proper care and consideration for the sensitivities of all segments of the population.

George J. Lawrence, Jr, MD
Chairman
AIDS Task Force
Medical Society of the State of New York

Contents

Part II. Overviews

Part III. Current Issues and Opinions

Part IV. Case Studies

Part V. Appendixes

Introduction

The epidemic of acquired immunodeficiency syndrome (AIDS) is now moving through its ninth documented year in the United States. Unlike other epidemics of this century, this one has posed unique problems because of the nature and characteristics of the causative viral agent, the relatively long incubation period from infection to clinical signs and symptoms, and the long period of communicability. It has appeared both in high technology societies such as those in the United States and Europe, and in developing areas, exemplified by sub-Sahara Africa. Vaccines for prevention and effective therapeutic agents for cure are still years away, forcing reliance on older methodologies of prevention and on high-technology supportive interventions for keeping patients with the disease alive. These basic characteristics plus the current social determinants of the disease have presented Americans with a number of social, medical, political, and economic issues that are now the focus of much public discussion and, in some instances, heated debate.

The contents of this book were originally published in various issues of the *New York State Journal of Medicine* during 1987 and 1988. They have now been pulled together and organized in a manner so as to provide easy access to them by a wide range of readers. The book is organized into 40 chapters which in turn are subdivided into four sections: Research Studies, Overviews, Current Issues and Opinions, and Case Studies. A final section consists of six appendices.

The chapters cover a broad range of topics and opinions contributed by a national authorship and reflect the complexity of the challenges posed by the disease. On the positive side, they demonstrate how inexorable has been the advance of our knowledge about AIDS and the high degree of societal commitment to dealing with the disease and all of the problems associated with it. From the perspective of 1989 this represents a marked advance forward from 1981 when the disease was first reported in the United States. It is useful to look backward briefly to remind ourselves about just how far we have come. For if the past is any predictor of the future, our advances in the several years ahead should be no less dramatic.

On June 5, 1981, the Centers for Disease Control (CDC) reported five cases of *Pneumocystis carinii* pneumonia among sexually active homosexual men.[1] The report stated that "All of the above observations suggest the possibility of a cellular-immune dysfunction related to a common exposure that predisposes individuals to opportunistic infections such as pneumocystosis and candidia-sis."[1] Within a short period of time the disease that had only been observed among homosexual men was found among other "at risk" groups, including intravenous (IV) drug users, recent Haitian immigrants, hemophiliacs, sexual partners of those who had the disease, recipients of blood transfusions, and infants of mothers with the disease or at risk for it.[2] In late 1982 the CDC promulgated a surveillance definition for AIDS.[3] The epidemic was underway.

Early on, several groups of medical scientists began what would prove to be a fruitful search for the causative agent of the disease. In 1983 research produced suggestive evidence that the agent might be a human retrovirus, which was later isolated and called by a variety of names, including LAV (lymphadenopathy-associated virus), HTLV-III (human T-cell lymphotrophic virus type III), and ARV (AIDS-associated retrovirus).[4,5] For a few years the combined acronyms HTLV-III/LAV were used in the medical literature to describe the virus. The term human immunodeficiency virus (HIV) was later proposed as a generic term as the various early isolates of the retrovirus were found to be closely related.[6] This term is now widely used for the causative agent of AIDS.

As of December 31, 1988, a total of 82,764 cases of AIDS had been reported to the CDC in the United States. Of these, 32,311 (28,432 men; 3,296 women; 583 children) had been reported in the previous 12 months. Fifty-six percent of all patients with AIDS had died by the end of 1988. Among those diagnosed before 1986, 85% had died.[7] Although the annual number of reported AIDS cases has increased, the rate of increase has generally declined. Among men with AIDS, 68% have had a history of homosexual/bisexual activity without intravenous (IV) drug abuse, 17% a history of IV drug abuse without homosexual/bisexual contacts, and 8% a history of homosexual activity and IV drug abuse.[7] Between 1987 and 1988, the proportion of men with homosexual/bisexual behavior histories and no IV drug abuse fell from 70% to 63%. Men with a history of IV drug abuse constituted 20% of AIDS cases in 1988.[7] Significant proportions of blacks and Hispanics are infected with AIDS because of IV drug abuse or because they are the sex partners or children of IV drug abusers.[7] Among the 6,983 women reported with AIDS as of December 31, 1988, 52% had histories of IV drug abuse and 18% had sex partners with histories of IV drug abuse.[7] As of March 21, 1988, 84,246 cases had been reported worldwide from 136 countries or territories. Of these, 10,973 had been reported from Africa, 61,602 from the Americas, and 10,616 from Europe.[8] The United States accounts for the vast majority of cases (90%) reported in the Americas.[8] Reported cases in many areas of the world are not a valid measure of the true incidence of the disease since under-reporting is common.

Several chapters in this book deal with the epidemiology of AIDS in Connecticut, New Jersey, New York City, and New York State. They reveal how different the pattern of the disease can be in contiguous geographic areas because of a variety of determinants.

The epidemiologic evidence gathered to date demonstrates that susceptibility to the disease may be general. The incubation period varies from a minimum of a few months after exposure to several years. Transmission primarily occurs from person to person through sexual contact, through the sharing of contaminated IV injection equipment, through the transfusion of blood or blood products, and transplacentally. Issues such as the role, if any, of either superinfection or reinfection in the clinical course of the disease have not yet been elucidated. Communicability probably exists from the start of the asymptomatic period through the development of the opportunistic diseases that characterize the clinical course of AIDS. The disease is now widely spread throughout the world and from the vantage point of 1989 it is likely that this spread will continue. The absence of cases in specific geographic areas may be more reflective of the failure to detect the disease and report it than to zero incidence.

In many countries of the third world and particularly in sub-Sahara Africa there is a reluctance to acknowledge the disease's existence. Yet this region of the world is the most affected by it. Denial has its roots in a complex web involving national pride, fear of being stigmatized and suffering economic repercussions (such as the loss of tourism), and concern about the local, social, and political consequences of admitting to a major problem for which remedial resources are unavailable. In some African countries such as Kenya, where studies of female prostitutes have shown that close to 60% are infected with HIV, citizens have been told to ignore what national leaders characterize as "malicious propaganda emanating from outside the country."[9] Yet in other countries such as Zaire there has been a frank recognition of the problem and constructive steps have been taken to deal with it.[10] In Kenya, with 600,000 foreign tourists a year, concern runs high about the economic, social, and political consequences of a reactive fall-off of visitors fearful of AIDS. Yet even there, where the disease is progressively spreading, positive public health efforts are being taken. Among these are universal screening of all blood donations for AIDS and large-scale health education programs.[9]

In this book Quinn provides an excellent overview of the problem of AIDS in Africa. He cogently notes the risk factors associated with the predominately heterosexual mode of transmission: sexual contacts with prostitutes, promiscuity, being a prostitute, and being a sexual partner of an infected person. However, the virus is also transmitted in Africa by blood transfusions and the use of contaminated injection equipment for medical purposes.[11] The primarily heterosexual transmission of HIV in Africa has

been viewed by some observers as a portent of epidemiological things to come in Europe and the United States. The obvious caveats of course are that the epidemiology of AIDS in Africa is at the midpoint of 1989 incompletely understood, and the fact that there may be other determinants in the African AIDS scenario that are not always present in the United States and Europe. These include large numbers of sexual partners and frequent unprotected prostitute contacts among heterosexual African AIDS patients, the widespread use of unsterile needles and syringes in clinics and hospitals, and the poorly understood process of HIV transmission enhancement by concurrent or antecedent sexually transmitted diseases.[11]

Heterosexual transmission of AIDS became a major focus of concern in 1987. By 1988 it was clear that the epidemiologic data did not support the contention of some that AIDS was becoming a major problem in the general heterosexual population in the United States. Largely confined now to high risk groups (homosexual and bisexual men and intravenous drug abusers) and their sexual partners, AIDS seems unlikely to move in a major way out of these groups into the general heterosexual population over the narrow bridges of bisexuality, transplacental spread from infected mothers, and heterosexual transmission from IV drug abusers and other infected persons. For in the infection-recipient groups on the other side of these bridges the crucial variable of multiple sex partners is often lacking. The suburban housewife who is infected with AIDS by a bisexual husband is not likely to have subsequent sexual contacts with a score or more of men as are her husband's male partners. Thus this form of heterosexual transmission leads the virus into a dead end from which it does not usually escape.

However, based on what is already known about the epidemiology of AIDS, it is probable that the number of HIV infections will increase among heterosexuals. This increase is likely to occur first in heterosexual subset populations that are closest to the existing transmission bridges from currently infected high-risk-behavior groups. The degree and rapidity of spread outside of this center will be directly related to the frequency of sexual contacts and the number of sexual partners, variables likely to be affected by public health education activities now underway. Of great concern is the level of HIV positivity among inner-city parturients and its implications for neonatal transmission.[12,13] In this book Hein underscores the vulnerability of certain groups of teenagers who, because of early age of first intercourse, choice of sexual partners, rates of sexually transmitted diseases, current contraceptive practices, and other factors, are at high risk for acquiring HIV infections. Many of these teenagers are on the other side of the AIDS transmission bridge from IV drug abusers and form a potential part of the epidemiologic center of the epidemic. Many of them are also found in inner city areas and should be the immediate focus of intense public health education activities.

The data on HIV infection rates among civilian applicants for military service presented in the chapters by Burke et al and Brundage et al may or may not sustain concern about spread to the general heterosexual population depending on one's interpretation of the data. One can cogently argue that the civilian applicants for military service who were screened are not representative of the universal population of which they are a part but rather may represent subsets whose prior behaviors may have put them at significant risk for HIV infection. If they are truly representative of the universe heterosexual population then one should see similar levels of HIV infection in this larger group. Yet initial studies to date of the larger universe population conducted on donated blood have only shown HIV prevalence rates of 0.38%.[14] There are limitations to the data generated from surveys of blood donated to blood banks just as there are limitations to data on HIV prevalence gathered at sexually transmitted disease clinics. What is needed are carefully designed, ongoing surveys of the general heterosexual population. These were called for at the February 1987 conference on AIDS sponsored by the CDC in Atlanta, Georgia.[15] Hopefully they will provide useful insights into the epidemiology of the disease in the heterosexual population. Meanwhile, current predictions as to what is likely to occur in the heterosexual population are largely derived from existing data which are far from complete.[16]

Far more complete are data on high-risk-behavior groups: homosexual men and IV drug abusers. Concerning the latter, Des Jarlais and his colleagues provide useful insights in their chapter into the relationship between IV drug abuse and the heterosexual transmission of HIV. Of significance is the finding that HIV-infected prostitutes in New York City have rarely transmitted the infection to clients. Des Jarlais and his colleagues put forth as one of the reasons for this the very credible explanation that prostitutes in the city have employed "safe sex" procedures, particularly the use of condoms, for a number of years as protection against other sexually transmitted diseases. They also underscore the close linkage between IV drug abuse and heterosexual transmission of HIV infection in the city.

The possible effectiveness of condoms in preventing the transmission of HIV infection has also been a prominent issue of the agenda for AIDS. There has been much heated discussion over the proposal to advertise condoms on television, a proposal that was at the time supported by the Surgeon General of the US Public Health Service, C. Everett Koop, MD.[17] Network television and some local stations have avoided these ads out of concern for offending the beliefs and convictions of a significant proportion of the American public that sees in them the potential for approving and promoting extramarital sexual relations, particularly among young people. Religious groups and former Secretary of Education William Bennett have advocated abstinence as the safest and best means of preventing HIV infection. The heated polemics that have characterized the discussion of this issue have centered more on moral, religious, and social issues than on the scientific one, namely, the effectiveness of condoms in preventing transmission of HIV. To date there are no extensive data documenting the level of prevention afforded by condoms against transmission under a variety of use circumstances.

There has been a strong call for public health education as one of the best means for preventing the transmission of HIV infection. Yet there are areas of disagreement about content, the debate over condom use being the best exam-

ple. The debate over prevention strategies continues and has tended to center more in the arena of heterosexual transmission than in those of homosexual and IV drug abuse transmission, where high prevalence rates of HIV infection should serve as a strong incentive for behavior modification. Three chapters in this book describe health education intervention strategies. Valdiserri and his colleagues describe small group intervention sessions with homosexual and bisexual men that show promise for reducing high-risk behavior. Echenberg describes two intervention strategies developed in San Francisco for both high- and low-prevalence groups. In addition to mass health education, the program employed by the San Francisco Department of Public Health utilizes contact notification in the low-prevalence group. This latter strategy is a very useful adaptation of that which has long been used to trace sexually transmitted disease partners. Both the program in Pittsburgh and the one in San Francisco demonstrate that public health education can go a long way at this stage of the epidemic. Ross and Carson in their chapter describe the effectiveness of distributing information on AIDS via six media in Australia and conclude that public media hold little advantage over informal information sources in reaching high risk groups.

How local communities deal with the AIDS epidemic in terms of public policy is clearly illustrated in the chapter by Arno and Hughes. They show how the contrasting public policy responses in New York City and San Francisco are attributable to a number of factors, prominent among which are the patient mix, the character of the public health and health care systems in each city, differences in the magnitude of the epidemic, and the role of risk groups and the local media and press in molding local response. This chapter focuses on another prominent issue that has received much attention, namely, that of the medical care costs involved in caring for patients with AIDS. Related to individual patient care costs and those of the aggregate is the issue of the impact of the epidemic on the health care system.

In another chapter O'Donnell and O'Donnell describe the results of an in-service educational program for AIDS among hospital workers. They found that among other things in-service education improved knowledge and satisfaction with the quality of care delivered. Howland et al present the results of a study they undertook to determine which variables determine the adaptation of AIDS teaching in public schools. None of the variables they studied proved significant, underscoring the need for further study in this area. In a related chapter, Siegel and Gibson discuss in detail some of the barriers to sexual behavior modification among heterosexuals at risk for AIDS and their health education implications.

The epidemic has already had a significant effect on the number and mix of beds in many hospitals. Three chapters in the book deal with issues related to the impact of the epidemic on the health care system. Raske provides sobering data on the impact of AIDS on New York City's not-for-profit hospitals. Young discusses the impact of AIDS on New Jersey's health care system, and Joseph discusses the impact on health care in New York City within the context of a number of other issues. As the numbers of patients with AIDS rise, pressures build to transfer them to municipal, generally teaching, hospitals, because of failure to receive adequate reimbursement from third-party payers. Educational programs for house staff and medical students have also been affected in teaching institutions by the number of inpatients with AIDS. Institutions struggle with their responsibility to treat AIDS patients while simultaneously trying to maintain a mix of patients with other disease states that helps assure both the comprehensiveness of educational content and its quality.[18] The attitudes of pre-clinical medical students towards caring for AIDS patients and performing internships and residencies in hospitals with significant numbers of such patients are presented in a chapter by this writer and his colleagues. In another chapter Nussbaum describes how AIDS can effectively be used for the medico-legal education of second year medical students.

As the number of patients with AIDS continues to grow there will be a need to provide a broad range of ambulatory and inpatient services. To meet these new service requirements health care planners must rethink pre-epidemic strategies and plans so as to permit rapid service responses to changing needs. Based on CDC prevalence estimates for AIDS, Scitovsky and Rice[19] estimate that the personal medical care costs for the disease will rise from the $630 million spent in 1985 to $8.5 billion in 1991. They estimate that indirect costs attributable to productivity loss among victims will rise to $55.6 billion in 1991, from $3.9 billion in 1985. Nonpersonal costs for research, education, screening, and general support services are expected to rise from $542 million for 1986 to $2.3 billion in 1991.[19]

The year 1989 witnesses a continued growth in our knowledge of the clinical course of AIDS and of means for dealing with the disease's many complications. Foster et al describe the therapeutic use of meclofenamate in patients with AIDS-related pulmonary involvement. Their study demonstrates that as necessity develops, as it frequently does in this disease, newer modalities are found and applied. However, therapeutic interventions have thus far been palliative at best. Much hope was attached to the introduction of azidothymidine (AZT) in late 1986.[20] At this writing it is too early yet to say how truly effective this drug will be as a therapeutic agent. Although AZT is easy to administer, its untoward effects require careful patient monitoring. DeHovitz[21] makes an important point in noting that this increased monitoring will translate into more frequent patient-physician contact which in turn will escalate medical care costs. Real breakthroughs in the development of other effective anti-HIV agents and vaccines appear hopeful but not imminent. As progress is made in the development of vaccines and therapeutic agents, basic science research on the virus itself continues to uncover new, important information. An example of this is the finding announced in June 1988 that the virus can remain hidden in the macrophage system and escape detection by commonly used screening tests.

As of this writing no other issue has seized the center of the debate platform as has that of mandatory testing for AIDS. The point of contention is not the testing itself but rather the confidentiality issue that is inextricably linked to it.[15] Instances have been reported in which the confidential nature of positive AIDS tests has been breached,

resulting in dismissal from employment; loss of housing; and cancellation of life, disability, and health insurance.[22] This issue was widely debated at the February 1987 conference on AIDS sponsored by the CDC, at which many cogent arguments against mandatory testing were put forth.[15] On the face of it mandatory testing appears to be an effective way of identifying those infected with HIV and of encouraging them not to engage in behaviors that would spread it. If the test were mandatory for all hospital admissions and for patients attending sexually transmitted disease clinics, significant numbers of HIV-infected individuals could be identified, their behavior modified, and the spread of the disease curtailed. In the absence of a cure or vaccine this appears to be a reasonable approach to prevention of spread.

However, there is some evidence that mandatory testing would drive those who are infected underground and away from preventive interventions, thus defeating the purpose of such testing.[23] The true magnitude of this impact has yet to be accurately documented. Given the current distribution of AIDS, which primarily occurs among homosexual men and IV drug abusers, it would probably not be cost effective to screen the 37 million Americans who are admitted to hospitals each year. The inducements for so doing would include a major change in the epidemiology of the disease in which very significant numbers of the general heterosexual population would become infected. Such an epidemiologic development does not appear imminent from the perspective of 1989. Also, a marked increase in the total number of cases might prompt reconsideration of mandatory testing.

DeHovitz and Landesman discuss in their chapter a number of issues related to HIV antibody testing and call for broader selective testing while rejecting mandatory testing. This view is in line with the consensus that has developed among public health officials in the United States that voluntary testing linked to counseling both before and after the test holds hope for preventing the spread of the disease.[24] It is this belief that underpins New York State's newly expanded program for counseling and testing. The degree of effectiveness of this approach in preventing the spread of HIV infection has yet to be demonstrated. Meanwhile, as long as the risks of discrimination in employment, housing, and insurance remain linked to possible breaches in confidentiality about positive test results, there will continue to be strong opposition to mandatory testing.[25] These concerns were heightened by the US Justice Department's ruling in June 1986 that denied HIV carriers the protection afforded by a federal law prohibiting discrimination against the handicapped. On March 3, 1987, the US Supreme Court ruled that recipients of federal monies could not discriminate against those who are physically or mentally impaired by contagious diseases.[26] Although the decision was handed down in the case of a Florida elementary school teacher who was dismissed in 1979 because of active tuberculosis, it affects those with AIDS. The immediate beneficiaries are children who are excluded from school because of AIDS and adults with the disease who are employed by employers receiving federal monies.[26] The critical issue of whether or not the federal 1973 Rehabilitation Act protects carriers of HIV who are asymptomatic was left undecided.[27] Although this decision affords less than complete protection to AIDS victims, it represents a major step forward.

There are numerous other issues related to AIDS, some of which are covered in several chapters in the section on Current Issues and Opinions. These reflect a range of social and philosophical challenges posed by the epidemic and provide some stimulating insights from authors who have given these issues serious thought.

AIDS has a broad spectrum of clinical presentations. Nine chapters deal with both common and unusual clinical complications encountered in the disease. Although this coverage is by no means exhaustive, it nonetheless provides some idea of the clinical range of disease states produced by AIDS.

The appendices consist of nationally promulgated guidelines and position papers from the American Medical Association, the Food and Drug Administration, and the United States Public Health Service Centers for Disease Control. These have been endorsed or approved by the Council of the Medical Society of the State of New York, some on the recommendation of the society's Committee on Preventive Medicine.

A number of individuals have been of great assistance in the preparation of the contents of this volume. Sincere thanks are extended to the staff of the *New York State Journal of Medicine*, to Ella Abney, Librarian, Mildred J. Arfmann, Editorial Assistant, Eleanor Burns, Assistant Librarian, Joseph G. Feldman, DRPH, Consultant in Biostatistics, and Vicki Glaser, Consulting Medical Writer. Carol L. Moore, the *Journal's* Managing Editor, and Elizabeth J. Somers, Secretary and Administrative Assistant to the *Journal* editor, performed a herculean task in editing, keyboarding, and formatting the content of this volume. I want to especially thank them for the skill and dedication which they have imparted to this effort. Special thanks are extended to Ernest Drucker, PHD, Associate Professor, Department of Epidemiology and Social Medicine, Montefiore Medical Center/Albert Einstein College of Medicine, for having made available a number of presentations from the 1987 and 1988 Montefiore symposia on AIDS. Thanks are also extended to the officers of the Medical Society of the State of New York, Mr Donald F. Foy, Executive Vice President of the society, and to Dr Milton Gordon, Chairman of the Committee on Publications, Library and Archives, and to the members of the committee for their support of this project. Special thanks are extended to Mary Safford, Senior Production Editor at Plenum Publishing, for her assistance and support in bringing this volume to fruition.

Predicting the course of any epidemic disease is extremely difficult because the expected often fails to happen and the unexpected occurs with regularity. There are many unforeseen variables and surprise developments that lay ahead on the road of AIDS prevention and treatment. From the vantage point of 1989, it is impossible to predict what they will be. What is more certain is that American society will have to continue to deal with the myriad problems associated with AIDS, many of which are comprehensively addressed in this volume.

PASCAL JAMES IMPERATO, MD
Editor
New York State Journal of Medicine

1. *Pneumocystis* pneumonia. *MMWR* 1981; 30:250–252.
2. Institute of Medicine, National Academy of Sciences: *Confronting AIDS, Directives for Public Health, Health Care and Research.* Washington, DC, National Academy Press, 1986, p 37.
3. Update on acquired immune deficiency syndrome (AIDS)—United States. *MMWR* 1982; 31:507–514.
4. Barre-Sinoussi F, Chermann JC, Rey F, et al: Isolation of a T-lymphotropic retrovirus from a patient at risk for acquired immune deficiency syndrome (AIDS). *Science* 1983; 220:868–871.
5. Gallo RC, Salahuddin SZ, Popovic M, et al: Frequent detection and isolation of cytopathic retroviruses (HTLV-III) from patients with AIDS and at risk for AIDS. *Science* 1984; 224:500–503.
6. Coffen J, Haase A, Levy JA, et al: Human immunodeficiency virus. *Science* 1986; 232:697.
7. Update: Acquired immunodeficiency syndrome—United States, 1981–1988. *MMWR* 1989; 38:229–236.
8. Acquired Immunodeficiency Syndrome (AIDS)—Worldwide. *MMWR* 1988; 37:286–288, 293–295.
9. Brooke J: Kenya is reacting bitterly as AIDS is highlighted. *NY Times,* February 24, 1987, p B4.
10. Brooke J: AIDS danger: Africa seems of two minds. *NY Times,* January 3, 1987, p 13.
11. Imperato PJ: The epidemiology of the acquired immunodeficiency syndrome in Africa. *NY State J Med* 1986; 86:118–121.
12. Landesman S, Minkoff H, Holman S, et al: Serosurvey of human immunodeficiency virus infection in parturients. *JAMA* 1987; 258:2701–2703.
13. Minkoff HL: Care of pregnant women infected with human immunodeficiency virus. *JAMA* 1987; 258:2714–2717.
14. Schorr JB, Berkowitz A, Cumming PD: Prevalence of HTLV-III antibody in American blood donors. *N Engl J Med* 1985; 313:384–385.
15. Altman LK: Mandatory tests for AIDS opposed at health parley. *NY Times,* February 25, 1987, pp 1, 16.
16. DeHovitz JA: A perspective on the heterosexual transmission of the acquired immunodeficiency syndrome. *NY State J Med* 1986; 86:117–118.
17. Werner LM: Koop urges TV condom ads to fight AIDS. *NY Times,* February 11, 1987, pp 1, A10.
18. Wachter RM: The impact of the acquired immune deficiency syndrome on medical residency training. *N Engl J Med* 1986; 314:177–179.
19. Scitovsky AA, Rice DP: Estimates of the direct and indirect costs of acquired immunodeficiency syndrome in the United States, 1985–1986 and 1991. *Public Health Rep* 1987; 102:5–17.
20. Barnes DM: Promising results halt trial of anti-AIDS drug. *Science* 1986; 234:15–16.
21. DeHovitz JA: Azidothymidine and human immunodeficiency virus infection. *NY State J Med* 1987; 87:7–8.
22. Altman LK: Privacy called vital to AIDS screening. *NY Times,* March 1, 1987, p E26.
23. Mandatory testing for AIDS? *US News and World Report* 1987; 102:62.
24. A new strategy against AIDS. *NY Times,* March 1, 1987, p E24.
25. Boffey PM: Homosexuals applaud rejection of mandatory tests for AIDS. *NY Times,* February 26, 1987, p B7.
26. Boffey PM: Laws urged to protect identities in AIDS testing. *NY Times,* February 25, 1987, p A18.
27. Taylor S Jr: Rights of disease victims backed; those with AIDS could benefit. *NY Times,* March 4, 1987, pp A1, A21.

Part I
Research Studies

Part I
Research Studies

Chapter 1

Demography of HIV infections among civilian applicants for military service in four counties in New York City

DONALD S. BURKE, MD; JOHN F. BRUNDAGE, MD; WILLIAM BERNER, MD; LYTT I. GARDNER, PhD; ROBERT R. REDFIELD, MD; JEFFREY GUNZENHAUSER, MD; JAMES VOSKOVITCH, MD; JOHN R. HERBOLD, DVM

ABSTRACT. During the period October 1, 1985, through July 31, 1986, serum specimens from 9,498 civilian applicants for military service from four New York City counties (New York, Kings, Queens, and Bronx) were tested for antibodies to the human immunodeficiency virus (HIV). Ninety-seven (1.03%) specimens were positive as confirmed by Western blot. Antibody prevalence was strongly associated with age. Among recruit applicants who were less than 18, 18–21, 22–25, and greater than 25 years old, HIV seroprevalence rates were 0.23%, 0.31%, 1.30%, and 2.95%, respectively. Among applicants of different racial groups, the rates of seroprevalence were as follows: whites, 19/2,553, 0.74%; blacks, 56/4,869, 1.15%; and others including Hispanic, 22/2,076, 1.06%. Rates among male applicants (84/7,938, 1.06%) and female applicants (13/1,560, 0.83%) were not significantly different ($p = 0.45$).

In October 1985 the US Department of Defense instituted a program for screening all civilian applicants for military service for evidence of infection with HIV. Data for the first six months of the program for the entire United States and its territories are summarized elsewhere.[1] Of the 14 counties with the highest seroprevalence rates in the continental United States, four were contiguous counties in the New York City area (New York, Kings, Queens, and Bronx). This chapter is a preliminary summary of current data on demographic factors associated with HIV infection in these four counties.

PATIENTS AND METHODS

Beginning October 1, 1985, blood samples for HIV testing were obtained as part of the medical examination conducted at 71 Military Entrance Processing Stations within the United States and its trust territories. Details of the methods used to detect HIV antibodies and to process demographic data are presented elsewhere (D.S. Burke, J.F. Brundage, W. Bernier, et al, unpublished manuscript, 1987). In brief, serum samples were screened by a contracting laboratory (Damon Laboratories) with a commercial HIV enzyme-linked immunoassay system (ELISA, Electronucleonics, Inc). All repeatable, positive samples were subsequently tested by Western blot. Blots were determined to be positive if antibodies to gp41 and/or p24+p55 were detected. Applicants who had positive samples were notified by a registered letter which also requested that they return to the examination station for counseling and repeat Western blot testing. In this report, applicants whose samples tested positive on a repeat blot, and applicants whose samples were positive on the first blot but did not submit a second specimen are considered antibody positive. All other applicants, including those positive by ELISA but negative by blot, are considered antibody negative. Data are analyzed for the ten-month period October 1, 1985–July 31, 1986. Data were tested for statistical significance using chi-square analysis for contingency tables and chi-square for assessing a linear trend.

RESULTS

Seroprevalence rates among civilian applicants for military service in the counties of New York, Kings, Queens, and Bronx are presented by county in Table I. Overall, 97 of 9,498 applicants were HIV seropositive (10.3/1,000). Rates by county ranged from 4.2/1,000 (10/2,400) in Queens to 17.1/1,000 (24/1,404) in Manhat-

TABLE I. HIV Seroprevalence Rates Among Military Recruit Applicants in Four Selected New York Counties, October 1, 1985–July 31, 1986

County	No. Positive	No. Tested	(Rate per 1,000)
New York	24*	1,404	17.1†
Kings	36	3,382	10.6
Queens	10	2,400	4.2
Bronx	27	2,312	11.7
Totals	97	9,498	10.3

* HIV seropositive as determined by Western blot.
† Rate HIV Western blot positive per 1,000 tested.

From the Walter Reed Army Institute of Research (Drs Burke, Brundage, Gardner, Redfield, and Gunzenhauser), the US Military Entrance Processing Command (Drs Berner and Voskovitch), and the Office of the Assistant Secretary of Defense (Health Affairs) (Dr Herbold).

The views of the authors do not reflect the positions of the Department of the Army or the Department of Defense.

TABLE II.   HIV Seroprevalence Rates Among Military Recruit Applicants in New York, Kings, Queens, and Bronx Counties, by Age, Sex, and Racial Group, October 1, 1985–July 31, 1986

Age (yr)	White M	White F	Black M	Black F	Other M	Other F	All Racial Groups M	All Racial Groups F
<18	0/115*	0/6	0/124	1/41	0/104	0/11	0/343	1/58
	0.0†	0.0	0.0	24.4	0.0	0.0	0.0	17.2
18–21	3/1,328	0/104	6/2,048	3/582	4/1,015	0/110	13/4,391	3/796
	2.3	0.0	2.9	5.1	3.9	0.0	3.0	3.8
22–25	3/495	2/57	15/896	2/255	5/381	1/61	23/1,772	5/373
	6.1	35.1	16.7	7.8	13.1	16.4	13.0	13.4
>25	11/389	0/59	25/700	4/223	12/343	0/51	48/1,432	4/333
	28.3	0.0	35.7	17.9	35.0	0.0	33.5	12.0
Totals	17/2,327	2/226	46/3,768	10/1,101	21/1,843	1/233	84/7,938	13/1,560
	7.3	8.8	12.2	9.1	11.3	4.3	10.6	8.3
	19/2,553		56/4,869		22/2,076		97/9,498	
	7.4		11.5		10.6		10.3	

* Number HIV Western blot positive/number tested.
† Rate HIV Western blot positive per 1,000 tested.

tan. Rates among applicants in these four counties in demographic subcategories of age, racial group, and gender are presented in Table II.

Among applicants who were less than 18, 18–21, 22–25, and greater than 25 years old, HIV seroprevalence rates were 2.3, 3.1, 13.0, and 29.5 per 1,000, respectively. Among applicants of different racial groups, the rates were as follows: whites, 19/2,553, 7.4/1,000; blacks, 56/4,869, 11.5/1,000; and others including Hispanic, 22/2,076, 10.6/1,000 ($p = 0.24$).

HIV seroprevalence among male applicants (84/7,938, 10.6/1,000) was only marginally greater than among female applicants (13/1,560, 8.3/1,000) ($p = 0.45$). Male and female seroprevalence rates were generally similar among each racial group: white males, 7.3/1,000 versus white females, 8.8/1,000 ($p = 0.88$); black males, 12.2/1,000 versus black females, 9.1/1,000 ($p = 0.49$); other racial group males, 11.3/1,000 versus other racial group females, 4.3/1,000 ($p = 0.51$).

When analyzed by age, male and female HIV seroprevalence rates were similar for applicants younger than 26 years (males, 36/6,506, 5.5/1,000; females, 9/1,227, 7.3/1,000) ($p = 0.31$). Among applicants 26 years old or older, HIV seroprevalence rates were greater among males (48/1,432, 33.5/1,000) than among females (4/333; 12.0/1,000) ($p = 0.06$). Overall, there was a significant trend of increasing prevalence by age in males ($p < 0.001$) but not in females ($p = 0.21$).

DISCUSSION

Although there are considerable data regarding the demography of AIDS cases in the United States,[1] to date there has been a dearth of comparable information about the early stages of infection with HIV, the causative agent of AIDS. Studies on HIV antibody prevalence have largely been confined to selected groups in locations with high AIDS incidence rates, such as male homosexuals in San Francisco (67% positive) or intravenous drug abusers in New York City (87% positive).[2,3] Data gathered from blood bank screening programs, where persons considered to be at high risk of infection are actively discouraged from donating, present the opposite extreme (0.04% positive).[4]

Data from the US Military Entrance Processing screening program provide new perspectives on the prevalence of HIV infection and the geographic and demographic factors associated with HIV infection. During the first six months of the program, more than 300,000 civilian applicants for military service were tested at 71 sta-

tions in the US and its territories.[1] HIV seroprevalence rates among recruit applicants in specific geographic localities were found to correlate closely with cumulative AIDS incidence rates in the general population in those localities. The overall seroprevalence rate among recruit applicants in the United States was 1.5/1,000. Seroprevalence rates among applicants from the New York City area were substantially higher than rates throughout the rest of the country.

For the current report, we analyzed data on HIV seroprevalence among applicants from four contiguous counties in New York City which had unusually high HIV infection rates. In these four counties, more than 1% of all applicants had serologic evidence of HIV infection. As was noted for the US at large, seropositivity was closely associated with increasing age. However, rates for any specified age group were four to ten times greater in these four counties than in the rest of the United States.

In this analysis we did not detect substantial differences in HIV seroprevalence rates between different racial groups. This finding differs from that for the nation at large, where black applicants have a 3.6-fold higher rate and applicants of other racial groups a 1.5-fold higher rate than white applicants (D.S. Burke, J.F. Brundage, W. Bernier, et al, unpublished data, 1987).

HIV seroprevalence rates among men and women in these four counties were surprisingly similar, suggesting that infection is occurring in the male and female populations at comparable rates. This observed sex ratio of close to 1:1 differs substantially from the ratio of 13:1 reported for AIDS cases.[1] When the male-to-female infection ratio was analyzed according to age or racial groups, rates were comparable in all subcategories except for applicants over the age of 25 years, for which the male-to-female ratio was 2.7:1.

We interpret these data to show that in the four counties in central New York City, HIV infections are highly prevalent among young adults. Risk of infection is not confined to any racial group and is not appreciably greater for men than for women, at least under age 26. Data on the probable mode of infection for each HIV-infected recruit applicant is not currently available. Although exposure through intravenous drug abuse cannot be ruled out, the high rates of infection observed among women suggest that heterosexual relations may be a significant mode of transmission in urban centers in the United States.

Young persons who apply for entry into the military may not be representative of the population at large. Nonetheless, these data suggest the possibility of a substantial change in the epidemiology of AIDS in the New York area within the next five to ten years.

REFERENCES

1. Peterman TA, Drotman DP, Curran JW: Epidemiology of the acquired immunodeficiency syndrome (AIDS). *Epidemiol Rev* 1985; 7:1–21.
2. Jaffe HW, Feorino PM, Darrow WW, et al: Persistent infection with human T-lymphotropic virus type III/lymphadenopathy-associated virus in apparently healthy homosexual men. *Ann Intern Med* 1985; 102:627–628.
3. Spira TJ, Des Jarlais DC, Marmor M, et al: Prevalence of antibody to lymphadenopathy-associated virus among drug-detoxification patients in New York [letter]. *N Engl J Med* 1984; 311:467–468.
4. US Public Health Service Workshop on human T-lymphotropic virus type III antibody testing. *MMWR* 1985; 34:477–478.

Chapter 2
Local policy responses to the AIDS epidemic: New York and San Francisco

PETER S. ARNO, PhD, ROBERT G. HUGHES, PhD

ABSTRACT. The epidemic of acquired immunodeficiency syndrome (AIDS) has been concentrated in a few large cities. Thus far, New York City and San Francisco have reported more AIDS cases than any other cities in the world. Together they account for 40% of the total number of cases reported in the United States through the end of 1986.

Both cities have expended an enormous amount of local resources in dealing with the epidemic, although the public policy response has been markedly different in each city. Although historically New York has had three times the AIDS caseload as San Francisco, it has consistently spent less money on public health education and other nonhospital-related health care services. The varied policy responses in each city can be attributed to several factors: differences in the magnitude of the epidemic; the patient mix; the role of risk groups in the political and economic life of each community; the scale of public health care systems, including the number of medical schools; the impact of local media; and the institutional roles of the respective health departments.

With the prospect of other cities facing an increasing number of AIDS cases, the New York and San Francisco experiences may prove useful. They indicate that each community's response to AIDS will probably reflect the underlying social, economic, and political characteristics of AIDS victims and the existing structure and organizational roles of traditional health care and community-based service providers.

From the Department of Health Care Administration, Bernard M. Baruch College/Mount Sinai School of Medicine, City University of New York (Dr Arno), and the School of Health Administration and Policy, Arizona State University (Dr Hughes).

This research was supported in part by fellowship grants from the Pew Memorial Trust. Earlier versions of this paper were presented at the Annual Meetings of the American Public Health Association, November 1985, in Washington, DC, and at the International Conference on AIDS in Paris, France, in June 1986.

Forty percent of the AIDS cases reported in the United States through 1986 have occurred in New York City and San Francisco. These two cities account for more cases than any other cities in the world. Yet the ways in which the epidemic has affected these two cities and their policy responses have been quite different. Early reports indicated that the average length of hospital stay for AIDS patients was four times longer in New York, and that services for AIDS patients, ranging from hospital care to housing and counseling, were organized differently in each city.[1-4]

The concentration of cases in these two cities, coupled with a federal policy preference for shifting responsibility for domestic social problems from the national to the local level, has made the experiences reported here important to an understanding of AIDS in the United States. This paper describes the AIDS epidemic in New York and San Francisco and examines the factors that have contributed to different policy responses in the two cities. This comparison illuminates the problems other cities are likely to face as AIDS continues to spread, and identifies those factors that are important in tailoring local responses to the epidemic.

To investigate the apparent differences between the two cities, we relied on a variety of data sources as well as the organizations that have been involved in coping with the epidemic in New York and San Francisco. We reviewed available published information, including congressional testimony, scientific literature, and newspaper reports, and also unpublished agency minutes and records from involved organizations. Finally, extremely valuable information was provided by numerous public officials, leaders of private AIDS-related organizations, and volunteers from agencies in both cities who discussed the responses to AIDS in their communities.

To place these cities in perspective, it is first useful to describe some of the basic economic and demographic characteristics of each city (Table I). For example, New

**TABLE I.   Demographic and Economic Characteristics:
New York City and San Francisco**

	New York City	San Francisco
Total population (1,000) (1982)	7,086	692
% Black (1980)	25.2	12.7
% Hispanic (1980)	19.9	12.3
Per capita income (1981)	$8,737	$11,026
Median family income (1979)	$19,268	$24,648
% Population below poverty level (1979)	19.7	13.4

Sources: US Department of Commerce: *Statistical Abstract of the United States*, 1985; US Department of Commerce: *1980 Census of Population*, 1983.

York is a far larger city, with ten times the number of people as San Francisco. Nearly twice the proportion of New York's population is black or Hispanic. San Francisco is a wealthier city, with a per capita income 26% higher than New York's, and fewer of its residents live in poverty. These general demographic and economic factors are reflected in the AIDS patient groups in each city and have influenced local policy responses to the epidemic.

NEW YORK AND SAN FRANCISCO: DIFFERENCES IN RESPONDING TO AIDS

New York and San Francisco have responded differently to the AIDS epidemic in the amount of money spent, the distribution of these funds among programs, the length of hospital stays of AIDS patients, and the array of services available. Initial policy attention, influenced by the predominant interest in controlling health care costs in this country, was directed at the cost of care for AIDS patients in the two communities.

Precise estimates of public spending on AIDS programs during the early years of the epidemic are difficult to assess, particularly in New York, where AIDS expenditures were not tracked and programs were split among several city agencies. These figures are therefore less reliable. In addition, figures describing the amount of public money spent on AIDS do not always include the local share of Medicaid funds spent at nonpublic hospitals. Thus, it is important to recognize not only the politically sensitive budget process in which these figures are often used, but that the figures may not be strictly comparable from year to year or from one city to another. Nevertheless, a sense of the magnitude of the resources devoted to AIDS can be ascertained from agency estimates of their own expenditures.

In 1985, the acting president of the New York City Health and Hospitals Corporation (NYCHHC, the municipal hospital system) estimated that $30 million was spent on inpatient health care delivery for AIDS patients in this public hospital system during fiscal year (FY) 1985.[5] During this time, the New York City Department of Health expended an additional $1.1 million on AIDS-related activities. These consisted mainly of disease surveillance and epidemiologic investigation, health education, and laboratory services.[6] Also in New York, the Human Resources Administration spent $600,000 for social services for persons with AIDS. In total, AIDS expen-

ditures of approximately $32 million have been identified for New York during FY 1985, but this fails to include public funds used to subsidize indigent care at private hospitals and a variety of other AIDS-related expenditures.

Expenditures of an estimated $25 million dollars for AIDS-related activities were made in San Francisco during FY 1985. The bulk of these funds ($17 million) was for inpatient care, which was financed primarily through private insurance and the Medi-Cal program.[7] The remaining $8 million was administered by the San Francisco Department of Public Health (SFDPH), more than 90% of which was derived from local taxes. Approximately 17% of these funds went for disease surveillance and epidemiologic investigations, 55% for assessments and medical care, 11% for social support services and housing, and 17% for public education and administrative coordination.[8]

As the epidemic grew, the expenditure of funds significantly increased in New York. An attempt was made by the New York City Office of Management and Budget to analyze the total amount and distribution of AIDS-related funds during FY 1986. Total spending in New York City was projected to range from $110 million to $148 million. New York City's tax levy support was estimated at approximately 38% of these figures. This included the city's contribution to inpatient medical care provided in municipal and voluntary hospitals, public health education, epidemiologic surveillance, and contracts for social service programs. The remaining balance included all other sources of reimbursement including federal and state funds and private insurers.[9]

This compares to a projected $37 million for total AIDS spending in San Francisco during this time (based on estimates).[8,10] Approximately 24% of this sum ($8.8 million) was derived from local tax revenues and was distributed to a similar range of activities as in the previous year. The remaining funds were primarily drawn from private insurers (37%) and the federal and state governments (18% and 13%, respectively).

By estimating the number of living persons with AIDS in each city during FY 1986, we calculated a per capita expenditure per AIDS patient: approximately $22,000 in San Francisco and $36,000 in New York.

A major part of overall costs in both cities is for inpatient care. The average daily cost of care in their municipal hospitals is quite similar, with estimates of $773 per day in San Francisco and $800 per day in New York—less than a 4% difference.[9,11] Yet the charges per admission are quite different: $20,320 in New York and $9,024 in San Francisco. As Table II indicates, the key difference in these charges is the number of days spent in the hospital.

The average length of stay for an AIDS patient in New York is more than twice as long as that in San Francisco.

TABLE II.   Hospitalization of AIDS Patients in Municipal Facilities, 1984: New York City and San Francisco

	New York City	San Francisco
Average length of stay (days)	25.4	11.7
Average charges per day ($)	800	773
Average charges per admission ($)	20,320	9,024

Sources: Based on data derived from references 9 and 11.

In addition, it appears that at least twice the proportion of AIDS patients are hospitalized at any given time in New York as in San Francisco. According to a 1985 survey,[5] approximately 22% of all living AIDS patients in New York were hospitalized. This compares to approximately 10% in San Francisco.[7] This finding is consistent with longer hospital stays in New York in general. Reasons for regional variations in length of stay, a pattern confirmed by AIDS patients, have been addressed elsewhere.[12]

A final difference between the two cities is in the earlier development in San Francisco of a relatively coordinated set of services for AIDS patients and citizens in major risk groups—from outpatient care, to housing and counseling, to prevention through community education. Not only were these services developed earlier in San Francisco, they were strongly supported by local public funds. This contrasts with the situation in New York in 1984, where one organization, the Gay Men's Health Crisis (GMHC), provided the bulk of AIDS-related community services. Only 3% of GMHC's resources were provided by New York City.[13] In contrast, the three largest organizations providing similar services in San Francisco—the Shanti Project, the San Francisco AIDS Foundation, and Hospice of San Francisco—received 62% of their financial resources from San Francisco City and County.[14]

EXPLAINING THE DIFFERENCES

Exploring possible reasons for the differences between the two cities, we found that they fall into three sets: epidemiologic factors, preexisting social and political structural characteristics, and policy responses in local agencies.

Many of these factors are related. Epidemiologic factors and the social organization of the risk groups, for ex-ample, influence each other, and both have important effects on policy responses. Thus, although we are presenting the three sets of factors separately, it should be recognized that they are related to each other within each city.

Epidemiologic Factors. Available data on the epidemiology of AIDS in New York, San Francisco, and the United States are summarized in Table III. The figures for the United States incorporate data for the two cities and are presented for reference. New York and San Francisco account for 30.4% and 9.5%, respectively, of the nation's AIDS cases.

Significant differences between the two cities can be seen in the total number of cases, the rate of cases in the population, the proportion of patients in various risk groups, the race and sex of patients, and the number of cases in children. Although New York has historically had more than three times as many AIDS cases as San Francisco, the rate of cases per 100,000 population is three times as great in San Francisco. This difference in the rate of cases between the two cities differs from the Centers for Disease Control (CDC) data. Their rates indicate a difference of less than 4% between New York and San Francisco.[15] Two reasons explain the differences in the rates we report and those of the CDC. First, the CDC uses Standard Metropolitan Statistical Areas (SMSAs) to measure the underlying population base, while we used data only for the cities. Second, the CDC data are based on AIDS cases by place of residence, and ours are by place of diagnosis. We chose these methods because our focus is on comparing the impact of the epidemic on the health care systems in these two cities.

The lower percentage of men affected in New York is due primarily to the larger number of affected intrave-

TABLE III. Reported AIDS Cases Through December 1986: New York City, San Francisco, and the United States

	New York City	San Francisco	United States
Total cases	8,847	2,760	29,137
% of US cases	30.4	9.5	100
Cases/100,000 population*	124.9	398.8	12.7
% Cases male	88.3	99.1	92.6
% Cases by race/ethnicity:			
White	44.8	86.2	59.6
Black	31.2	5.8	25.0
Hispanic	23.4	6.6	14.4
Other/unknown	0.6	1.3	1.0
Number of pediatric cases†	166	7	410
% Cases by transmission category:			
Gay or bisexual men‡	61.1	97.0	72.2
Intravenous (IV) drug users	29.1	1.2	16.8
Transfusion with blood or blood products	0.9	0.8	2.0
Hemophilia/coagulation disorder	0.2	0.1	0.9
Heterosexual contact§	2.1	0.4	3.8
Child of parent with AIDS or at increased risk for AIDS	1.7	0.1	1.1
None of the above/other	4.9	0.4	3.2
Total	100	100	100

Sources: New York City Department of Health, Office of Epidemiologic Surveillance and Statistics; San Francisco Department of Public Health, Bureau of Communicable Disease Control; Centers for Disease Control, US AIDS Program, Center for Infectious Diseases.
* Cases/100,000 are based on 1982 populations for each city.
† Pediatric cases refer to patients under 13 years of age at time of diagnosis.
‡ Eight, 13, and 11 percent of gay and bisexual men in New York, San Francisco, and the United States, respectively, also reported having used IV drugs.
§ Heterosexual contact refers to sexual relations with a person with AIDS or at risk for AIDS.

nous (IV) drug users in that city, compared to the predominance of gay men in San Francisco. Female IV drug users and women infected by their sexual partners who are IV drug users represent a much larger proportion of AIDS cases in New York than in San Francisco.

AIDS cases also vary significantly by race and risk group. San Francisco's AIDS patients are more likely to be white, whereas New York's are more likely to be black or Hispanic. This reflects general demographic differences in these cities. Compared to all AIDS patients in the US, patients in San Francisco are much more likely to be homosexuals, whereas patients in New York consist of a larger proportion of IV drug users.

Heavy incidence among IV drug users affects another patient group—children. In New York, where IV drug use and sharing of contaminated needles is more common than in the rest of the country, 79% of children with AIDS were presumably infected during pregnancy by mothers who were either IV drug users themselves or who had been infected by IV drug users.[16] The proportion of IV drug-related AIDS cases among children is likely to rise because of the continued spread of AIDS among drug users and the decline in the number of cases transmitted through contaminated blood and blood products (as a result of improved screening of the nation's blood supply).

Two patient groups remain hospitalized longer than others—IV drug users and children with AIDS. Both groups are concentrated in New York City. There have been 2,570 AIDS cases among IV drug users and 166 cases of pediatric AIDS reported in New York City through 1986. This represents 52% and 40% of the nation's cases in the respective groups. Only 33 IV drug-related and seven pediatric cases were reported in San Francisco during this time. (The figures for both cities do not include approximately 8–13% of cases among homosexual or bisexual men who also report using IV drugs.)

The municipal hospitals in New York are overwhelmed with IV drug users, a group which comprises 60% of all AIDS patients hospitalized there.[9] These patients are generally indigent, have poor underlying health status, have fewer sources of social support, and are more likely to be homeless than other patient groups. The primary AIDS diagnosis for many IV drug users is *Pneumocystis carinii* pneumonia (PCP). In general, this opportunistic infection is more debilitating and requires longer and more frequent hospital stays than other AIDS-related conditions, the most common of which is Kaposi's sarcoma, which is often treated on an outpatient basis.[17] In a study of AIDS patients at San Francisco General Hospital (SFGH), the average length of stay for AIDS patients with Kaposi's sarcoma was 7.6 days, compared to 18.1 days for those with PCP.[11] Furthermore, during 1984, Kaposi's sarcoma accounted for 13.3% of the total AIDS admissions at this hospital, as compared to only 3.5% of AIDS admissions in the public hospitals in New York City.[9] All these factors increase the likelihood of a longer hospital stay and an increased direct cost of care for AIDS patients in New York.

Hospitalization of children with AIDS has not been a major problem in San Francisco, since there have been so few cases. New York, by contrast, has had to address issues arising from pediatric AIDS, including the unusually long length of stay for these patients. As discussed above,

more than three quarters of the pediatric AIDS patients in New York have parents who are or have been IV drug users. Many of these parents may be ill, and some have died from AIDS. In addition, there is a lack of alternative facilities to care for children outside the hospital, and it has been extremely difficult to place children with AIDS in foster care. Again, this is consistent with the situation confronting adult AIDS patients, who, in New York's tight housing market, also face difficulty in finding available space in nursing homes, and thus are likely to have prolonged hospital stays. A one-day survey conducted in New York's municipal hospitals found nine pediatric AIDS patients awaiting nonhospital placement. All were homeless, and all were candidates for home care. Three of these patients had been on an alternate level of care status (ie, those patients who no longer require acute care hospital services and are ready for placement in nonhospital settings) for 12, 14, and 18 months.[18] Thus, overall, the AIDS epidemic is quite different in New York than in San Francisco. New York is confronted with approximately three times the number of cases, and the patients are more heterogeneous than those in San Francisco with respect to race, age, sex, income, and major risk factors. In effect, the differences in scale and diversity of patients in New York, when compared to San Francisco, present local policy makers with two quite different epidemics of the same disease.

Preexisting Social and Political Structures. The local responses to the epidemic did not occur in a vacuum. They grew out of and were influenced by the social and political structures already existing in each community. Each city's historical development—in size, number, and type of institutions providing health services; methods of payment for health care; and the roles of public agencies—set the stage for what could happen in the epidemic. We differentiate two components in the preexisting social and political structures: one is related to the community and its institutions, especially the structure of health and human service organizations; the other is related to the social and political structures of those persons in the major risk groups.

The scale and complexity of health and human service organizations is far greater in New York than in San Francisco. The difficulties associated with a larger scale in New York range from the simple logistics of epidemiologic case monitoring to the institutional complexities of developing a response in 11 acute care municipal hospitals and over 70 other private and voluntary hospitals scattered unevenly throughout five boroughs. This contrasts with the one city health care facility and 13 other hospitals in San Francisco. In addition, the existence of a single medical school in San Francisco has fostered a relatively unified response to the epidemic, while in New York there is a history of competition in selected areas among the seven medical schools, making a similar response much more difficult.

The cities are similar in having a complex role in the financing of health care for part of their populations. These roles have been illuminated by the AIDS epidemic and the enormous resources needed to cope with it. One of the major differences in the two cities is how local tax monies have been allocated. One report estimated that more than 90% of New York City AIDS funds are spent on inpatient hospital care, largely through the city government's 25% share of Medicaid expenditures, and direct subsidies to the NYCHHC and voluntary hospitals providing indigent care.[19] This results in sizable expenditures of local funds in New York because of the large number of AIDS patients who are enrolled in the Medicaid program. In comparison, in San Francisco only approximately 25% of municipal AIDS funds are spent on inpatient care. The large difference is due in part to San Francisco's local government not contributing to the Medicaid program. This reduces the cost of hospitalization to the city, while increasing the cost to the state of California.

These differences point out the importance of local-state relationships in responses to AIDS, especially in funding. In New York, the state health department has increased its influence vis-a-vis the New York City Health Department through its statutory responsibilities in Medicaid and in voluntary hospital financing in general. In addition, following the fiscal crisis of the 1970s, the state assumed other responsibilities that were formerly the province of city agencies. For example, administrative control over substance abuse programs was shifted to the state during the late 1970s, and it is these agencies that are trying to cope with the growing epidemic among IV drug users.[20]

Both cities help pay for the costs of hospitalizing medically indigent patients who are not covered by any third-party payers. This has been an especially acute problem with AIDS patients, many of whom are treated with experimental drugs because no efficacious drug regimen is available. Third-party payers, both private and public, have been reluctant to pay for hospital care when experimental drugs are used in treatment. Thus, both local governments have been forced to subsidize treatment costs. Even more important for the cities' budgets is the fragmented mix of policies that have resulted in a large number of AIDS patients joining millions of other Americans who "fall through the cracks" and have inadequate health insurance coverage. It is estimated that more than 55 million people in this country have little or no health insurance at all.[21] These patients, who are generally confined to municipal hospitals, are subsidized by local tax revenues in both cities.

The payer mix for AIDS patients in the municipal hospitals of each city is quite similar (Table IV). In the municipal hospitals, those patients not covered by private insurance, Medicaid, or Medicare usually have no other insurance coverage and are subsidized by local government. In San Francisco's nonmunicipal hospitals, Kaiser Permanente, a health maintenance organization, covers at least 50% of those patients in the "other" category, reducing the overall level of uncompensated care to approximately 13% of the total AIDS inpatient caseload in that city.

The budgets of the cities in the years preceding the epidemic also may have influenced the extent to which each committed financial resources to the epidemic. The ability of local government in San Francisco to respond to the AIDS crisis with substantial funds as early as 1983 was made easier by the existence of a budget surplus that existed during the early 1980s (but is now gone). In contrast, New York was just coming out of a protracted period of financial crisis and near bankruptcy in the late 1970s.

Another factor that existed before the epidemic and influenced local responses was the different roles of the local health departments. In San Francisco, the health department incorporated traditional public health functions, outpatient clinics, and San Francisco General Hospital under one bureaucracy. This strengthened local public health decision makers in their position that the health department should take the lead in responding to the AIDS epidemic through direct action and active coordination, funding, and support of other organizations. In New York, the health department's functions were separate from hospital services, which fell within the bureaucracy of the NYCHHC. Thus, the health department in general "should provide those services that others have not, will not, should not, or cannot provide," [22] ie, its role is to fill the gaps in the system. In an early response to the AIDS epidemic, the department called a meeting of all interested parties in the city and defined its role as "seeking not to direct, but to provide a neutral meeting ground." [22]

A further difference lies in the difficulties of coordinating the diversity of services that can be used to address the AIDS epidemic. In New York, three large, separate city bureaucracies, the Health Department, the Health and Hospitals Corporation, and the Human Resources Administration, each developed programs to deal with AIDS, with little formalized central coordination. In San Francisco, these functions were under the authority of one agency, and this allowed extensive health department organizational resources to be used to encourage the integration of community-based, ambulatory, and institutional programs.

The preexisting social and political structures of persons in the major risk groups are a second component that helps explain the differences in the two cities. In San Francisco, AIDS has predominantly affected white, middle-class, homosexual men. In New York, at least half the cases are reported among minorities, and almost a third are known IV drug users—an impoverished, highly stigmatized, and politically powerless stratum of society.

In a 1984 survey, the number of openly homosexual or bisexual men in San Francisco was estimated to be approximately 69,000, or 24% of all men aged 15 years and older.[23] The homosexual community was also found to be relatively affluent and well-educated, with 44% having

TABLE IV.   Percent of AIDS Patient Discharges by Payer Source: San Francisco and New York Hospitals, 1985

	Medicaid	Medicare	Private Insurance	Other
San Francisco				
Municipal hospital	64%	2%	17%	17%
Nonmunicipal hospital	16	2	57	25
New York City				
Municipal hospital	65	1	13	21
Nonmunicipal hospital	45	3	36	16

Sources: Based on data derived from references 9 and 10 and from Kaufman and Kelly: *AIDS Reports from New York City*, memorandum to Steve Anderman, Deputy Director, Division of Health Care Financing, New York State Department of Health, December 10, 1985.

pre-tax earnings of $25,000 or more, 57% having college degrees, and 21% having postgraduate degrees. A preliminary survey in New York indicates a similar socioeconomic background for homosexual men.[24] However, given the distribution of cases in other patient groups (eg, IV drug users) and by race, AIDS has afflicted a poorer and less educated population in New York.

The roles of the risk groups in the economic and political life of these communities are markedly different. The homosexual community is a well-organized, visible, and powerful political force in San Francisco, with openly gay representatives holding elective office in local government since the late 1970s. There is no comparable group of gay political power in New York. Thus, in San Francisco, the major identified risk group has been represented by organized spokesmen who were an integral component of the local political establishment even before the AIDS epidemic began.

Such visibility and political power for the major risk group in San Francisco is probably reflected in the differences in newspaper coverage of AIDS by *The New York Times* and *The San Francisco Chronicle*. Although these two papers play somewhat different roles, in that the *Chronicle* is viewed as more locally oriented than the *Times* (and therefore would be expected to put more emphasis on a locally important issue), the more extensive AIDS coverage by the *Chronicle* is still noteworthy. Between June 1982 and June 1985, 442 articles about AIDS appeared in the *Chronicle*, of which 67 were front-page stories. This compares to 226 articles published in the *Times*, of which seven were page-one news. The extensive nature of coverage by the *Chronicle*, aside from providing a degree of health education not found in New York, helped to sustain a level of political pressure on local government and health officials to respond to the AIDS crisis. The difference in coverage is also probably a reflection of the relative importance of the AIDS epidemic among other local issues. In San Francisco, AIDS was clearly a top issue; in New York, it had to compete for attention with a multitude of other issues.

Thus, the preexisting social and political structures of the institutions and major risk groups reinforced the differences in the epidemiology of AIDS in the two cities. In New York, the complexity of coping with AIDS was heightened by the heterogeneity of the risk groups and their diffuse political and social organization, by the number and diversity of organizational actors in the health and human services sector, by the roles of public agencies in financing health care and in responding to the epidemic, and by the relative importance of AIDS as a local policy issue. In San Francisco, on the other hand, both the epidemiology and the social and political factors put fewer constraints on those agencies that responded to the epidemic. Indeed, the conditions were that a well-educated, highly organized, and politically active group of citizens were at risk of AIDS in a city with relatively well-coordinated relationships among the major public health care institutions. The epidemiology and the social and political factors contributed, directly and indirectly, to some of the differences between the two cities through their influence on the cities' policy responses.

Policy Responses in New York and San Francisco. In both cities, the AIDS epidemic has generated a largely unanticipated need for a variety of medical, public health, social, and educational resources. For example, active disease surveillance and epidemiologic investigations have been necessary to track the epidemic, to establish routes of transmission, and to plan for future health care resources to service the needs of those afflicted. AIDS patients require hospital care, outpatient services, social support and, in many cases, housing and food. Members of high-risk groups need public health education, counseling, and specific guidelines regarding behavior to prevent transmission of the disease. The population outside the main risk groups needs education to understand the risks and how the disease is transmitted in order to reduce unwarranted fears, to promote support for effective programs, and to prevent further spread of the epidemic. The policy responses in the two cities, as reflected in agency behavior, followed paths that were consistent with the differences in epidemiologic factors and social and political structures.

In 1982, the San Francisco Department of Public Health (SFDPH), through its Office of Lesbian and Gay Health, began to coordinate efforts to plan and develop services to deal with AIDS. By 1983, in efforts to avoid duplication of services by a growing number of organizations and to coordinate the city and county's responses, a separate AIDS Activity Office was established within the SFDPH with the following specific purposes: to better coordinate and link the continuum of services related to the AIDS epidemic; to identify service gaps and develop plans for addressing these needs; to oversee, monitor, and support AIDS-related contract services; to anticipate funding requirements and justify new funding requests; and to develop and maintain the department's liaison with certain external funding and service agencies, community groups, and education programs. However, significant local funding for AIDS programs in San Francisco did not begin until FY 1984, when expenditures increased to $4.3 million from $180,000 the previous year.[8]

During the early years of the epidemic in New York (1981–1984), there was no centralized governmental response. Although an Office of Gay and Lesbian Health existed within the Department of Health since 1982, it was an advisory body with no policy-making authority. More importantly, it had less political power than the comparable office in San Francisco due to its location within the health department and its inability to influence other city bureaucracies that deal with AIDS in New York.

In November 1984, at the direction of the mayor, an AIDS Policy and Planning Committee was formed. Its first order of business was to send a fact-finding delegation to San Francisco (January 1985) to study that city's response and to make recommendations for improving New York's services to AIDS patients.

The delegation's foremost recommendation was to improve administrative coordination among all city agencies dealing with the AIDS crisis through the Policy and Planning Committee. This body was formalized in March 1985, and its charge was to oversee planning, coordination, monitoring, and evaluation of all the AIDS services provided by the city directly or by contract. Other recommendations called for increased resources for the surveillance efforts of the health department, and enhancement of acute and chronic medical services (including outpatient services), the provision of housing and social services, and educational programs. Most of these recommendations and other AIDS programs were implemented by the beginning of 1986, with a large increase in city appropriations during FY 1986.[9]

In San Francisco, the existence of an office within the health department devoted to gay and lesbian health issues provided a natural organizational focus for AIDS issues as the epidemic developed. The relatively small scale of the city, the recognized importance of homosexuals in local politics, the relatively high educational and income levels of the gay community, and its social organization all contributed to the development of an integrated system of outpatient and community-based services for AIDS patients. These services not only provide an important part of the care for AIDS patients, they have a financial impact on the local health care system by allowing many patients to remain outside the hospital for longer periods and, once admitted, to be discharged earlier. The range of community services available include outpatient clinics, public health education, hospice care, legal services and entitlements advocacy, psychosocial counseling, substance abuse services, and practical support and housing for AIDS patients.

While these services now exist in each city, the timing of their development and sources of funding differed. For example, outpatient clinical services for AIDS patients have been available at SFGH since September 1981. In the fall of 1982, SFGH established a special multidisciplinary clinic (infectious diseases, oncology, psychiatry, psychology, nursing, dermatology, and social work). At the University of California in San Francisco (UCSF), another outpatient clinic for AIDS patients opened in August 1984. During 1985, the clinics at SFGH and UCSF averaged approximately 1,000 patient visits per month.[8]

In New York City, the first outpatient clinic for AIDS patients was opened at Kings County Hospital in early 1984. During 1985, it was open two afternoons per week and handled between 120 and 175 patient visits per month. The first full-time AIDS ambulatory care clinic was opened in Manhattan in the spring of 1985. Slowness in providing comprehensive AIDS outpatient services in New York has probably increased the level and expense of hospitalization there.

The diversity of AIDS patients in New York makes the process of developing a useful range of services far more difficult. Developing services appropriate for both IV drug users and children with AIDS has obviously been much more of a problem for New York than for San Francisco. On the other hand, the highly successful, specialized inpatient AIDS ward at San Francisco General Hospital, where most patients are middle class gay men, has benefited from the homogeneity of its patients and extensive support from the gay community. Attempts to develop such a ward in a setting where the majority of patients are substance abusers would obviously entail difficulties. Other community-based programs in San Francisco, such as the Shanti AIDS Residence Program, which provides long-term housing for AIDS patients (and thereby helps keep patients out of the hospital), are not designed to accommodate patients with substance abuse problems, and, in fact, Shanti does not accept such patients into its program. Thus, the ability of San Francisco to develop a range of successful community-based services is due not only to good planning and a commitment of local resources, it is a reflection of the strength and importance of the gay community, whose members comprise the majority of patients and those at risk.

To support its community-based services, New York City has relied more on state and private funding and less on local funds compared to San Francisco. This may be due to the transfer of responsibility for various services from New York City to New York State government after the fiscal crisis of the 1970s, or it may be due to a paucity of local political power among the groups at risk. It may also reflect the enormous management and planning difficulties—rooted in the complexity of the epidemic in New York—of local government officials as they attempted to develop programs. For example, a city-funded program for home attendant services to persons with AIDS provided care to only a fraction of those in need. An audit of this program found that from its inception in December 1983 through February 1985 a total of only 80 clients had received service, although it was designed to serve a 200-client caseload.[25] The report elaborated a series of reasons for the program's failure to meet its goals, including poor contract planning, lack of needs assessment, enrollment limited to those who were eligible for Medicaid, excessive processing time, lack of housing, and poor community outreach.

Nevertheless, community-based AIDS organizations have played a key role in responding to the epidemic in both cities. They have provided an important and otherwise missing dimension to patient care and have been instrumental in developing and disseminating risk reduction strategies. At the same time, they have had an important financial impact on the local health care systems by keeping patients out of the hospital.

One reason government support for community-based organizations is a cost effective strategy is the heavy reliance on volunteer labor in these groups, which allows for a greater production of services per dollar expended than would be possible if government provided these services directly. However, a significant level of financial support is still necessary to develop administrative structures and to pay staff who can recruit, train, supervise, and support volunteers. According to one national survey,[26] nearly 80% of services provided by community-based AIDS groups around the country were performed by volunteers. In New York and San Francisco, the magnitude of donated labor is enormous, conservatively estimated at more than 100,000 hours in each city (Table V). The amount of donated labor at the Gay Men's Health Crisis in New York is similar to the combined total of the Shanti Project and the San Francisco AIDS Foundation. However, the ratio of unpaid staff hours to paid staff hours is twice as large in New York, indicating a greater reliance on volunteers and lesser funding by local government there.

CONCLUSIONS

The large number of AIDS cases in New York and San Francisco has had a significant impact on the local health

TABLE V. Hours Worked, Largest Community-based AIDS Organizations: New York and San Francisco, 1984–1985

	Volunteer Staff Average Total Hours/Month	Paid Staff Average Total Hours/Month	Ratio Volunteer/ Paid Hours
San Francisco			
AIDS Foundation	3,807	1,976	1.93
Shanti Project	6,852	3,900	1.76
New York			
Gay Men's Health Crisis	8,834	2,427	3.64

Sources: Based on data derived from references 13 and 14.

care systems. It is likely that as the epidemic spreads it will place increasingly greater strains on other health care systems in cities and counties with growing numbers of cases, as well as on public and private sources of health care financing. While the absolute number of AIDS cases continues to grow in metropolitan areas, there is convincing evidence that the disease is spreading across the country. According to the Centers for Disease Control, the four cities with the largest number of AIDS cases—New York, San Francisco, Los Angeles, and Miami—accounted for 73% of all reported cases in September 1982. This figure declined to 65% by September 1983, and, by February 1987, their proportion of the nation's total had fallen to 50%. In other words, the proportion of total AIDS cases not based in these four metropolitan areas has increased by more than 85% during this time period.

The availability of outpatient and community-based care facilities and programs and the relatively low charges per AIDS admission in San Francisco may give an important clue to the direction other communities should follow in a rational planning policy for the treatment of AIDS patients. The average length of hospitalization for AIDS patients in San Francisco is far shorter than in New York and in most other cities. This is due in part to the variations in patient groups, case mix, and practice patterns that are found in different regions of the country. However, an integrated system of health care delivery which is subsidized by local government in San Francisco and includes outpatient clinics, home health and hospice care, housing, and other social support services, allows patients to be discharged from the hospital earlier than in other cities where such services are not as readily available. The success of San Francisco's response to the epidemic does not, however, mean that other cities should attempt to respond in exactly the same way. New York's example illustrates how one city, confronted with complex problems, considered a variety of local conditions rather than merely adopting another city's model. Each community should develop its own response in light of its own epidemiologic circumstances and social and political structures, learning from the experiences of San Francisco and New York City.

The investment of public funds in community-based services affords better quality care for AIDS patients. It is also a rational fiscal response that helps reduce the economic impact of the epidemic by reducing the need for inpatient care. This lowers private health insurance expenditures, Medicaid outlays, and local tax revenues that must be spent when Medicaid or other third-party reimbursement is unavailable or below costs.

Aside from financial support from the public sector, the viability of community-based AIDS organizations depends on a large, steady stream of unpaid labor. If the patient mix shifts further away from homosexual men towards IV drug users, as it slowly appears to be doing, it is unclear whether the level of voluntarism can be maintained. In low incidence regions, there may not be an identified at-risk population from which to draw volunteers. Thus, unless further financial support is forthcoming, gaps in services to AIDS patients, already experienced by many of these communities, may become more severe as the epidemic continues to spread geographically.

New York City and San Francisco illustrate that the AIDS epidemic may manifest itself quite differently in various cities and can trigger diverse responses based on local conditions. With the likely prospect of other cities facing large increases in the number of those afflicted with AIDS, the experiences of New York and San Francisco may prove useful. They indicate that each community's response to AIDS will probably reflect the underlying social, economic, and political characteristics of AIDS victims and the existing structure and organizational roles of traditional health care and community-based service providers. They also indicate the intrinsic limits to the current dependency on unpaid labor and the contributions from private charity and local government, increasing the pressure for additional state and federal support for community-based services and the care of AIDS patients.

Acknowledgment. The authors thank the many people in New York City and San Francisco who generously provided their time and expertise in helping to gather and interpret the data from each community.

REFERENCES

1. Arno PS: Statement before the Subcommittee on Health and the Environment, Committee on Energy and Commerce, US House of Representatives, July 22, 1985.
2. Hardy AM, Rauch K, Echenberg D, et al: The economic impact of the first 9,000 cases of acquired immunodeficiency syndrome in the United States. Presented at the International Conference on AIDS, Atlanta, Georgia, April 17, 1985.
3. Shilts R: AIDS crisis hits an unprepared New York. *San Francisco Chronicle*, February 1985; 14:1.
4. Leishman K: San Francisco. A crisis of public health. *Atlantic Monthly*, October 1985, pp 18–41.
5. Boufford JI: Statement before Intergovernmental Relations and Human Resources Subcommittee of the Committee on Government Operations, US House of Representatives, September 13, 1985.
6. Botnick V: New York City's Response to AIDS. Memo to Edward Koch, Mayor, and Stanly Brezenoff, Deputy Mayor for Operations, City of New York, March 27, 1985.
7. West Bay Hospital Conference: *Monthly AIDS Hospital Utilization Report*. San Mateo, California, October 25, 1985.
8. San Francisco Department of Public Health: *San Francisco's Response to AIDS: Status Update*. October 8, 1985.
9. Sencer DJ, Botnick VE: *Report to the Mayor: New York City's Response to the AIDS Crisis*. Office of the Mayor, City of New York, December 1985.
10. West Bay Hospital Conference: *Quarterly AIDS Utilization Report*, San Mateo, California, March 5, 1986.
11. Scitovsky AA, Cline M, Lee PR: Medical care costs of patients with AIDS in San Francisco. *JAMA* 1986; 256:3103–3106.
12. Knickman J, Foltz AM: Regional differences in hospital utilization. How much can be traced to population differences? *Med Care* 1984; 22:971–986.
13. Gay Men's Health Crisis: 1984 Annual Report, New York, 1985.
14. Arno PS: The nonprofit sector's response to the AIDS epidemic. Community-based services in San Francisco. *Am J Public Health* 1986; 76:1325–1330.
15. Centers for Disease Control: *AIDS Weekly Surveillance Report*. US AIDS Program, Center for Infectious Diseases, Atlanta, Georgia, January 5, 1987.
16. New York City Department of Health: *AIDS Surveillance Update*. Office of Epidemiologic Surveillance and Statistics, January 1987.
17. Volberding PA: The clinical spectrum of the acquired immunodeficiency syndrome. Implications for comprehensive patient care. *Ann Intern Med* 1985; 103:729–733.

18. Boufford JI: Statement before Subcommittee on Health and Environment, Committee on Energy and Commerce, US House of Representatives, November 1, 1985.

19. New York State Comptroller. *Review of New York City's Proposed Financial Plan for Fiscal Years 1986 through 1989.* Report No. 30-86, December 11, 1985.

20. Imperato PJ: *The Administration of a Public Health Agency.* New York, Human Sciences Press, 1983, pp 100–105.

21. Farley PJ: Who are the underinsured? *Milbank Memorial Fund Quarterly/Health and Society* 1985; 63:476–503.

22. Sencer DJ: Major urban health departments: The ideal and the real. *Health Affairs* 1983; 2:88–95.

23. Research and Decisions Corporation: *Designing an Effective AIDS Prevention Strategy for San Francisco; Results from the First Probability Sample of an Urban Gay Male Community.* Prepared for the San Francisco AIDS Foundation, December 3, 1984.

24. Martin JL: *The Impact of AIDS on New York City Gay Men: Development of a Community Sample.* Presented at the Annual Meetings of the American Public Health Association, Washington, DC, November 21, 1985.

25. New York City Comptroller: *Report on the New York City Human Resources Administration of the American Red Cross AIDS Home Attendant Program,* ML 85-504, April 15, 1985.

26. US Conference of Mayors: *Local Responses to AIDS: A Report of 55 Cities.* Washington, DC, November 1984.

Chapter 3

The effect of group education on improving attitudes about AIDS risk reduction

RONALD O. VALDISERRI, MD; DAVID W. LYTER, MD; LAWRENCE A. KINGSLEY, DrPH; LAURA C. LEVITON, PhD; JANET W. SCHOFIELD, PhD; JAMES HUGGINS, MSW; MONTO HO, MD; CHARLES R. RINALDO, PhD

ABSTRACT. Four hundred sixty-four homosexual and bisexual men, recruited from a cohort of 1,700 men enrolled in a study of the natural history of acquired immunodeficiency syndrome (AIDS), participated in a peer-led, small-group educational session promoting AIDS risk reduction. Although levels of knowledge about AIDS and human immunodeficiency virus (HIV) transmission were uniformly high prior to intervention, at least 60% of the men reported having engaged in unprotected, receptive anal intercourse with more than one partner in the preceding six months. Prior to intervention, a substantial number of the men had mixed feelings about AIDS risk reduction or endorsed negative attitudes about AIDS risk reduction. After attending the session, attitudes improved significantly in five of the six areas surveyed.

The ability of a group educational session to influence attitudes about AIDS risk reduction in a positive way suggests that this type of intervention may be effective in enabling homosexual and bisexual men to adopt low-risk sexual activities by influencing the nonhealth motives of sexual behavior, especially peer norms about safe sex. Long-term follow-up of this cohort will test for maintenance of this attitudinal change and, more importantly, will evaluate whether this attitudinal change is predictive of future changes in sexual behavior and HIV seroconversion rates. The authors stress the importance of incorporating existing health promotion research findings into the design and evaluation of AIDS risk reduction programs.

AIDS is the most dramatic and devastating consequence of the ongoing epidemic of human retroviral infection. In response, public health officials are attempting to prevent or decrease the sexual transmission of HIV among all risk groups, including homosexual and bisexual men, by urging the adoption of safer sexual practices. Although some officials have pointed to decreasing rates of rectal gonorrhea as evidence that homosexual men are themselves modifying high-risk behavior,[1] others have argued that such behavioral changes may have a minimal impact on the incidence of AIDS, because of the high seroprevalence rate of HIV antibody among the urban homosexual male population.[2]

There are few published evaluations of the efficacy of health promotion campaigns for AIDS risk reduction in the homosexual community. Therefore, it is important to utilize existing research and theory about health behavior derived from the design and evaluation of other risk reduction programs in designing and implementing AIDS risk reduction programs for homosexual and bisexual men. A review of the salient health promotion literature supports the hypothesis that simply acquiring more knowledge about risky activity may be inadequate to change behavior in many individuals. This has been demonstrated in efforts to encourage smoking cessation,[3-6] nutrition education,[7] seat belt use,[8] and breast self-examination.[9]

Among persons for whom information alone is not adequate to induce behavioral change, specific skills dealing with how to change and experiences that reinforce successful change may be essential. Support for this hypothesis is found in the literature that describes diabetes education,[10] smoking cessation and prevention of smoking onset,[6] and occupational safety training.[11] Specifically, the nonhealth motives of health-related behavior must be addressed if unhealthy behavior is to be modified. These

From the Department of Pathology (Drs Valdiserri and Rinaldo), Department of Medicine (Dr Lyter), and Division of Infectious Diseases (Dr Ho), University of Pittsburgh School of Medicine; the Department of Epidemiology (Dr Kingsley) and the Department of Health Services Administration (Dr Leviton), University of Pittsburgh School of Public Health; the Department of Psychology (Dr Schofield), University of Pittsburgh; and the Persad Center, Inc (Mr Huggins).

Portions of this paper were presented at the International Conference on AIDS, Paris, France, June 25, 1986. This research was supported by a grant from the Centers for Disease Control (DHHS Grant No. U62/CCU3001060-01) and the Pitt Men's Study (Contract No. AI-32513, NIH).

nonhealth motives are often influenced by peer norms and existing social support systems,[10,12,13] and as such may be modified by group process.

Preliminary information concerning sexual behaviors among male homosexuals at risk for AIDS supports these assertions. In 1983, when McKusick et al[14] surveyed 655 homosexual men in San Francisco, they found that although men "were uniformly well-informed about the prescribed behavior for AIDS risk reduction," many displayed discrepancies between what they believed and their reported sexual behavior. Others have stressed the inadequacy of "warn and scare tactics" in preventing the transmission of HIV,[15] and, in terms of efficacy, some researchers have noted parallels to adolescent smoking prevention programs, in which social influence models using peer-led group discussions have been more effective than fear-based media and educational campaigns.[3,16]

Research in other areas of health promotion has documented that context may be just as important as content in terms of inducing health-related behavioral change.[17] This also implies that a group format may be more successful at promoting AIDS risk reduction among homosexual and bisexual men than media-based campaigns or individual counseling sessions, because such a format can affect group social norms. Supplying accurate information about HIV risk reduction in conjunction with social influence could promote behavioral change among homosexual men in three ways: by providing a coping mechanism for fear arousal;[18] by increasing feelings of self-efficacy;[19] or by decreasing feelings of perceived vulnerability.[20] Using peers (other homosexual men) to deliver the information may also increase efficacy, as has been observed in smoking prevention programs for adolescents.[3,21]

SUBJECTS AND METHODS

In September 1983, the University of Pittsburgh received funding from the National Institutes of Health to conduct a prospective study of the natural history of HIV infection in homosexual and bisexual men. To date, the "Pitt Men's Study" (PMS) has enrolled more than 1,700 men from western Pennsylvania, Ohio, and West Virginia in a baseline study of the epidemiology of HIV infection. From this population, 1,062 self-selected men have agreed to participate in a more extensive study that represents the Pittsburgh cohort of the Multicenter AIDS Cohort Study (MACS). Members of both groups are tested for antibody to HIV at six-month intervals and provide information about sexual behavior and other health matters via questionnaire. The MACS group also has periodic physical examinations. The results of antibody tests are not released to volunteers without their express consent.

Beginning in September 1985, these 1,700 men were invited by mail to participate in an educational session (known as the AIDS Prevention Project) as part of the process of learning their HIV antibody status. In addition to this direct mail invitation, the AIDS Prevention Project (APP) was also promoted within the male homosexual community. Volunteers already enrolled in the PMS were encouraged to participate in the APP, while men who had not joined either study were recruited for both studies simultaneously. Recruitment efforts consisted of flyers, brochures, and a poster stressing the preventability of AIDS through appropriate sexual precautions. Numerous mailings and community presentations were also undertaken stressing the importance of prevention as a practical alternative to anxiety and fear. Although earlier recruitment efforts were closely linked to the process of learning HIV antibody results, ongoing recruitment efforts have emphasized that individuals can participate in the risk reduction program even if they do not wish to learn their HIV antibody status.

Intervention. The intervention consists of an informal group educational session led by a male health educator who is also homosexual. Groups consist of five to ten participants and last 60–75 minutes, including questions after the presentation. The goals of this session are as follows: to increase individual knowledge about the transmission, incubation period, and spectrum of clinical diseases related to HIV; to increase individual understanding of the relative HIV transmission risk associated with specific sexual practices; to instruct participants in the appropriate use of condoms; and to educate participants about interpreting HIV antibody tests.

Data Collection and Analysis. Data are collected at three points in this project: before the intervention (pre-test); one to two weeks after the intervention (post-test); and four to six months after the intervention (long term). They are obtained from self-administered questionnaires that assess knowledge, attitude, and self-reported sexual behavior. Sexual behavior is reported only at pre-test and long term; attitude and knowledge are assessed at all three points. After an individual calls to schedule an appointment for the educational session, the pre-test questionnaire is mailed to him, with instructions that he is to bring the completed form with him on the day of his session. The post-test questionnaire is handed to participants immediately after they have completed a session, with the instructions that they are to return it by mail (a pre-stamped envelope is provided) within two weeks. Appointments for disclosure of antibody test results are scheduled separately, after the intervention. Antibody test results are released to individual volunteers by a study clinician. Long-term questionnaires are mailed to participants four to six months after they have completed a session, with instructions that they are to return the questionnaire, in person, at their next Pitt Men's Study visit.

The knowledge assessment instrument consists of 17 multiple choice items dealing with HIV transmission, HIV incubation period, manifestations of HIV infection, interpretation of HIV antibody test results, and currently recognized AIDS risk groups. The attitude assessment tool consists of 38 items for which responses are recorded on a 5-point Likert scale with 1 representing "strongly disagree," 3 representing "mixed feelings," and 5 representing "strongly agree;" there is also an option for "not applicable." The attitude assessment surveys feelings and beliefs about high- and low-risk sexual practices, condom use, number of sexual partners, anonymous sexual partners, perceived vulnerability to AIDS, and perceptions about the acceptance of safer sexual practices by peers. The 38 statements in this instrument are written with emphasis on the following: intention to act in a specified manner; willingness to alter sexual habits; and individual, subjective perceptions about safer sexual practices. Positive statements describe the intention to refrain from high-risk sexual practices, to engage in low-risk sexual practices, to use condoms regularly, to decrease the number of sexual partners, to refrain from anonymous sexual encounters, and to discuss AIDS prevention with sexual partners. Finally, in regard to peer acceptance, a positive response would be defined as one in which a subject agrees with statements describing the acceptance of AIDS risk reduction by homosexual friends and acquaintances. The sexual behavior questionnaire focuses on the number of partners, types and frequency of sexual practices, including anal intercourse, and the frequency of use of condoms and spermicides (as antiviral agents).

All individuals who formally declined participation in the intervention (105 subjects) completed knowledge, attitude, and sexual behavior questionnaires, so that these data are available for pretest or baseline comparison to individuals who agreed to participate. Comparable data are not available for those who failed to respond.

RESULTS

Pre-Intervention Assessment. Of the 1,700 individuals contacted

TABLE I. Comparison of Groups at Baseline (N = 1,700)

	No Response	Declined	Accepted
No. (% total)	1,050 (62%)	105 (6%)	545 (32%)
Mean age (years)	31	32	33
College degree	54%	58%	66%*
HIV seropositive	19%	22%	19%

* $p < 0.001$, chi-square test.

through May 31, 1986, 1,050 (62%) failed to respond, 105 (6%) declined to participate, and 545 (32%) accepted the invitation to participate in an educational session prior to learning their HIV antibody status. Table I shows comparative demographic data on these three groups at baseline. Although the mean age and percent of seropositivity for HIV antibody does not differ significantly across groups, individuals who agreed to participate were more likely to have a college education than those who failed to respond ($p < 0.001$).

Table II compares high-risk sexual practices of the groups at baseline—prior to intervention. Although similar data are not available for the nonresponders, it is apparent that a majority of individuals in both the "decline" and "accept" groups were still participating in high-risk sexual activities prior to this intervention. At least 60% of both groups had engaged in unprotected receptive anal intercourse with more than one partner in the six months prior to the assessment. Of the 545 men who were willing to participate in this group educational session, 464 were actually enrolled in sessions from September 1985 through May 1986.

As seen in Tables III and IV, knowledge at baseline about a variety of topics related to HIV infection or AIDS was uniformly high in both the 464 session participants and the 105 men who declined. Also, no significant differences in knowledge about HIV were noted in these two groups. Men from both groups scored lowest (77% mean correct response) on two questions about the local prevalence of HIV infection, with nearly equal percentages over- and under-estimating prevalence.

Based on their content, attitude statements were categorized and assigned to one of the following six categories: sexual practices; condom use; number of partners/anonymous partners; perceived vulnerability to AIDS; discussion of AIDS prevention with partners; and perceptions about peer acceptance of AIDS risk reduction. Tables V and VI describe the attitudes held by individuals who declined and those who participated in the intervention, at the time of the pretest. No substantial attitudinal differences were noted between the two groups. Although a majority of respondents endorsed atti-

TABLE II. Comparison of Sexual Practices Prior to Intervention

Total Number of Sex Partners, Last Six Months	Declined (N = 105)	Accepted (N = 545)
1	26%	24%
2–5	44%	48%
6–25	27%	25%
26+	3%	4%
% reporting receptive anal intercourse, last six months, >1 partner	61%	60%
Mean no. partners for RAI,* last six months (range)	1.7 (1–15)	1.9 (1–100)

* RAI, receptive anal intercourse, for those with ≥1 partner, mean is expressed as log base 10.

TABLE III. Knowledge About AIDS in Individuals Who Declined Participation (N = 105)

Subject of Multiple Choice Questions (Number of Questions)	Mean % Correct Response (Range)
Transmission of HIV (5)	90% (76–99%)
AIDS risk groups (1)	97%
HIV incubation period (1)	96%
Manifestations of HIV infection (3)	92% (91–94%)
Local AIDS prevalence (2)	77% (67–86%)
Interpretation of HIV antibody results (5)	88% (80–94%)

tudes that correspond to AIDS risk reduction, a sizable minority did not, or had "mixed feelings" on the matter. Of interest is the fact that the highest overall endorsement (combined mean percent response frequency of "strongly agree" and "agree") among both decliners and accepters was associated with the category of statements dealing with attitudes about decreasing the number of sexual partners (76% for decliners and 71% for participants).

Compared to other categories, items related to discussing AIDS prevention with partners received the lowest overall endorsement. Individuals who declined participation scored 53% in this category, and those who agreed to participate scored 48%. This may indicate that although homosexual men may know how to reduce the risks of transmitting HIV sexually, they are uncertain of how to approach the issue with a partner.

Post-Intervention Assessment. Within two weeks after completing the intervention, participants were asked to return a follow-up questionnaire that assessed knowledge and attitude. The assessment of knowledge one to two weeks after the intervention (Table VII) demonstrated scores that were quite similar to pre-intervention ratings. This finding is not surprising given the high levels of knowledge noted prior to the intervention. The only exception is that scores improved for the two questions that deal with the local prevalence of HIV antibody and HIV-related disease.

Table VIII shows the distribution of responses to the attitudinal statements of 464 men after their participation in the group educational session. The greatest change away from "mixed feelings" and the endorsement of unhealthy behaviors occurred in the area of atti-

TABLE IV. Knowledge About AIDS in Individuals Who Participated, Prior to Intervention (N = 464)

Subject of Multiple Choice Questions (Number of Questions)	Mean % Correct Response (Range)
Transmission of HIV (5)	86% (71–99%)
AIDS risk groups (1)	95%
HIV incubation period (1)	95%
Manifestations of HIV infection (3)	92% (85–96%)
Local AIDS prevalence (2)	77% (65–90%)
Interpretation of HIV antibody results (5)	87% (75–97%)

TABLE V.   Attitudes Held by Individuals Who Declined Participation (N = 105)

Subject of Attitudinal Statements (Number of Statements)	Mean % Response Frequency (Range)				
	Strongly Agree	Agree	Mixed Feelings	Disagree	Strongly Disagree
Sexual practices (10)	42% (33–63%)	29% (21–37%)	18% (8–27%)	8% (1–16%)	4% (1–9%)
Condom use (7)	42% (27–66%)	23% (14–28%)	17% (8–24%)	12% (1–20%)	7% (0–16%)
Number of partners/ anonymous partners (8)	55% (43–76%)	21% (18–25%)	13% (5–20%)	7% (0–14%)	4% (0–8%)
Perceived vulnerability to AIDS (5)	41% (24–63%)	23% (19–29%)	26% (11–38%)	6% (1–11%)	5% (3–7%)
Discussing AIDS prevention with partners (4)	33% (18–55%)	20% (7–34%)	20% (15–28%)	17% (7–28%)	12% (1–30%)
Perceptions about peer acceptance of AIDS risk reduction (4)	27% (25–30%)	46% (34–56%)	23% (10–35%)	4% (2–5%)	1% (0–2%)

tudes about condom use (mean change, 10%) and discussing AIDS prevention with a partner (mean change, 9%)—both areas in which specific behaviors should lead directly to greater prevention. The smallest change away from "mixed feelings" and the endorsement of unhealthy behaviors occurred in the category of statements about number of partners/anonymous partners.

Of major importance is the fact that the post-intervention attitude scores differed significantly from pre-intervention scores on the basis of a Wilcoxon matched-pairs signed-ranks test (Table IX). In all categories of statements except one, a majority of statements within each category demonstrated significant change in a positive direc-

tion (away from the endorsement of unhealthy behaviors and toward the endorsement of healthier behaviors) at a significance level of $p <$ 0.05. However, no significant change was found in pre-intervention versus post-intervention scores for any of the eight statements that assessed attitudes about numbers of partners and anonymous contacts.

DISCUSSION

Data from the initial phase of a project designed to promote AIDS risk reduction have been analyzed to deter-

TABLE VI.   Attitudes Held by Individuals Who Participated, Prior to Intervention (N = 464)

Subject of Attitudinal Statements (Number of Statements)	Mean % Response Frequency (Range)				
	Strongly Agree	Agree	Mixed Feelings	Disagree	Strongly Disagree
Sexual practices (10)	42% (29–64%)	28% (22–35%)	16% (6–25%)	9% (3–13%)	5% (3–7%)
Condom use (7)	40% (19–65%)	25% (19–33%)	22% (8–35%)	10% (1–15%)	5% (1–7%)
Number of partners/ anonymous partners (8)	47% (33–73%)	24% (17–28%)	16% (7–23%)	9% (2–15%)	6% (2–8%)
Perceived vulnerability to AIDS (5)	40% (22–64%)	27% (23–31%)	22% (7–34%)	7% (3–11%)	4% (3–7%)
Discussing AIDS prevention with partners (4)	27% (9–53%)	21% (10–24%)	24% (14–32%)	16% (6–30%)	13% (4–30%)
Perceptions about peer acceptance of AIDS risk reduction (4)	26% (23–32%)	44% (40–50%)	25% (17–32%)	3% (2–4%)	1% (1%)

TABLE VII. Knowledge About AIDS After Participation in an Educational Session (N = 464)

Subject of Multiple Choice Questions (Number of Questions)	Mean % Correct Response (Range)
Transmission of HIV (5)	94% (87–99%)
AIDS risk groups (1)	96%
HIV incubation period (1)	94%
Manifestations of HIV infection (3)	94% (92–97%)
Local AIDS prevalence (2)	84% (79–89%)
Interpretation of HIV antibody results (5)	91% (81–98%)

mine whether group educational sessions are capable of influencing knowledge and attitudes about AIDS in the immediate post-intervention period. Participants were homosexual and bisexual men recruited from an ongoing study of the natural history of AIDS. The participants agreed to attend an educational session as a prerequisite for learning their HIV antibody serostatus, which had been previously determined as part of the natural history study protocol. The study group described here consisted of 464 men who attended one of these sessions.

The fact that a majority of individuals (1,050) failed to respond to this invitation may have important implications for public health officials who wish to link AIDS risk reduction programs with disclosure of antibody results. In fact, all the data obtained from this study must be interpreted with the understanding that in the pilot phase of the program, enrollment was a prerequisite for obtaining HIV antibody results. This introduces a degree of selection bias, in that individuals who participated in the intervention may have been more motivated and therefore more capable of change than individuals who declined or failed to respond, because they did not wish to learn their antibody status.

Seroprevalence rates for all three groups—nonresponders, those who declined, and those who accepted—were equivalent, ranging from 19% to 22%. These data suggest that rates of infection are no different among those who agreed to participate in the intervention than among those who did not. The three groups were also quite similar in regard to age. The only statistically significant difference detected was that individuals who agreed to participate in the intervention were more likely to have a college degree than those who failed to respond.

An analysis of the sexual practices of the two groups (those who declined and those who accepted) prior to intervention demonstrated remarkable similarities regarding the total number of different sexual partners in the previous six months. Among both groups, nearly two thirds reported engaging in unprotected receptive anal intercourse with more than one partner in the preceding six months. This finding is particularly noteworthy when correlated with the extraordinarily high level of knowledge about AIDS and its transmission demonstrated by both groups prior to intervention. As has been noted by other investigators,[14,22] accurate knowledge of high-risk sexual activities, such as unprotected receptive anal intercourse, may not be predictive of sexual behavior.

Although a majority of individuals endorsed positive attitudes about AIDS risk reduction prior to the intervention, in all areas surveyed, there was still a sizable minority of at-risk men who did not endorse positive attitudes about AIDS risk reduction or who had "mixed feelings" on the matter. One of the goals of this intervention is a

TABLE VIII. Attitudes Held by Individuals After Participation in an Educational Session (N = 464)

Subject of Attitudinal Statements (Number of Statements)	Mean % Response Frequency (Range)				
	Strongly Agree	Agree	Mixed Feelings	Disagree	Strongly Disagree
Sexual practices (10)	48% (34–72%)	28% (21–39%)	14% (4–21%)	8% (2–11%)	4% (2–6%)
Condom use (7)	48% (23–83%)	25% (15–35%)	17% (1–36%)	7% (1–12%)	3% (1–5%)
Number of partners/ anonymous partners (8)	48% (34–72%)	24% (21–27%)	15% (5–22%)	8% (1–14%)	5% (1–7%)
Perceived vulnerability to AIDS (5)	48% (24–77%)	24% (16–31%)	17% (2–27%)	6% (2–11%)	5% (2–8%)
Discussing AIDS prevention with partners (4)	34% (10–63%)	22% (13–31%)	19% (9–24%)	15% (5–31%)	10% (2–28%)
Perceptions about peer acceptance of AIDS risk reduction (4)	31% (26–34%)	44% (40–47%)	22% (17–28%)	3% (2–3%)	1% (1%)

TABLE IX.   Pre-Intervention Versus Post-Intervention
Attitude Change (N = 464)

Subject of Attitudinal Statements	Number of Statements	Number of Statements with Positive Change
Sexual practices	10	7* (70%)
Condom use	7	5* (71%)
Number of partners/ anonymous partners	8	0
Perceived vulnerability to AIDS	5	3* (60%)
Discussing AIDS prevention with partners	4	3* (75%)
Perceptions about peer acceptance of AIDS risk reduction	4	3* (75%)

* $p < 0.05$, by Wilcoxon matched-pairs signed-ranks test.

reduction of this minority and of the risky behaviors that may correlate with these attitudes.

Prior to intervention, the lowest percentage of agreement for both the men who declined and those who subsequently participated was found among the statements concerning the discussion of AIDS prevention with sexual partners. This may indicate that for some men, accurate knowledge about HIV transmission is, by itself, inadequate to promote risk reduction behavior. The highest percentage of endorsement prior to intervention was found in association with statements about reducing the numbers of sexual partners and anonymous contacts. This may correlate with the observations of others that many homosexual men have already responded to the AIDS epidemic by decreasing their sexual activity.[1,23,24] If this is so, it follows that homosexual and bisexual men would tend to recognize reduction in the number of sexual partners as a positive or beneficial adaptation, even before this intervention program.

Although there was little overall change in the levels of knowledge after the intervention (Table VII), this is not surprising given the extremely high levels of knowledge recorded at pre-test. Attitude scores, however, improved significantly after the educational intervention. Positive attitudinal changes were noted in response to a majority of statements dealing with sexual practices, condom use, perceived vulnerability to AIDS, the intention to discuss AIDS prevention with future sexual partners, and perceptions of peer acceptance of safer sexual practices (Table IX). Attitudes about condom use and the discussion of AIDS prevention with partners showed the greatest change away from "mixed feelings" and the endorsement of risky practices toward the endorsement of risk reduction practices.

No significant change was detected in the post-test responses to any of the eight attitudinal statements dealing with numbers of sexual partners, including anonymous contacts. Although it is possible that this intervention program is not capable of influencing these attitudes, this is unlikely since significant positive change was achieved in all other areas surveyed. An alternate explanation may be that homosexual and bisexual men who are capable of reducing or willing to reduce their sexual contacts have already done so as a result of the prominent association of AIDS with promiscuity, as reported by the media. Although this is a positive change and should continue to be reinforced by health officials, it may also promote the dangerous misconception that most sexual acts are safe if performed by individuals who are not promiscuous or with non-anonymous partners. Because of the extremely long incubation period of this virus, monogamy per se does not guarantee that an individual will not become infected.

The ability of the group educational session to positively change attitudes about AIDS risk reduction in the immediate post-intervention period provides evidence that this type of intervention may be successful at influencing the nonhealth motives of sexual behavior in homosexual and bisexual men, by affecting group norms. Research from other health promotion efforts would suggest that the ability to influence these motives would result in more effective and, perhaps, more permanent behavioral change.[10,12,13,25] Regarding AIDS risk reduction, it has been suggested that emphasizing the social acceptability of safer sexual practices might be more effective at persuading homosexual and bisexual men to change sexual behaviors than merely stressing the dangers of unsafe sexual practices.[22,25] The process of discussing sexual practices and AIDS risk reduction among a group of homosexual and bisexual men may, in fact, serve to validate the notion of safe sex for group participants.

The long-term follow-up of this cohort will test whether these immediate changes in attitude are predictive of future sexual behavior. The problems of predicting behavior from attitude are well known, and attitude may or may not be related to subsequent sexual behavior in this group. However, the pattern of results described here suggests that behavioral change is likely to follow. Furthermore, many of the attitudinal items surveyed reflect specific intentions to act, rather than global attitudes toward sex. Such specific items appear to be more highly correlated with actual behavior.[26]

The long-term follow-up of participants in this project will also determine whether attitudinal change is maintained over time, and whether there is a relationship between attitudes and subsequent sexual behavior, through both self-report and clinical indicators such as HIV seroconversion rates. The AIDS Prevention Project is ongoing; in the future, an additional intervention program is planned—one that has a skills training component in addition to the group educational session. This will enable an evaluation of the differential efficacy of each component.

Finally, these results demonstrate the importance and appropriateness of applying existing health promotion theory and research findings to the field of AIDS risk reduction.

Acknowledgments. The authors thank Mr Kerry Stoner, Mr Tony Silvestre, and Ms Diane Bell for their assistance.

REFERENCES

1. Judson FN: Fear of AIDS and gonorrhea rates in homosexual men. *Lancet* 1983; 2:159–169.
2. Handsfield HH: Decreasing incidence of gonorrhea in homosexually active men—minimal effect on risk of AIDS. *West J Med* 1985; 143:469–470.
3. McAlister AL, Perry C, Maccoby N: Adolescent smoking: Onset and prevention. *Pediatrics* 1979; 63:650–658.
4. McAlister AL, Puska P, Salonen JT, et al: Theory and action for health promotion: Illustrations from the North Karelia project. *Am J Public Health* 1982; 72:43–50.
5. Perry C, Killen J, Telch M, et al: Modifying smoking behavior of teenagers: A school-based intervention. *Am J Public Health* 1980; 70:722–725.
6. Leventhal H, Cleary PD: The smoking problem: A review of research and theory in behavioral risk modification. *Psychological Bull* 1980; 88:370–405.
7. St Pierre RG, Cook TD, Staw RB: An evaluation of the nutrition education and training program: Findings from Nebraska. *Evaluation and Program Planning* 1981; 4:335–344.
8. Ware A, Bigelow B, Sleet D: Safety belt use at the worksite. *Corporate Commentary* 1984; 1:16–27.
9. Parkinson R, Denniston RW, Baugh T, et al: Breast cancer: Health education in the workplace. *Health Educ Q* 1982; 9:61–72.
10. Steiner G, Lawrence PA: *Educating Diabetic Patients*. New York, Springer-Verlag, 1981.
11. Samways MC: Cost-effective occupational health and safety training. *Am Ind Hyg Assoc J* 1983; 44:A6–A9.
12. Levine DM: Health education for behavioral change—clinical trial to public health program. *Johns Hopkins Med J* 1982; 151:215–219.
13. Diesenhaus H: Current trends in treatment programming for problem drinkers and alcoholics, in *Alcohol and Health Monographs: Prevention, Intervention and Treatment: Concerns and Models*. Washington, Public Health Service NIAAA, 1982.
14. McKusick L, Horstman W, Coates TJ: AIDS and sexual behavior reported by gay men in San Francisco. *Am J Public Health* 1985; 75:493–496.
15. Coates TJ, Temoshok L, Mandel J: Psychosocial research is essential to understanding and treating AIDS. *Am Psychol* 1984; 39:1309–1314.
16. Thompson EI: Smoking education programs, 1960–1976. *Am J Public Health* 1976; 687:250–257.
17. Worden JK, Costanza MC, Foster RS, et al: Content and context in health education: Persuading women to perform breast self-examination. *Prev Med* 1983; 12:331–339.
18. Leventhal H, Meyer D, Gutmann M: The role of theory in the study of compliance to high blood pressure regimens, in Haynes RB, Mattson MW, Tilmer OE (eds): *Patient Compliance to Prescribed Antihypertensive Medication Regimens: A Report to the National Heart, Lung and Blood Institute*, US Dept of Health and Human Services publication No. (NIH) 81-2102, 1980.
19. Bandura A: Self-efficacy: Toward a unifying theory of behavioral change. *Psychol Review* 1977; 84:191–215.
20. Rosenstock IM: Historical origins of the health belief model. *Health Education Monographs* 1974; 2:328–335.
21. Vartiainen E, Palonen V, McAlister A, et al: Effects of two years of education intervention on adolescent smoking. *Bull WHO* 1983; 61:529–532.
22. Designing an effective AIDS prevention strategy for San Francisco. San Francisco, Research and Decisions Corporation, 1984.
23. Schechter MT, Jeffries E, Constance P, et al: Changes in sexual behavior and fear of AIDS. *Lancet* 1984; 1:1293.
24. Puckett SB, Bart M, Bye LL, et al: Self-reported behavioral change among gay and bisexual men—San Francisco. *MMWR* 1985; 34:613–615.
25. McKusick L, Conant M, Coates T: The AIDS epidemic: A model for developing intervention strategies for reducing high-risk behavior in gay men. *Sex Trans Dis* 1985; 12:229–233.
26. Fishbein M, Ajzen I: *Belief, Attitude, Intention and Behavior*. Reading, Mass, Addison-Wesley, 1975.

Chapter 4

Hospital workers and AIDS: Effect of in-service education on knowledge and perceived risks and stresses

LYDIA O'DONNELL, EdD, CARL R. O'DONNELL, ScD, MPH

ABSTRACT. Hospital workers were surveyed in 1985 and again in 1986, after the institution of in-service training programs, regarding their knowledge about AIDS and their perceptions of the risks and stresses of AIDS patient care. The study found that in-service training was associated with reductions in workers' reported stress, perceived risks, and negative attitudes, and with improvements in knowledge and satisfaction with the quality of care provided.

In the six years since acquired immunodeficiency syndrome (AIDS) was first described, clinical and impressionistic accounts have documented the existence of "AIDS-anxiety" among health-care providers.[1-6] It is often assumed that these concerns have been lessened by mounting evidence that AIDS is not easily transmitted, greater experience with the disease, and increased public awareness and acceptance of those persons who have AIDS. However, since medical personnel are being called upon to treat an increasing number of patients with AIDS, their initial apprehensions may have been compounded or supplanted by the demands of providing more AIDS-related care. Hospitals have been advised to establish AIDS committees and to devote considerable resources to AIDS-related education programs. To date, the need for such programs, given the widespread media attention and public education about the disease, is not fully documented. We report on a longitudinal study of a hospital staff's knowledge about AIDS, as well as their perceptions of the risks and stresses associated with the care of AIDS patients. We evaluated the extent to which attendance at in-service programs is associated with improvements in AIDS-related knowledge and with decreases in negative attitudes.

METHODS

In April 1985 we surveyed professional and technical employees at the major AIDS treatment center in Massachusetts, a 500-bed teaching hospital to which approximately 60 AIDS patients had been admitted by the time of the survey. The sampling pool consisted of employees in departments and on floors most likely to be providing care to patients with AIDS. A total of 227 participants, or 71% of those contacted, completed questionnaires. In the spring of 1985, the hospital established an AIDS Education Committee, which initiated a coordinated effort to provide sup-

From the Department of Medicine, New England Deaconess Hospital, Boston, Mass, and the Wellesley College Center for Research on Women, Wellesley, Mass.

port and education to staff members. In-service education programs were available to hospital employees throughout the next year. Information was provided on the biology and epidemiology of AIDS, its clinical course and treatment, and infection control. There was explicit discussion of high-risk activities and risk groups. In June 1986, by which time more than 130 AIDS patients had been admitted, employees in these same areas were resurveyed. A total of 208 staff members, or 65% of those contacted, completed questionnaires. More than half of these (52%) had participated in the previous survey. Of those who did not complete the original survey, 52% were new employees. In the first survey year, 50% of the participants were registered nurses (RNs), 19.4% were technicians, 14.1% were house officers, 11.9% were licensed practical nurses (LPNs) or aides, and 8.8% were social service personnel. In the second survey year, 49.5% of the participants were RNs, 17.3% were technicians, 14.9% were house officers, 9.6% were LPNs and aides, and 8.7% were social service personnel.

Information was collected on the employees' degree of contact with AIDS patients, knowledge of modes of transmission, and (for the second survey year) attendance at in-service education programs. Employee and nursing grand rounds were charted, as well as classes with supervisors and unit teachers, infection control personnel, and the AIDS health educator. Attendance at in-service programs was voluntary, and programs were provided for all shifts. (Programs were not designed for house officers, so they were excluded from this part of the analysis.) Respondents were asked to report on how comfortable, stressed, and at-risk they felt while working with AIDS patients. They also assessed the adequacy of their knowledge and the job they performed.

Responses to individual questions were cross-tabulated by survey year, job category, and class attendance. Chi-square tests were used to assess differences in proportions. Differences were considered significant at the 0.05 probability level; all reported differences are significant unless otherwise specified.

RESULTS

From 1985 to 1986, there were overall reductions in how employees perceived the risks and stresses of care of AIDS patients, despite an increase in the number of patients seen. The percentage of those who worked with AIDS patients "sometimes" or "often" rose from 65.7% to 74.6%, and the average number of AIDS patients seen over the course of the year increased from 10.8 to 17.3. However, rather than increasing with patient load, the percentage of time staff perceived they spent with AIDS patients decreased from 8.1% to 6.6%. The percentage of those who reported that dealing with AIDS patients was one of the more stressful parts of their job decreased from 48% to 34.6%.* The percentage indicating that they were uncomfortable with AIDS patients went down from 35.5% to 26%.* More staff members felt they had sufficient knowledge of patients' physical needs (75.5% compared to 61.6%), emotional needs (52% compared to 42%), and infection control procedures (the percentage without sufficient knowledge decreased from 33.6% to 9.9%). Furthermore, in 1986 only 14.5% assessed as "not good" how their fellow workers dealt with patients' physical needs, compared to 54.5% in 1985. There was a small but not significant decrease (23.9% to 20.2%) in the percentage of those who felt at high risk of getting AIDS because of their jobs.* There was a similar decline in how many assessed as "not good" the job their fellow workers did with patients' emotional needs (42.7% to 35.5%). The percentage of staff who reported that AIDS could be transmitted in each of ten different ways (Table I) also decreased.

Twenty-two percent of the respondents had attended no classes, 32.7% attended one class, and 45.3% attended two or more classes. Attendance at in-service education programs was associated with reductions in stress, perceived risk, and discomfort around patients (Table II). Class attendance did not vary by frequency of contact with AIDS patients or by length of employment. The degree of risk,

* Indicated by a score of 3 or 4 on a 1-to-4 scale.

TABLE I. Changes in Knowledge About AIDS Transmission

Can AIDS be transmitted in the following ways?	% Answering Yes*	
	1985 (N = 227)	1986 (N = 208)
1. by blood transfusion	93	83
2. being stuck by a needle from AIDS patient	69	63
3. giving CPR	58	36
4. kissing an individual with AIDS	44	23
5. sharing eating utensils	38	15
6. airborne transmission	26	11
7. emptying bedpans	20	9
8. changing bed linens	14	5
9. shaking hands with AIDS patient	5	1
10. being in same room with AIDS patient	5	0

* All differences are significant at the <0.05 level except for item 2.

stress, and discomfort reported by nonattenders of classes was greater than that reported by class attenders, and also exceeded that reported by all those surveyed in 1985.

LPNs/aides and technicians were least likely to attend any education programs. Reductions in stress and perceptions of risk and discomfort were consistent across all job categories except that of LPNs/aides, who reported slight increases in stress and discomfort (from 35% to 45%, and from 48% to 55%, respectively). Although in the same direction as the sample as a whole, reductions were smallest for technicians. Among all respondents, those who had attended two or more classes were less likely to report that AIDS could be transmitted through a needlestick injury or by changing bedpans, giving CPR, receiving blood, or sharing eating utensils.

DISCUSSION

From 1985 to 1986, staff members showed significant improvements in knowledge about AIDS transmission and reductions in the perceived stresses and risks of providing AIDS-related care, despite a more than two-fold increase in AIDS patient admissions. These changes were not experienced by those who did not attend hospital in-service programs. A sizable minority of staff continued to experience AIDS-related difficulties.

In-service programs can make a difference in how staff members respond to the demands of AIDS patient care.

TABLE II. Hospital Employees' AIDS-related Stress, Perceived Risk, and Discomfort, as Related to Attendance at In-service Education Programs

Survey Question	Sample (N=153)*	No. of Classes Attended (%)			
		0	1	2+	Chi-Square
Is working with AIDS one of the more stressful parts of your job?	35.2%†	51.5	25.0	35.3	6.36‡
How much risk do you think you have of getting AIDS because of your job?	20.9%	36.3	19.2	14.7	6.41‡
How uncomfortable are you with AIDS patients?	28.8%	54.5	26.9	17.1	15.04§

* Excludes responses of 31 house officers, and 24 staff members who provided incomplete survey data (these employees had little or no contact with AIDS patients).
† Percentages indicate those selecting response of "3" or "4" on a 1-to-4 scale.
‡ $p < 0.05$.
§ $p < 0.005$.

Such programs are useful despite public and media attention to AIDS and consequent reductions in initial "AIDS-anxiety." Program developers should encourage participation by all employees, and pay particular attention to the needs of technical and nursing-support staff.

Acknowledgments. The authors acknowledge the efforts of Alison Sneider, Suzanne Holloran, Janet Bath, and Julie White of the New England Deaconess Hospital AIDS Education Committee.

REFERENCES

1. AIDS: A time bomb at hospitals' door. *Hospital* 1986; 60(1):54–61.
2. Ellis M: Guidelines on AIDS in bid to quell fears. *RCN Nurs Stan* 1983; 9(6):343.
3. Mather AD: AIDS update: Halting the "epidemic of fear." *Inf Rep* 1985; 2:1–3.
4. O'Donnell L, O'Donnell C, Pleck J, et al: Psychosocial responses of hospital workers to the acquired immune deficiency syndrome. *J Appl Soc Psych* (in press).
5. Phillips JL: As a nurse, I want to find out what the facts are on AIDS. *Critical Care Update* 1983; 10(9):37.
6. Wachter RM: The impact of the acquired immunodeficiency syndrome on medical residency training. *N Engl J Med* 1986; 314:177–180.

Chapter 5

Cyclooxygenase inhibition and improved oxygenation in patients with pulmonary complications of AIDS

STEVEN H. FOSTER, MD; ROBERT C. GARRETT, MD[†]; HENRY M. THOMAS III, MD

ABSTRACT. Pulmonary involvement related to acquired immunodeficiency syndrome (AIDS) compromises oxygenation, by both ventilation-perfusion mismatch and increased shunt. In animal studies, meclofenamate, a cyclooxygenase inhibitor, decreases shunt and improves oxygenation. Oral meclofenamate (200 mg) was given to seven patients who had AIDS with pulmonary involvement (*Pneumocystis carinii* pneumonia or Kaposi's sarcoma) and abnormal gas exchange.

Arterial PO_2 was measured 30 and 0 minutes before and 45 and 60 minutes after administering meclofenamate, and the shunt fraction (venous admixture) was estimated. In all patients, arterial PO_2 increased, shunt decreased, and PCO_2 and pH did not change after meclofenamate therapy.

Cyclooxygenase inhibition appears to have strengthened hypoxic vasoconstriction and decreased the shunt fraction, possibly by eliminating prostacyclin-induced vasodilation in diseased lung regions. Cyclooxygenase inhibition may be of benefit in the management of hypoxemia associated with AIDS and warrants further investigation.

Hypoxemia is a frequent and serious complication of the pulmonary abnormalities that occur in patients with AIDS. Supplemental oxygen may not substantially increase arterial oxygenation levels because of increased blood flow through abnormal shunt pathways in the lung.

Oxygenation is improved by the diversion of blood flow away from regions of the lung in which gas exchange is impaired. Pulmonary arteries constrict in response to regional hypoxia, but the hypoxic vasoconstriction is not strong enough to prevent substantial perfusion of hypoxic regions, with resultant hypoxemia. An additional factor that may contribute to hypoxemia in these patients is the production of prostacyclin, a potent vasodilator. Prostacyclin synthesis is continuous in the lung[1] and may be increased by hypoxia.[2,3] Its vasodilatory effect opposes the ability of hypoxic vasoconstriction to divert blood flow from hypoxic regions and may further increase perfusion of the abnormal shunt pathways.

Using an animal model of regional hypoxia, it has been shown that preventing prostacyclin-induced vasodilation by inhibiting the cyclooxygenase pathway uniformly reduces perfusion of hypoxic lung tissue by as much as 40%.[4] Reported here are the results of a preliminary study of the effects of inhibition of cyclooxygenase in seven patients with hypoxemia due to pulmonary complications of AIDS.

PATIENTS AND METHODS

All patients had the diagnosis of AIDS by Centers for Disease Control (CDC) criteria[5] and had diffuse pulmonary involvement as indicated by an abnormal chest film and a calculated venous admixture greater than 10% while breathing an inspired oxygen concentration of 40% or more. In this series, pulmonary involvement was documented by fiberoptic bronchoscopy to be caused by either *Pneumocystis carinii* pneumonia (six patients) or Kaposi's sarcoma (one patient). Exclusion criteria included allergy to nonsteroidal anti-inflammatory agents, unstable cardiorespiratory status, history of peptic ulcer disease, bleeding in the upper gastrointestinal tract, and a serum creatinine level greater than 3 mg/dL. Informed consent was obtained from the subjects after the nature of the procedures had been fully explained. The investigation was approved by the Institutional Review Board of Cornell University Medical College.

An indwelling arterial needle was placed in each of these patients. For measurement of PO_2, PCO_2, and pH, a 3-mL blood sample was drawn into a heparinized syringe and was immedi-

From the Will Rogers Pulmonary Research Laboratory, Cornell University Medical College, White Plains and New York, NY.

This work was supported by the Will Rogers Institute, the Stony Wold-Herbert Fund, Inc, and the Potts Foundation.

† Deceased.

ately transported to the laboratory. Measurements were made on a Radiometer ABL1 blood gas machine within five minutes of blood sampling. The ABL1 was calibrated with an automatic internal calibration system (Radiometer) and was within the specifications of a quality control system (General Diagnostics, Blood G.A.S. Control).

The patients were started on 40% inspired oxygen; two patients required higher concentrations of 50% and 80%. A 20-minute interval was allowed for equilibration. Arterial PO_2 was measured 30 minutes before and just prior to oral administration of 200 mg of meclofenamate. Arterial blood gas measurements were repeated at 15-minute intervals for the next hour. Vital signs were monitored. Since there were no significant differences in blood gas values 30 minutes before and just prior to meclofenamate administration, values of each variable were averaged to give a premeclofenamate value; likewise, similar values at 45 and 60 minutes after meclofenamate administration were averaged to give a postmeclofenamate value. Changes produced by meclofenamate were analyzed using the paired t-test.[6]

RESULTS

Figure 1 shows the arterial PO_2 data before and after meclofenamate administration. Arterial oxygenation increased in each patient from a mean PO_2 level of 92 ± 33 mm Hg (standard deviation) (12.2 ± 0.7 kPa) to 116 ± 45 mm Hg (15.5 ± 6.0 kPa) (t = 2.6, $p < 0.05$).

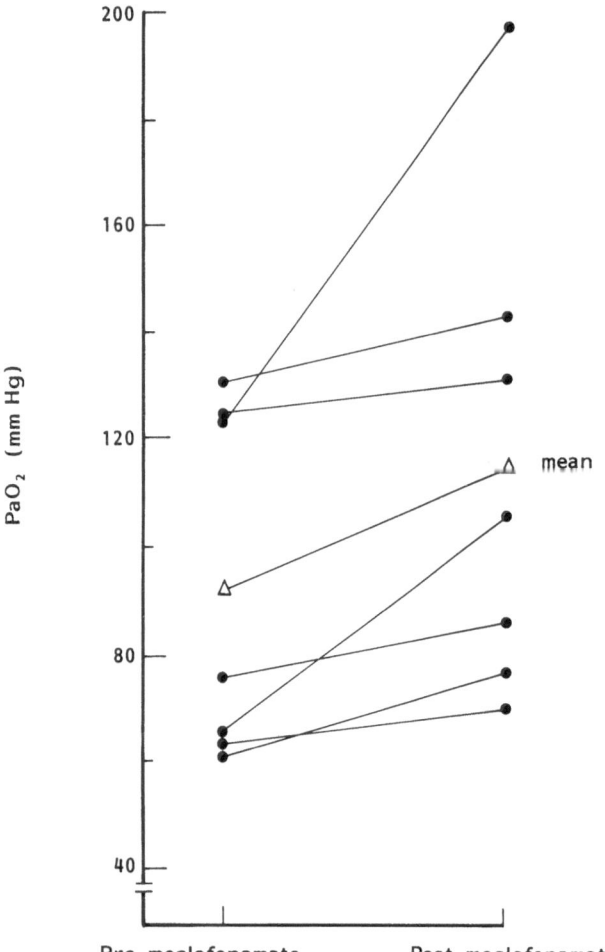

FIGURE 1. Arterial PO_2 in seven patients with pulmonary complications of AIDS, before and after administration of 200 mg meclofenamate. The mean increase is statistically significant (t = 2.6, $p < 0.05$).

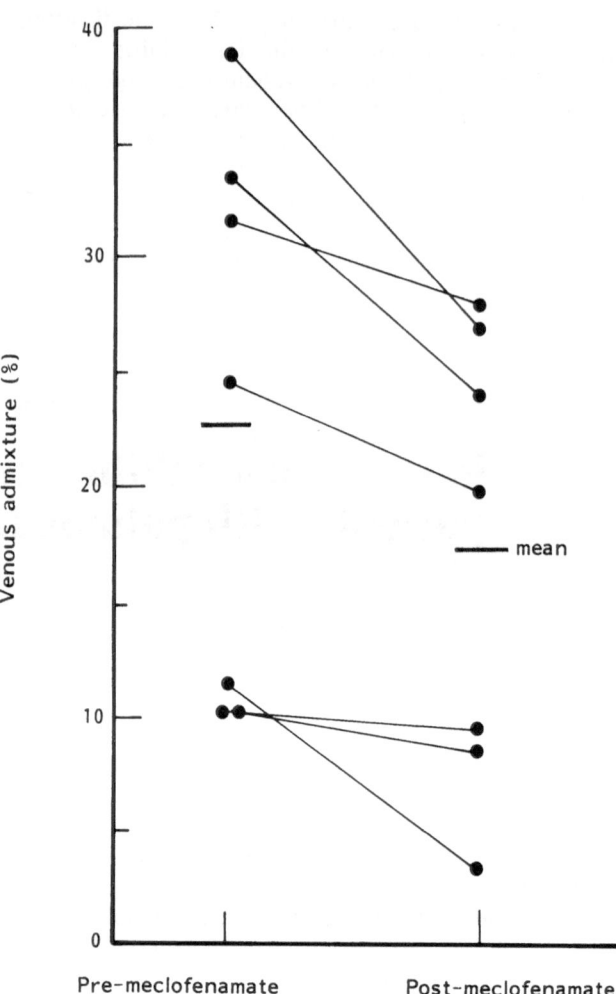

FIGURE 2. Shunt fraction (venous admixture) in seven patients with pulmonary complications of AIDS, before and after administration of 200 mg meclofenamate. The mean decrease is statistically significant (t = 3.7, $p < 0.01$).

To obviate any undue statistical influence of high PO_2 values on the flat portion of the oxyhemoglobin dissociation curve and to standardize the data for two patients on FIO_2 greater than 40%, the arterial oxygenation data are expressed in terms of estimated venous admixture. The shunt fraction (venous admixture) was calculated from measured values of PO_2, hemoglobin, and an assumed arteriovenous oxygen content difference. Estimated venous admixture decreased in each patient from a mean of $22.8 \pm 12.2\%$ to $17.1 \pm 9.9\%$ (t = 3.7, $p < 0.01$; Fig 2). The shunt fraction was, on average, one fourth smaller after meclofenamate therapy.

The increase in PO_2 had a time course appropriate for oral administration of meclofenamate (Fig 3). There was little increase in PO_2 at 15 minutes (+4 mm Hg; +0.5 kPa) and 30 minutes (+7 mm Hg, $p < 0.05$; +0.9 kPa), and then a substantial rise at 45 minutes (+25 mm Hg, $p < 0.10$; +3.3 kPa) and one hour (+24 mm Hg, $p < 0.05$; +3.1 kPa).

The values of pH and PCO_2 were not affected by meclofenamate. Mean pH was 7.43 ± 0.04 before and 7.43 ± 0.03 after therapy; PCO_2 was 29.8 ± 4.9 mm Hg (4.0 ± 4.4 kPa) before and 30.7 ± 4.7 mm Hg (4.1 ± 0.6 kPa) after drug administration. Furthermore, heart rate, respiratory rate, blood pressure, and temperature were unchanged.

DISCUSSION

These preliminary results are encouraging. The arterial

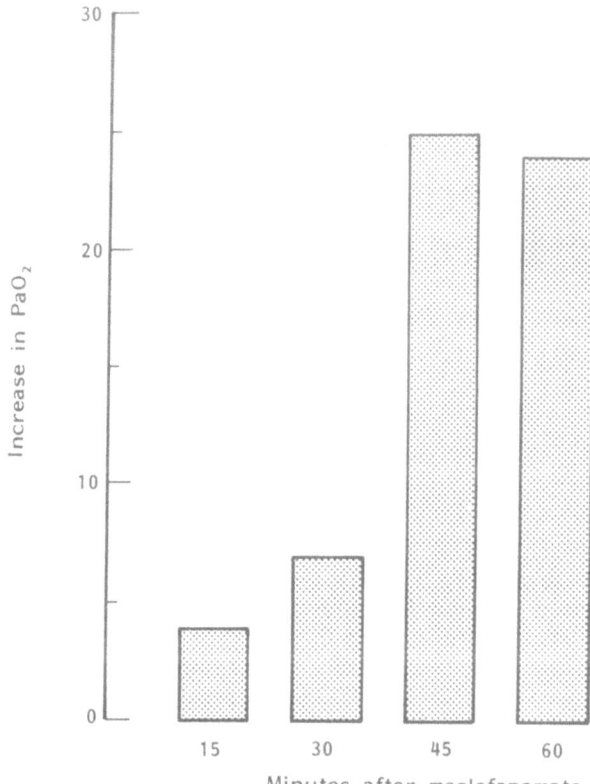

FIGURE 3. Time course of change in arterial Po_2 after administration of meclofenamate. Values are means for seven patients.

Po_2 level rose and the venous admixture fell in all seven patients. The inhibition of cyclooxygenase probably improved oxygenation by increasing the resistance to blood flow through hypoxemic lung regions.

In the absence of measurements of cardiac output and mixed venous Po_2, one cannot fully analyze the mechanism of improvement in oxygenation; for example, if cardiac output falls, shunt fraction may also fall, with a resultant elevation of Po_2.[7,8] However, in studies of anesthetized animals that received a 2-mg/kg bolus of meclofenamate, the cardiac output and mixed venous Po_2 were found to be stable.[4]

In the present study, the increase in arterial oxygenation does not appear to be due to improvement in the pathologic process in the lung: patients were selected for stability over a 24-hour period, and arterial Po_2 was then shown to be stable during the 30-minute period preceding the administration of meclofenamate.

It is possible that the effects observed are due to a property of meclofenamate not related to cyclooxygenase inhibition. However, in animal studies, several chemically un-related cyclooxygenase inhibitors have been shown to augment the strength of hypoxic vasoconstriction and redistribute blood flow from vessels in hypoxic lung regions to vessels in normoxic lung regions.[4,9] These results suggest that in the present study, inhibition of the cyclooxygenase pathway is the most likely mechanism.

The venous admixture calculation with 40% inhaled oxygen primarily measures perfusion of shunt pathways. Diffusing capacity is frequently reduced in patients with pulmonary complications of AIDS, and it is possible that long diffusion pathways, such as those seen in the adult respiratory distress syndrome,[10,11] may produce a gas exchange abnormality almost as severe as shunt. Perfusion of low V/Q regions may also contribute to calculated venous admixture. Although the precise combination of oxygenation abnormalities in patients with AIDS is not known, reducing blood flow to regions of abnormal gas exchange appears to be beneficial.

These data suggest that in patients with AIDS who have hypoxemia, the production of vasodilator prostanoids such as prostacyclin opposes hypoxic vasoconstriction in the lung and contributes to the development of the hypoxemia. Elimination of the vasodilatory effect of prostacyclin appears to strengthen hypoxic vasoconstriction and improve oxygenation. We do not believe that these results are restricted to patients with AIDS, and they may be of value in any acute lung disease with significant shunt pathways, such as the adult respiratory distress syndrome or pneumonia. The clinical benefit to be obtained by cyclooxygenase inhibition in pulmonary complications of AIDS warrants further investigation.

REFERENCES

1. Bakhle YS, Ferreira SH: Lung metabolism of eicosanoids: Prostaglandins, prostacyclin, thromboxane, and leukotrienes, in *Handbook of Physiology, Section 3: The Respiratory System. Circulatory and Nonrespiratory Functions*. Bethesda, American Physiological Society, 1985, vol 1, pp 365–386.

2. Garrett RC, Thomas HM 3d: Relation of prostanoids to strength of hypoxic vasoconstriction in dogs with lobar atelectasis. *J Appl Physiol* 1985; 59:72–77.

3. Stephenson AH, Sprague RS, Brash DW, et al: Effects of cyclooxygenase inhibition on the renal hemodynamic response to acute hypoxia. *Fed Proc* 1986; 45:659.

4. Garrett RC, Thomas HM 3d: Meclofenamate uniformly decreases shunt fraction in dogs with lobar atelectasis. *J Appl Physiol* 1983; 54:284–289.

5. Update: Acquired immunodeficiency syndrome (AIDS)—United States. *MMWR* 1983; 32:389–391.

6. Snedecor GW, Cochran WG: *Statistical Methods*. Ames, Iowa, Iowa State University Press, 1973.

7. Smith G, Cheney FW Jr, Winter PM: The effect of change in cardiac output on intrapulmonary shunting. *Br J Anaesth* 1974; 46:337–342.

8. Breen PH, Schumacker PT, Sandoval J, et al: Increased cardiac output increases shunt. Role of pulmonary edema and perfusion. *J Appl Physiol* 1985; 59:1313–1321.

9. Hales CA, Rouse ET, Slate JL: Influence of aspirin and indomethacin on variability of alveolar hypoxic vasoconstriction. *J Appl Physiol* 1978; 45:33–39.

10. King TK, Weber B, Okinaka A, et al: Oxygen transfer in catastrophic respiratory failure. *Chest* 1974; 65:40S–44S.

11. Lamy M, Fallat RJ, Koeniger E, et al: Pathologic features and mechanisms of hypoxemia in adult respiratory distress syndrome. *Am Rev Respir Dis* 1976; 114:267–284.

Chapter 6

Medical students' attitudes towards caring for patients with AIDS in a high incidence area

Pascal James Imperato, MD; Joseph G. Feldman, DrPH; Kamran Nayeri, MA; Jack A. DeHovitz, MD, MPH

ABSTRACT. Second-year medical students (N = 174) at a medical school located in an area of high incidence for acquired immunodeficiency syndrome (AIDS) were surveyed for their attitudes and perceived risk of different degrees of contact with AIDS patients. Fifty percent of the class were surveyed prior to a 60-minute lecture on the epidemiology of AIDS; the other half were surveyed immediately thereafter. Data were analyzed by multivariate and univariate analyses of covariance and logistic regression. The lecture had no measurable impact on students' attitudes and perception of risk. More than 60% of students believed that drawing blood from an AIDS patient carried a moderate to high risk. More than 22% thought that performing a physical examination was associated with a moderate to high risk. Perceptions of risk associated with various types of patient contact generally correlated with views supporting the prerogative of declining care to AIDS patients. A large number of students expressed the view that physicians in private practice should have the prerogative of declining to care for new patients with AIDS (48.3%) and for longstanding patients who develop AIDS (41.4%) provided that care is insured elsewhere. Perception of risk correlated with choice of location of future residency training programs. These data suggest that medical students in the early years of training may have misperceptions of the risk of acquiring human immunodeficiency virus (HIV) infection not corrected by merely receiving scientific facts. These misperceptions may influence both career choices and site of graduate training if not modified by subsequent corrective experiences in the third and fourth years of medical school.

As of February 1988, some 52,000 cases of acquired immunodeficiency syndrome (AIDS) had been reported to the US Centers for Disease Control.[1] Of these, 13,000 cases (25%) occurred in New York City, the two boroughs of Manhattan and Brooklyn accounting for the majority

of cases.[1-3] While homosexual/bisexual men still account for the majority of cases in the city, intravenous (IV) drug abusers account for close to 30%.[4] Of the estimated 200,000 IV drug abusers in New York City, close to 60% are thought to be seropositive for the human immunodeficiency virus (HIV).[5] AIDS is currently the leading cause of death in New York City among men aged 25–44 years and women aged 25–34 years.[6]

HIV-infected IV drug abusers have progressively spread their infections to their heterosexual and/or homosexual sex partners.[7] A large number of women of childbearing age in New York City who contract AIDS do so by sharing contaminated injection equipment during drug abuse or by sexual contact with a male drug user.

From late November 1987 through late December 1987, the New York State Department of Health tested the blood of every infant born in the state for HIV.[8] A total of 19,157 infants were tested, and overall 164 were found to be positive. Of the 9,047 infants born in New York City during the month-long period, 148 were positive.[8] Thus the rate of positivity for New York City was 1.64%, or 1 in 61.[8] The highest rate of positivity was in the borough of the Bronx (2.24%) followed by Manhattan (1.96%), Brooklyn (1.74%), Queens (0.81%), and Staten Island (0.76%).[8] These rates of positivity are thought to reflect the rate of HIV infection among the city's drug users and their sexual partners.

The State University of New York Health Science Center at Brooklyn (SUNY HSCB) is geographically located in a high AIDS incidence area in the city. Its major teaching hospital affiliate, Kings County Hospital Center (KCHC), is a 1,200-bed municipal hospital situated across the street from the SUNY HSCB. Both institutions are situated in an inner city minority area where intravenous drug abuse is a very significant problem.

There are a total of 5,000 deliveries a year at KCHC and an equal number of planned abortions.[9] Some 500 deliveries (10%) are among Haitian women.[9] In a recent study at KCHC it was found that 12 (2%) of 602 core blood samples were HIV positive.[9] Approximately half of the beds on the medical service at KCHC are currently occupied by AIDS patients.[10]

The high incidence of AIDS in the community served by SUNY HSCB has greatly increased the frequency

From the Department of Preventive Medicine and Community Health, State University of New York Health Science Center at Brooklyn, Brooklyn, NY.

with which physicians, house staff, and clinical clerks must care for patients who have the disease or who are HIV positive. The presence of large numbers of AIDS patients on a teaching service creates numerous medical, legal, ethical, and social issues which must be dealt with by these medical practitioners on an ongoing basis.

Other investigators have reported on medical students' attitudes towards AIDS and homosexual patients in a geographic area of low incidence.[11] However, the current study evaluated both attitudes and perceived personal risks associated with the care of AIDS patients as well as projected medical care behavior in one of the highest incidence areas in the United States. The study had several purposes, among which were to document second-year medical students' attitudes towards AIDS patients, to assess their perceptions of risk to self in caring for these patients, to examine correlations, if any, between risk perception and projected medical care behavior, and to see if a detailed lecture on AIDS and its risks would alter preexisting perceptions of risk to self in providing medical care.

METHODS

The survey was conducted among second-year medical students in December 1987. This is a time in the curriculum when the students have not yet received any systematic training in the clinical sciences. The questionnaire contained 25 questions that were of the fixed-alternate type, with space being provided for individual open-ended responses at the end. The survey instrument was administered during the final small group seminar session of the second-year course in preventive medicine and community health. Student participation was completely voluntary, and students were told not to identify themselves on the survey in any manner. To insure anonymity, students collected the questionnaires and brought them to the departmental offices. A total of 174 of 209 (83.2%) students completed the questionnaire. In order to assess the impact, if any, of the AIDS lecture, responses provided by 62 students on a Tuesday, two days before the lecture, were analyzed separately from those of 77 respondents who completed the questionnaire the afternoon following the lecture on Thursday. The course offered several seminars, two of which included discussions on some topics related to AIDS. All seminars consisted of eight two-hour weekly sessions. A total of 35 students were enrolled in these two seminar groups, and were excluded from the evaluation of the lecture.

Analysis of covariance was used to compare the Thursday lecture group with the Tuesday lecture group. Both multivariate and univariate analyses of covariance were used to assess differences in perceived risk of various behaviors and to ascertain a pattern of consistent responses. The impact of perceived risk on behaviors and attitudes was assessed using a polytomous logistic regression model with three outcomes: yes, no, or maybe.[12] Perceived risk was based on the sum of risk scores assigned to taking a medical history, performing a physical exam, performing invasive procedures, drawing blood, or being in the same room with an AIDS patient. The summary score could range from 5 to 30, with 30 indicating a very high perceived risk for each of the behaviors, and 5 indicating no risk associated with any of them.

RESULTS

Descriptive Data. The first four questions solicited basic information on age, sex, marital status, and number of children. Of the total group 77.0% were single, 12.6% were married, and 9.8% were engaged. Of the 174 students, 52.3% had personally seen a patient with AIDS, and 25.9% knew of someone (neighbor, acquaintance, relative, student, etc) with AIDS or who had died of AIDS. Results for the five questions that elicited perceptions of risk associated with a variety of activities are shown in Table I. The lowest perceived risk behavior was being in the same room with an AIDS patient, 93.1%

TABLE I. Medical Students' Perceived Risk of AIDS Transmission by Activity (N = 174)

Activity	Perceived Risk (%)						
	Very High	High	Moderate	Low	Very Low	None	Don't Know
Taking medical history	1.2	0.6	6.9	7.5	20.1	63.2	0.6
Performing physical examination	2.9	4.0	15.5	21.8	40.2	14.9	0.6
Performing invasive procedures	13.8	17.8	35.1	18.4	11.5	1.1	2.3
Drawing blood	12.6	17.8	31.6	22.4	13.8	1.7	0.1
Being in same room	1.7	1.1	2.9	4.0	17.8	71.3	1.1

rating this risk as low, very low, or none. The next lowest risk behavior was rated as taking a medical history from an AIDS patient, 90.8% rating this risk as low, very low, or none. By contrast, 76.9% rated performing a physical examination in these categories and 22.4% responded that performing a physical examination carried a very high, high, or moderate risk. Performing invasive procedures was rated as carrying the greatest risk, with 66.7% responding that this activity carried a very high, high, or moderate risk. This was followed by 62.0% who rated drawing blood as carrying a very high, high, or moderate risk (Table I).

With regard to whether students would allow their own children to be in the same room as AIDS patients, 41.4% said yes, 17.8% said no, 26.4% said maybe, and 13.8% said they didn't know.

Medical students' beliefs regarding their prerogatives relating to medical care behaviors are presented in Table II. The two activity areas of concern to students were drawing blood and performing surgical procedures. With regard to the former, 31.6% replied yes and 14.9% replied maybe that they should have the prerogative of declining to draw blood. For surgical procedures the figures are 43.1% and 23.0%, respectively. Even with regard to performing physical examinations on AIDS patients, 13.8% said yes and 17.2% said maybe concerning the prerogative of declining to do so.

Whereas 21.8% of respondents were unsure or thought that medical students should have the prerogative of declining to take a medical history from an AIDS patient, only 10.9% thought interns and residents should (Table III). With regard to interns and residents not performing physical examinations, 5.2% said yes and 12.6% said maybe, much lower than the respective figures of 13.8% and 17.2% for medical students (Table II). While 31.6% of students thought they should have the prerogative of declining to draw blood from AIDS patients, only 14.4% thought interns and residents should (Table III). Yet 25.3% said interns and residents should be able to

TABLE II. Medical Students' Beliefs About Their Prerogatives Relating to the Care of AIDS Patients (N = 174)

Activity	Belief				
	Yes	No	Maybe	Don't Know	No Answer
Decline to take medical histories	6.9	78.2	10.9	3.5	0.6
Decline to perform physical examination	13.8	66.1	17.2	0	2.9
Decline to draw blood	31.6	50.0	14.9	3.5	0
Decline to perform surgical procedures	43.1	28.7	23.0	4.6	0.6

TABLE III.   Medical Students' Beliefs About the Prerogatives of Interns and Residents Relating to the Care of AIDS Patients (N = 174)

Activity	Yes	No	Maybe	Don't Know	No Answer
			Belief		
Decline to take medical histories	3.5	89.1	6.3	0.6	0.6
Decline to perform physical examination	5.2	79.9	12.6	1.7	0.6
Decline to draw blood	14.4	71.3	10.3	2.9	1.2
Decline to perform surgical procedures	25.3	49.4	20.7	3.5	1.2

decline performing surgical procedures on AIDS patients and 20.7% said maybe (Table III). Overall, significantly more students thought that they should have the prerogative of declining to perform these activities compared to interns and residents.

When asked about the relative infectivity of AIDS patients and persons who are HIV positive, 27.0% replied that AIDS patients pose a greater risk, 56.9% said they posed the same risk, 14.9% did not know, and 1.6% gave no answer.

In response to whether a large census of AIDS patients in a teaching hospital would reduce the scope and value of training offered to interns and residents, 40.2% said yes and 28.5% said maybe. When asked about the effect of a high proportion of AIDS patients in a hospital respected for the quality of its teaching programs, 45.4% said it would make the hospital less appealing for training. Only 4.0% said it would make it more appealing and 37.9% said it would have no influence.

Students were asked if physicians in private practice should have the prerogative of declining to care for AIDS patients. This question was framed with regard to both new patients with AIDS and longstanding patients who develop AIDS. Concerning new patients, 10.3% said that physicians should have the prerogative of declining care outright with no questions asked. Only 4.0% gave this response for longstanding patients who subsequently develop AIDS. For new patients, 48.3% responded that physicians should have the prerogative of declining care provided the patient is insured care elsewhere. This response was given by 41.4% with regard to longstanding patients. Male and female students did not vary in their perceptions of risks or predicted behaviors.

Impact of the Lecture. There were no significant differences in perceptions of risk or beliefs regarding prerogatives relating to the care of AIDS patients between the students who received the one-hour lecture on AIDS and those who did not. The largest difference

TABLE IV.   Perceived Risk as a Percent of Maximum Risk Score by Beliefs Regarding Medical Students' Prerogatives

Prerogative to Decline for AIDS Patients:	Yes	No	Maybe	Probability	Change in the Probability* of Response = No[†]
		Belief			
Taking medical histories	60.2	42.4	55.1	0.001	−2.9%
Performing physical examination	57.5	41.1	51.9	0.001	−4.0%
Drawing blood	51.3	41.2	47.7	0.05	−3.4%
Performing surgical procedures	48.1	42.7	44.8	NS[‡]	

* Adjusted for sex and personal knowledge of an AIDS patient.
[†] Per unit increase in risk score.
[‡] NS, not significant.

TABLE V.   Perceived Risk as a Percent of Maximum Risk Score by Beliefs Regarding Interns' and Residents' Prerogatives

Prerogative to Decline for AIDS Patients:	Yes	No	Maybe	Probability	Change in the Probability* of Response = No[†]
		Belief			
Taking medical histories	61.1	44.6	50.6	NS	
Performing physical examination	56.3	43.5	53.6	0.01	−1.9%
Drawing blood	50.6	42.8	53.2	0.01	−2.4%
Performing surgical procedures	48.8	43.2	46.1	NS[‡]	

* Adjusted for sex and personal knowledge of an AIDS patient.
[†] Per unit increase in risk score.
[‡] NS, not significant.

between groups was for perceived risk of being in the same room with an AIDS patient, which 8.1% of the nonlectured group viewed to be of moderate to higher risk compared to 3.9% of the lectured group ($p < 0.07$).

Influence of Perceived Risk on Predicted Behavior. The associations of perception of risk with students' beliefs regarding prerogatives to decline different types of contact with AIDS patients are shown in Tables IV–VI. The average risk score is indicated according to whether the student believed that medical practitioners should have the prerogative of declining service. The last column shows the percentage increase in the probability of a negative response for every unit increase in the risk score. Overall, the perception of risk score was 45.6% of the possible maximum.

There were significant differences in beliefs about medical student prerogatives in declining to take a medical history, perform a physical examination, and draw blood. In each instance, those students with a higher perception of risk were more likely to think that medical students in general should have the prerogative of declining care ($p < 0.01$). The exception was participation in surgical procedures where the trend was similar but the difference was not significant. Here, the majority thought that medical students should (43.1%) or maybe should (23%) have the prerogative to decline participation. With minor exception (being in the same room) the beliefs of the students carried over to expectations for interns and residents (Table V). Once again, the performance of surgery on AIDS patients was thought to carry high risk by a large number of students and was not influenced by the students' perception of risk score. There was no association between the risk score and beliefs about the prerogatives of private physicians to decline caring for an AIDS patient (Table VI).

Students who would not allow one of their own children in the same room with an AIDS patient had an average score of 61.7% compared to 39.6% for those who would ($p < 0.001$) (Table VII).

Students with a higher risk score thought that the presence of

TABLE VI.   Average Percent Risk of Maximum Score* by Beliefs Regarding Private Practitioners' Prerogatives

Prerogative to Decline:	Unqualified Yes	Yes, if Alternative Care Is Assured	No	Probability
	Belief			
Care for new AIDS patients	48.4	45.4	44.3	NS[†]
Care for patients of some years who develop AIDS	51.3	44.7	46.4	NS

* Adjusted for sex and personal knowledge of an AIDS patient.
[†] NS, not significant.

TABLE VII. Perceived Risk as a Percent of Maximum Score by Attitudes Concerning AIDS Patients

	Belief				Change in the *Probability of
	Yes	No	Maybe	Probability	Response = No[†]
Allow own children to visit AIDS patients	39.6	61.7	44.9	0.001	3.0%
Risk of transmission is the same for AIDS patients and HIV-positive individuals	48.6	43.7	45.9	NS[‡]	
A large AIDS patient load would reduce the scope and value of postgraduate training	48.9	44.3	41.6	0.01	2.3%—Yes
A large AIDS patient load at a well-respected teaching hospital would make it less appealing for postgraduate training	48.4	44.3	42.9	0.01	2.6%

* Adjusted for sex and personal knowledge of an AIDS patient.
† Per unit increase in risk score.
‡ NS, not significant.

many AIDS patients reduced the scope and value of residency training and noted that this would make an otherwise acceptable training program less appealing.

DISCUSSION

The results of this study indicate that second-year medical students have definite perceptions of the risk of acquiring AIDS through various types of patient contact. These perceptions frequently correlated with beliefs regarding prerogatives related to medical care behavior. Neither the perceptions of risk nor beliefs were influenced by a lecture on AIDS which carefully set forth the epidemiology of the disease and the risks associated with various types of contact. Those students who expressed a higher perception of risk with regard to taking a medical history, performing a physical examination, or drawing blood were more likely to think that they should have the prerogative of declining care.

Students viewed the performance of invasive surgical procedures and the drawing of blood as carrying the greatest risks. Large numbers of students (43.1%) thought that they should have the prerogative of declining to participate in the performance of surgical procedures or the drawing of blood (31.6%). It is noteworthy that student views for these activity prerogatives for interns and residents were 25.3% and 14.4% respectively (Tables II, III). These differences may in part be explained by some of the subjective comments made by students on their response sheets. A number of them expressed the concern that they, unlike interns and residents, are not yet skilled in the performance of these procedures. Therefore they perceive that they would be more likely to accidentally infect themselves. Thus, declining to participate in these procedures with AIDS patients may reflect a concern about greater risk due to a lack of requisite skills. Such views might well change as students acquire these skills in their third year of training.

Medical educators have become increasingly concerned about the impact of the presence of large numbers of AIDS patients on teaching services. These concerns relate to recruitment of house officers and maintaining a mix of patients manifesting a broad scope of disease problems necessary for their education. It is clear from this study that many students (40.2%) think that having significant numbers of AIDS patients in a teaching hospital reduces the scope and value of training offered to house staff. Similarly, 45.4% were of the opinion that such hospitals would be less appealing for training. If these views persist throughout subsequent years of medical school, they may have an important influence on the choice of hospital for postgraduate training. This has very important implications for teaching hospitals in high AIDS incidence areas.

The refusal of a few private practice physicians to treat AIDS patients has in part led a number of professional organizations and regulatory bodies to reaffirm the legal and ethical responsibilities of physicians to treat these patients. In November 1987, the American Medical Association's (AMA) Council on Ethical and Judicial Affairs published a report, *Ethical Issues Involved in the Growing AIDS Crisis.*[13] The report addressed a range of issues and firmly stated that "a physician may not ethically refuse to treat a patient whose condition is within the physician's current realm of competence." [13-15] A number of other professional organizations have taken similar stands.[16]

The Associated Medical Schools of New York, a professional organization that represents all of New York State's 13 medical schools, took a strong stand on this issue in December 1987. In a statement, the association recommended that any student, resident, or intern who refused to treat HIV infected individuals should be dismissed.[17]

The New York State Department of Health, which is responsible for ensuring the care and treatment of all members of the public in facilities and programs licensed under New York State law, has also issued a strong policy statement on discrimination against AIDS patients.[18] The department does not officially recognize AIDS as either a sexually transmitted disease or as a communicable disease, but as "a physical impairment closely associated with the human immunodeficiency virus (HIV)." The reasons for this position relate to concerns that a sexually transmitted disease or communicable disease classification would require the implementation of public health measures (eg, contact tracing) which would lead to discrimination against AIDS patients in housing, employment, insurance, etc. In November 1987, the New York State Court of Appeals, the highest court in the state, ruled that AIDS is a communicable disease.[19] However, this ruling has limited application to the conjugal visits for prisoners who are HIV positive.

Invoking the provisions of the Federal Rehabilitation Act of 1973, the department has the statutory legal authority to prosecute and punish any medical facility that refuses to treat a patient solely by reason of their AIDS handicap.[18] Despite these position statements and the force of law, it is still possible for physicians in private practice to avoid treating AIDS patients if they so wish. Surgical specialists, at generally higher risk than primary care practitioners because of the procedures they perform, can simply decline referrals on the grounds of being over-booked. There are a number of anecdotal reports of surgical specialists using this mechanism.

It is significant that 48.3% of students stated that physicians in private practice should have the prerogative of declining to care for new patients with AIDS provided care was insured elsewhere; the figure for longstanding patients was 41.4%. Far fewer students gave interns and residents this prerogative (Table III), perhaps in part because of the perception that house staff have few options in the matter. It is noteworthy that these opinions were expressed at a time when the ethical issue of physician refusal to treat AIDS patients was prominent in the popular press.

The data from this study suggest that early in training students may have misperceptions of the risk of acquiring HIV infection which are not corrected by simply transmitting the facts. These misperceptions may influence subsequent career choice and site of graduate training if they persist into the clinical years of medical school training. It is possible that subsequent experience with the care of AIDS patients during the third and fourth years of medical school may correct both the perceptions of risk and projected behaviors expressed by second-year medical students.

REFERENCES

1. Centers for Disease Control, Atlanta, Ga, February 1988.
2. Joseph SC: AIDS policy and prevention in New York City. *Bull NY Acad Med* 1987; 63:659–678.
3. Novick L: New York State in the AIDS Epidemic. *Bull NY Acad Med* 1987; 63:692–712.
4. Weinberg DS, Murray HW: Coping with AIDS. The special problems of New York City. *Engl J Med* 1987; 317:1469–1472.
5. Spira TJ, Des Jarlais DC, Marmor M, et al: Prevalence of antibody to lymphadenopathy associated virus among drug detoxification patients in New York. *Engl J Med* 1984; 311:467–468.
6. New York City AIDS Surveillance Data. New York City Department of Health, December 1987.
7. Des Jarlais DC, Wish E, Friedman SR, et al: Intravenous drug use and the heterosexual transmission of the human immunodeficiency virus: Current trends in New York City. *NY State J Med* 1987; 87:283–286.
8. Lambert B: One in 61 babies in New York City has AIDS antibodies, study says. *NY Times*, January 12, 1988, pp 1, B4.
9. Landesman S, Minkoff H, Holman S, et al: Serosurvey of human immunodeficiency virus infection in parturients. *JAMA* 1987; 258:2701–2703.
10. Personal communication, Department of Medicine, KCHC, January 1988.
11. Kelly JA, St Laurence JS, Smith S, et al: Medical students' attitudes toward AIDS and homosexual patients. *J Med Educ* 1987; 62:549–556.
12. Wilkinson L: *Systat: The System for Statistics. Logit. A Supplementary Module.* Evanston, Ill, Systat, Inc, 1986.
13. *Ethical Issues Involved in the Growing AIDS Crisis*, Report of the Council on Ethical and Judicial Affairs, Chicago, American Medical Association, 1987.
14. Staver S: Unethical to refuse to treat HIV-infected patients. *Am Med News*, November 20, 1987, pp 1, 43.
15. Pear R: A.M.A. rules that doctors are obligated to treat AIDS. *NY Times*, November 13, 1987, p A14.
16. Position Statement: Physicians and the Medical Care of Patients with AIDS. New York, New York County Medical Society, December 14, 1987.
17. Sullivan R: 13 medical colleges say staffs must treat AIDS. *NY Times*, December 9, 1987, p B3.
18. Policy Statement on Discrimination Based upon Acquired Immune Deficiency Syndrome (AIDS). Albany, New York State Department of Health, October 2, 1987.
19. Opinion, State of New York Court of Appeals, *In the matter of John and Jane Doe vs Thomas A. Coughlin, III, Commissioner, New York State Department of Correctional Services et al*, November 24, 1987.

Chapter 7

Geographic and demographic features of the AIDS epidemic in New York City

JOHN MILBERG, MPH; PAULINE THOMAS, MD; RAND STONEBURNER, MD, MPH

ABSTRACT. Extensive surveillance and epidemiologic investigations of acquired immunodeficiency syndrome (AIDS) have enabled the New York City (NYC) Department of Health (DOH) to plan and focus prevention and education efforts. While the DOH manages a number of support and counseling services, many such programs are administered by local community groups. In order to provide appropriate services and keep their communities properly informed, agencies require epidemiologic information specific to their geographic areas. Using surveillance and vital record data, this report analyzes basic epidemiologic features of AIDS in NYC, stressing racial/ethnic and geographic patterns. Borough-specific incidence rates indicate that Manhattan has been affected most severely, with a rate more than 2.5 times that of the borough with the next highest rate, the Bronx. Manhattan is the only borough in which whites have the highest incidence of AIDS; rates in blacks and Hispanics are higher in every other borough and citywide. The disproportionate racial/ethnic impact of AIDS is also evident in mortality rates. Compared to whites, blacks and Hispanics, particularly women, are at a considerably increased risk of dying of AIDS. Mortality rates in small geographic units are also presented in order to provide a more detailed picture of AIDS in NYC.

From the Office of Epidemiology, Surveillance and Statistics (Mr Milberg), the AIDS Surveillance Unit (Dr Thomas), and the Office of AIDS Research (Dr Stoneburner), New York City Department of Health, NY.

Data for this analysis were provided by the AIDS Surveillance Unit and the Bureau of Health Statistics and Analysis of the New York City Department of Health.

Since the first reports of acquired immunodeficiency syndrome (AIDS) in New York City in 1981, the principal

TABLE I. Cumulative AIDS Incidence Rates per 10,000 Population By Borough of Residence and Race/Ethnicity, 15–64-Year-Olds Only, New York City, 1981–1986

Borough	Race/Ethnicity			
	White	Black	Hispanic	Total*
Manhattan	49.7 (2,684)†	48.9 (972)	34.3 (799)	43.5 (4,455)
Bronx	6.1 (151)	19.7 (458)	24.6 (626)	16.7 (1,235)
Brooklyn	6.2 (441)	18.7 (854)	15.5 (383)	11.7 (1,678)
Queens	4.3 (341)	16.7 (382)	12.0 (217)	7.5 (940)
Staten Island	3.7 (77)	14.1 (22)	15.7 (19)	4.9 (118)
Total	14.9 (3,694)	23.7 (2,688)	21.0 (2,044)	18.0 (8,426)

* Not included are 53 cases of other or unknown race/ethnicity.
† Rate (cases).

risks and routes of transmission of this disease have been well established.[1] Extensive surveillance and epidemiologic investigation have enabled the New York City (NYC) Department of Health (DOH) to focus its prevention and education efforts.[2] While the DOH supports a wide variety of AIDS services and itself provides an information hotline, counseling service, and anonymous human immunodeficiency virus (HIV) testing clinics, many support programs active in NYC are run by local community groups. In order to provide appropriate services and keep their communities properly informed, agencies require epidemiologic information specific to their own treatment areas.

METHODS

In this study, two sources of data, the AIDS surveillance registry and NYC death certificates, were used to analyze geographic and demographic patterns of AIDS in NYC. Borough-specific incidence trends were assessed using the surveillance registry; mortality rates in small geographic units (health districts) were obtained from death certificates. Together these data provide a comprehensive picture of AIDS epidemiology in NYC.

Surveillance data, collected since 1981, are the major source of demographic and patient risk information on cases of AIDS in adults (patients aged 13 years and older) in NYC. The case definition used for surveillance (through August 1987) is that established by the Centers for Disease Control,[3] and includes only those persons with severe (pathologically confirmed) opportunistic infections attributable to HIV infection. The surveillance system is fully described in other reports.[2,4] This analysis includes cases diagnosed from 1981 through 1986 and reported through April 1987. Mortality data are derived from death certificates maintained by the Bureau of Vital Records in the Department of Health. Data accumulated for this period are nearly complete;

90% of AIDS cases identified through surveillance are reported within six months of diagnosis (NYC Department of Health AIDS Surveillance, unpublished data). Deaths are coded using ICD-9 criteria for underlying cause of death. Deaths in which a history of narcotics use is confirmed by the medical examiner are also noted on certificates and are classified as "narcotics-related." All mortality data presented here include 15–64-year-old residents of NYC only. Incidence and mortality rates are generated using 1980 NYC census data.

RESULTS

Compared to all other boroughs, cumulative incidence rates in Manhattan are the highest in all racial/ethnic groups (Table I). However, this is the only borough in which whites have the greatest incidence of AIDS; rates among blacks and Hispanics exceed those of whites in all other boroughs and in total, citywide incidence.

The distribution of risk groups for AIDS differs considerably by borough of residence (Table II).[5] In Manhattan, cases among nonintravenous-drug-using homosexual or bisexual men account for 74.4% (3,341) of all cases diagnosed in this borough from 1981 through 1986. This proportion has been fairly consistent since 1982, the first complete year of reporting (Table III). The incidence of AIDS among intravenous (IV) drug users, as among homosexual men, has increased steadily since 1981. IV drug users have consistently accounted for about 22% (1,006) of Manhattan cases. Finally, 51 cases of AIDS in women attributed to heterosexual contact with a male IV drug user or a bisexual man have been reported in Manhattan. The rate of such cases has remained at just over 1% of Manhattan cases. Because of the high proportion of cases among homosexual men in this borough, the male-to-female ratio of AIDS cases is high: 16:1 vs 9:1 citywide.

The distribution of cases in the Bronx contrasts greatly with that of Manhattan: A majority of cases in this borough (773, or 62%) are attributable to IV drug use, and only 26% (318) to homosexual contact. These proportions have also been fairly steady since 1982. Cases acquired by male-to-female heterosexual transmission comprise 6% (73) of all cases of AIDS in the Bronx. This is the highest such proportion of all the boroughs, and (in addition to the large proportion of AIDS in the Bronx among women) is reflected in the lowest borough-specific male-to-female case ratio in the city, 4.9:1. Interestingly, 60% of heterosexually acquired disease has occurred among Hispanics, as has a nearly identical proportion of IV-drug-related AIDS cases in this borough. This similarity in the racial distribution of AIDS among male IV drug users and women in whom it was heterosexually acquired is present in all boroughs (Table IV). There are only five cases in NYC of men for whom heterosexual contact with a woman is considered the principal source of HIV infection.

Brooklyn and Queens are the only boroughs to have experienced an increase in the proportion of cases occurring among homosexual men. These accounted for 28% of all Brooklyn cases in 1982 and for 39% in 1986. In this period, the proportion of IV-drug-related cases declined from 52% to 45%. Nearly 15% of the cases reported from Brooklyn occurred among persons of Haitian origin; citywide, 75%

TABLE II. Cumulative AIDS Incidence By Borough and Patient Group, New York City, 1981–1986

Borough	Patient Group				
	Homosexual/ Bisexual	Intravenous Drug User*	Male-to-Female Transmission	Other†	Total
Manhattan	74.4 (3,341)‡	22.4 (1,006)	1.1 (51)	2.1 (95)	53.0 (4,493)§
Bronx	25.7 (318)	62.4 (773)	5.9 (73)	6.0 (74)	14.6 (1,238)
Brooklyn	35.6 (599)	46.7 (786)	3.4 (57)	14.4 (242)	19.9 (1,684)
Queens	46.8 (443)	43.5 (412)	2.9 (27)	6.8 (64)	11.2 (946)
Staten Island	41.5 (49)	50.0 (59)	0.8 (1)	7.6 (9)	1.4 (118)
Total	100.0 (4,750)	100.0 (3,036)	100.0 (209)	100.0 (484)	100.0 (8,479)

* Includes homosexual/bisexual IV drug users.
† Includes blood-product-related cases, persons from countries where risks are unclear, and those with no identified risk.
‡ Row % (cases).
§ Column % (cases).

TABLE III.   Percent Distribution of AIDS Cases by Year, Borough, and Major Patient Groups, New York City, 1982–1986

| Borough | Patient Group | Year of Diagnosis | | | | |
		1982	1983	1984	1985	1986
Manhattan	Homosexual/bisexual	78.0*	73.1	76.9	74.6	72.2
	IV drug user	20.0	24.6	19.6	22.6	24.1
	Male-female transmission	1.0	0.3	0.9	1.0	1.6
	Total (N)	241	529	875	1290	1567
Bronx	Homosexual/bisexual	20.9	29.1	25.6	26.3	24.1
	IV drug user	62.8	63.3	65.0	62.8	62.1
	Male-female transmission	6.9	3.6	4.4	7.0	6.2
	Total (N)	43	110	226	369	494
Brooklyn	Homosexual/bisexual	27.9	29.3	36.4	34.0	39.6
	IV drug user	52.4	45.7	47.2	49.7	44.2
	Male-female transmission	0	4.9	1.8	3.3	4.2
	Total (N)	61	164	324	453	689
Queens	Homosexual/bisexual	36.8	45.3	49.4	39.6	49.6
	IV drug user	50.0	39.5	41.3	52.0	40.8
	Male-female transmission	2.6	2.3	2.3	2.5	3.4
	Total (N)	38	86	174	275	385
Staten Island	Homosexual/bisexual	25.0	50.0	33.0	44.7	39.1
	IV drug user	75.0	40.0	47.6	44.7	54.3
	Male-female transmission	0	0	0	0	6.5
	Total (N)	4	10	21	38	46

* Column percent.

TABLE IV.   Racial/Ethnic Distribution (Percent) of Male Intravenous Drug and Female Heterosexually Acquired AIDS By Borough,* New York City, 1981–1986

| | Manhattan | | Bronx | | Brooklyn | | Queens | |
	IV Drug Use	Heterosexual	IV Drug Use	Heterosexual	IV Drug Use	Heterosexual	IV Drug Use	Heterosexual
White	19.0	20.4	7.9	8.3	16.4	17.9	25.1	20.0
Black	48.1	40.8	33.9	32.0	50.1	48.2	52.1	64.0
Hispanic	33.7	36.7	58.0	59.7	32.1	33.9	22.4	16.0

* Only two male-to-female cases have been reported from Staten Island.

of all Haitians with AIDS are from Brooklyn. (According to the NYC Department of Planning, 63% of Haitian-born immigrants reside in Brooklyn and 27% live in Queens.) After the Bronx, Brooklyn has the lowest male-to-female case ratio, 6.2:1.

While whites and blacks comprise between 35% and 40% of AIDS cases in Queens, the cumulative incidence rate among blacks (17/10,000) is four times that of whites (4/10,000), while the rate among Hispanics (12/10,000) is three times that of whites. Furthermore, within each racial/ethnic group, the distribution of cases by risk group differs considerably. Among blacks, for example, 61% of cases are IV drug related and 31% occur among homosexual men. These proportions are reversed in whites. Again, the racial group with the greatest proportion of male IV drug users (in this case blacks) also has the largest number of heterosexually acquired cases in women. The male-to-female ratio of cases in this borough is 8.5:1.

Only 118 cases of AIDS were diagnosed in Staten Island between 1981 and 1986. This represents 1.4% of all NYC cases, and a cumulative incidence rate of 4.9 per 10,000 population, the lowest in the city. Reflecting the racial distribution of this borough, 63% (77) of the patients are white and nearly 50% (36) are homosexual men. The male-to-female ratio of AIDS cases in this borough is 9.5:1.

Mortality Rates.   The following refers only to 15–64-year-old white, black, and Hispanic residents of NYC who died in 1986 and whose underlying cause of death is recorded as AIDS on the death certificate. AIDS mortality and proportional mortality rates in 1986 by age, sex, and race/ethnicity are presented in Table V. From a previous link of death certificates and the AIDS surveillance registry, three ICD-9 codes were found to be the most sensitive indicators of AIDS deaths.[6] These codes are 279.1 (deficiency of cell-mediated immunity); 136.3 (pneumocystosis); and 173.9 (malignant neo-

plasm of the skin, site unspecified). There were 2,441 AIDS-related deaths among NYC residents 15–64 years of age during 1986, yielding a crude mortality rate of 52.0 per 100,000 population.* Racial/ethnic data were missing or unknown in 169 cases; eight deaths occurred among Asians.

In all racial groups, mortality rates among 25–44-year-old males far exceeded the levels in the younger (15–24 years) and older (45–64 years) age groups. Mortality rates, reflecting incidence rates, were highest in blacks and Hispanics.

Compared to whites, blacks in the 25–44-year age group had a 2.2 times greater risk, and Hispanics a 1.5 times greater risk, of dying of AIDS. While the AIDS mortality rate among men 25–44 years of age was lowest among whites, AIDS did account for the highest proportion of deaths (35.2%) in this group. This indicates that black and Hispanic males in this age group are at greater risk of dying of other, non-AIDS-related causes.[7]

As in males, AIDS mortality rates in females are highest in 25–44-year-olds of all racial/ethnic groups. Furthermore, the rate is again highest in blacks and Hispanics. Compared to white women, the relative risk of dying of AIDS was elevated in black women (5.1) and Hispanic women (3.7). This disproportionate racial/ethnic elevation in the risk of death due to AIDS was originally reported in 1984.[6]

Health District Rates.   AIDS mortality among males within each health center district, and the proportion associated with nar-

_____

* Using ICD-9 code 279.1 only, the Bureau of Health Statistics and Analysis reported 2,407 AIDS deaths among New York City residents aged 15 to 64 in 1986. This represents a crude mortality rate of 51.3 per 100,000 population. These rates do not reflect, of course, the degree of underaccounting of AIDS deaths which occurs due to misclassification of underlying cause of death.

TABLE V.   AIDS Mortality Rates (per 100,000) and Proportional Mortality* By Sex, Age, and Race/Ethnicity, New York City, 1986

| | Race/Ethnicity† | | | | | |
| | White | | | Black | | Hispanic | |
	Rate (No.)	PM‡	Rate (No.)	PM	Rate (No.)	PM
Males						
15–24 years	7.7 (20)	10.4	14.5 (22)	6.2	13.6 (18)	7.8
25–44 years	108.5 (553)	35.2	236.3 (500)	25.4	167.0 (421)	30.4
45–64 years	49.91 (212)	5.4	104.6 (136)	5.2	81.5 (77)	6.6
Total	65.8 (785)	13.6	113.6 (658)	13.2	107.8 (516)	18.6
Females						
15–24 years	1.1 (3)	4.4	6.3 (11)	10.0	4.0 (6)	8.4
25–44 years	9.3 (48)	9.0	47.6 (134)	14.8	34.1 (80)	19.8
45–64 years	0.8 (4)	0.2	7.7 (14)	0.8	4.0 (5)	0.8
Total	4.3 (55)	1.8	24.9 (159)	5.4	18.0 (91)	8.2

* The proportion of all deaths in the specified age, race, and sex group that was attributed to AIDS.
† 169 AIDS deaths occurred in other or unknown racial/ethnic groups and there were eight deaths among Asians.
‡ PM, proportional mortality (%).

TABLE VI.   Age- and Race-Adjusted* AIDS Mortality Rates per 100,000, Males 15–64 Years Only, By Health Center District of Residence, New York City, 1986

Borough	District	Number of Deaths	Adjusted Rate	% Narcotics Related
Manhattan	Central Harlem	73	76.1	64.4
	East Harlem	59	157.6	45.8
	Kips Bay	73	150.4	2.8
	Lower East Side	156	205.7	23.0
	Lower West Side	349	299.3	6.4
	Riverside	131	171.1	9.2
	Washington Heights	55	89.1	31.0
	Total	896		
Bronx	Fordham	48	77.2	43.8
	Morrisania	54	295.7	64.8
	Mott Haven	46	92.8	67.4
	Pelham	41	67.2	39.0
	Tremont	56	74.5	49.6
	Westchester	69	81.8	49.2
	Total	314		
Brooklyn	Williamsburg	37	128.4	67.6
	Bay Ridge	14	22.9	28.6
	Bedford	66	95.9	51.6
	Brownsville	64	69.8	59.4
	Bushwick	46	89.7	76.0
	Flatbush	74	49.5	24.4
	Fort Greene	56	117.0	44.6
	Gravesend	26	65.8	46.2
	Red Hook	39	104.7	25.6
	Sunset Park	25	79.1	40.0
	Total	447		
Queens	Astoria	35	79.1	28.6
	Corona	52	64.5	27.0
	Flushing	23	39.6	13.0
	Jamaica East	78	46.9	53.8
	Jamaica West	38	42.8	34.2
	Maspeth-Forest Hills	18	18.7	5.0
	Total	244		
Staten Island		30	38.9	33.4
Total New York City		1,932		32.6

* Direct method using 1980 New York City census data.

cotics use, are shown in Table VI. A map of the number of deaths attributed to AIDS by zip code of residence appears in Figure 1. Age- and race-adjusted mortality rates were calculated to control for the different race and age compositions in the districts. Because of the relatively small number of deaths among females, and the degree of stratification necessary for the adjustment, we were unable to calculate adjusted rates for females.

Four of the five highest adjusted rates are in Manhattan. Morrisania, in the South Bronx, has the second highest adjusted rate after the Lower West Side. In Manhattan, three areas with high AIDS mortality rates are readily visible from the map. Most prominent, in the southern portion of the island, are five zip codes within the health districts of the Lower East and West Sides. The Upper West Side (Riverside) and East Harlem, with respective mortality rates of 171 and 157 per 100,000 population, have also been affected severely.

The health districts of Morrisania and Mott Haven, which constitute the South Bronx, have the highest adjusted mortality rates in this borough, and the largest proportion of deaths (66%) that were narcotics related. Three contiguous health districts along the western portion of Brooklyn—Williamsburg, Fort Greene, and Red Hook—have the highest adjusted mortality rates in this borough. Districts with the largest number of deaths—Flatbush, Bedford, and Brownsville—are in central Brooklyn. Although Astoria and Corona, in the western portion of Queens, have the highest adjusted AIDS mortality rates in this borough, East Jamaica had the greatest number of deaths and the highest proportion of deaths (54%) attributable to IV drug use.

DISCUSSION

This study briefly describes the demographic impact of AIDS in NYC, stressing racial/ethnic and geographic features of the epidemic. A descriptive analysis can be useful to community groups and organizations providing education and support services to those already infected and to those at increased risk of infection. Incidence and mortality rates enable one to compare the impact of AIDS among health districts, and to draw a detailed picture of AIDS epidemiology within a specific neighborhood.

At least three factors influence the distribution of AIDS: varied racial/ethnic, age, and sex compositions within the city; different degrees and types of risk-associated behavior practiced therein; and different underlying

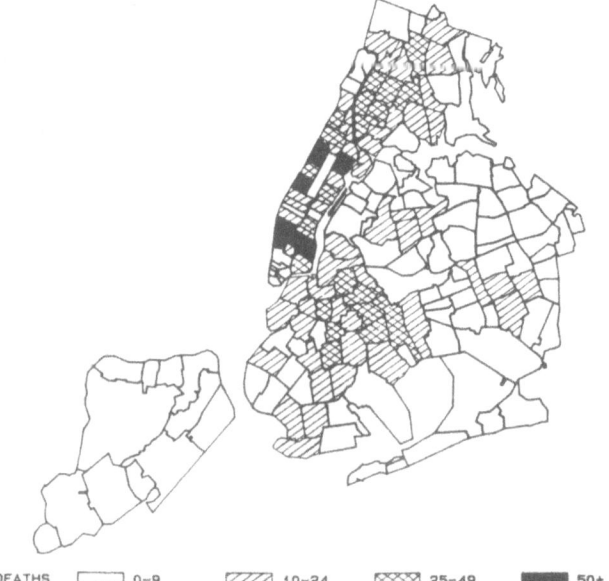

DEATHS ☐ 0–9   ▨ 10–24   ▩ 25–49   ■ 50+

FIGURE 1.   Geographic distribution of AIDS mortality in New York City, 1986, by zip code of residence.

seroprevalence levels of the virus. As is clear from the figures presented here, the epidemiology of AIDS is quite different across the five boroughs of NYC and within the boroughs themselves.

In the six-year period analyzed, Manhattan has been affected most severely. The cumulative incidence of AIDS in this borough is more than 2.5 times that of the next highest, the Bronx. Furthermore, transmission patterns in these boroughs differ dramatically. The early and large impact among homosexual men in Manhattan—accounting for 75% of all cases in that borough—has persisted through 1986. Similarly, IV drug use has consistently accounted for 22% of Manhattan cases. These proportions are nearly reversed in the Bronx.

The high seroprevalence of HIV and incidence and prevalence of AIDS among homosexual men in specific areas of Manhattan indicates the continuing need for health care, psychological support services, and education for those affected, as well as for preventive education for new entrants to this population. The reason for the proportional increase in cases among homosexual men in Brooklyn and Queens is unclear, but suggests a growing need for specific services in these boroughs, particularly if individuals are not being reached by agencies located in Manhattan.

The need to reach the Hispanic and black population is especially clear from the figures (Table I) which indicate that incidence rates in these groups exceed those among whites in all boroughs except Manhattan. Moreover, compared to whites, Hispanics and blacks, particularly women, are at increased risk of dying of AIDS.[6] In these racial/ethnic groups AIDS is also disproportionately transmitted by the sharing of intravenous drugs, and IV-drug-related AIDS accounts for the largest proportion of cases in the Bronx, Brooklyn, and Staten Island. Narcotics-related AIDS mortality is especially high in Morrisania and Mott Haven in the South Bronx, and in Williamsburg, Brownsville, and Bushwick in Brooklyn (Table VI). The need for greatly expanded services for intravenous drug users has been widely emphasized.[5,8]

Intravenous drug use is also the principal source of direct infection in women, and of indirect infection through heterosexual contact with male drug users.[9] Because of the geographic and racial/ethnic patterns of IV drug use, black and Hispanic women constitute the large majority of victims of heterosexually acquired AIDS in all boroughs. Furthermore, children born to black and Hispanic women constitute more than 90% of the pediatric AIDS cases in New York City.[10] Clearly, services for current IV drug users and potential future users should be sensitive to these demographic features and trends.[8,9]

City and community services for persons with AIDS and those at increased risk for AIDS have expanded considerably in NYC since the recognition of this epidemic. The current analysis suggests the important role epidemiologic surveillance can play in providing a detailed demographic picture of AIDS, and how this information can assist in monitoring the impact and need for support and preventive services.

REFERENCES

1.   Selik RM, Haverkos HW, Curran JW: Acquired immune deficiency syn-

drome (AIDS) trends in the United States, 1978–1982. *Am J Med* 1984; 76:493–500.

2. New York City Department of Health AIDS Surveillance: The AIDS epidemic in New York City, 1981–1984. *Am J Epidemiol* 1986; 123:1013–1025.

3. Centers for Disease Control: Revision of the CDC surveillance case definition for AIDS. *MMWR* 1987; 36(suppl 1S).

4. Chamberland ME, Allen JR, Monroe JM, et al: Acquired immunodeficiency syndrome in New York City. Evaluation of an active surveillance system. *JAMA* 1985; 253:383–387.

5. Joseph SC, Schultz S, Stoneburner R, et al: AIDS policy and prevention in New York City. *Bull NY Acad Med* 1986; 63:659–672.

6. Kristal AR: The impact of the acquired immunodeficiency syndrome on patterns of premature death in New York City. *JAMA* 1986; 255:2306–2310.

7. Bureau of Health Statistics and Analysis: *Summary of Vital Statistics 1985.* New York City Department of Health.

8. Weinberg DS, Murray HW: Coping with AIDS: The special problems of New York City. *N Engl J Med* 1987; 317:1469–1472.

9. Castro KG, Lieb S, Jaffe HW, et al: Transmission of HIV in Belle Glade, Florida: Lessons for other communities in the United States. *Science* 1988; 239:193–197.

10. New York City Department of Health AIDS Surveillance Update, December 31, 1987.

Chapter 8

HIV infection among young adults in the New York City area

Prevalence and incidence estimates based on antibody screening among civilian applicants for military service

JOHN F. BRUNDAGE, MD; DONALD S. BURKE, MD; LYTT I. GARDNER, PhD; ROBERT VISINTINE, MD; MICHAEL PETERSON, DVM; ROBERT R. REDFIELD, MD

ABSTRACT. Since October 1985, the Department of Defense has screened civilian applicants for military service for antibody to the human immunodeficiency virus (HIV). Among young adult applicants from 15 New York and New Jersey counties in the New York City region, the overall seroprevalence rate was 7.1 per 1,000 (314/44,139). Seroprevalence rates were higher among men than women (male-female ratio, 1.4:1) and higher among black/non-Hispanic applicants than applicants from other racial/ethnic groups, and they increased almost linearly with age from the late teens through the twenties. Male-specific prevalence rates exceeded 0.5% in nine of the 15 counties, while female-specific prevalences exceeded 0.5% in seven. In Manhattan, the Bronx, and Brooklyn, there were geographic foci associated with significantly increased seroprevalences. Despite potential biases, applicant screening data provide unique insights into the current state and the dynamics of the HIV infection epidemic among young adults. Differences of infection risk based on demographic and geographic factors provide empirical bases for allocating prevention, intervention, and clinical services in the region.

Although it has been approximately six years since end-stage human immunodeficiency virus (HIV) infection was first reported in the New York area, the HIV infection epidemic is at least twice as old in the region. Because of the long and variable period from the time of infection to clinical presentation of end-stage disease, and because the infection epidemic has spread beyond its initial urban epicenters and behaviorally defined risk groups, acquired immunodeficiency syndrome (AIDS) case reports do not reflect the current state of the HIV infection epidemic. Serial prevalence surveillances, based on broad geographic and demographic sampling, are required to assess current infection prevalences and the dynamics of the infection epidemic.

Since October 1985, the Department of Defense has screened more than 1.2 million civilian applicants for military service for antibody to HIV. In this report, data from the applicant screening program are summarized to estimate the concentration and the rate of spread of the virus among young adults living in the New York City metropolitan region.

METHODS

Screening Program and Algorithm. The applicant screening program and the algorithm used to determine antibody positivity have been previously described.[1,2] Briefly, blood is drawn from each applicant at the time of the routine preinduction medical examination. Sera are sent to a single contracting laboratory for analysis. All sera are initially tested by enzyme-linked immunosorbent assay (ELISA). Specimens that are initially ELISA positive are retested in duplicate. Specimens that are repeatedly ELISA positive are further analyzed using the Western blot method. Specimens with either a gp41 band or multiple other HIV-specific bands are considered antibody positive. Applicants who submit specimens that are repeatedly ELISA and Western

From the Department of Epidemiology, Division of Preventive Medicine (Drs Brundage and Gardner), and the Department of Virus Diseases, Division of Communicable Diseases and Immunology (Drs Burke and Redfield), Walter Reed Army Institute of Research, Washington, DC; the United States Military Entrance Processing Command (Dr Visintine), North Chicago, Illinois; and the Office of the Assistant Secretary of Defense (Health Affairs) (Dr Peterson), Washington, DC.

The opinions or assertions contained herein are the private views of the authors and are not to be construed as official or as reflecting the views of the Department of the Army or the Department of Defense.

blot positive are notified and asked to submit a second specimen for repeat Western blot analysis. An applicant is therefore considered antibody positive when sera are repeatedly ELISA positive on a single specimen and repeatedly Western blot positive on duplicate specimens. For this analysis, applicants who declined to submit a second specimen were considered antibody positive after a single specimen was repeatedly positive on ELISA and Western blot screening.

New York Area Applicant Population. During the first 21 months of screening, there were 44,139 applicants for military service from the New York metropolitan region—Bronx, Kings, Nassau, New York, Queens, Richmond, Suffolk, and Westchester counties in New York; Bergen, Essex, Hudson, Middlesex, Monmouth, Passaic, and Union counties in New Jersey. Applicants were young adults (44% younger than 21 years; 81% younger than 26 years); predominantly male (86%); and represented the following racial/ethnic groups: black, non-Hispanic (40%), white, non-Hispanic (40%), Hispanic (10%), and other (10%).

RESULTS

Prevalence Estimates

Overall and Sex-Specific Prevalences. Among all applicants, the seroprevalence rate was 7.1/1,000 (314/44,139). The prevalence was 7.4/1,000 (280/37,838) among males and 5.4/1,000 (34.6/6,301) among females. The overall male-to-female prevalence ratio was 1.4:1. Figure 1 shows sex-specific prevalences and male-to-female prevalence ratios during each of the first seven calendar quarters of routine applicant screening.

Race/Ethnicity. Of six subgroups defined by race/ethnicity (black/non-Hispanic, white/non-Hispanic, Hispanic/other) and gender, black males had the highest overall seroprevalence rate (12/1,000; 162/14,008). Black females had the next highest prevalence (7.5/1,000; 28/3,732). Prevalence rates among white males and white females were relatively low: 3.7/1,000 (60/16,225) and 1.8/1,000 (3/1,626), respectively. Prevalence rates among Hispanic/other applicants were intermediate: males, 6.7/1,000 (58/8,605) and females, 3.2/1,000 (3/943). The male to female prevalence ratio was lower among black applicants than among white or Hispanic/other applicants (Fig 2).

Age. Seroprevalence rates consistently increased with age from the late teens through the twenties. Age-prevalence trends were similar among males and females, and male-to-female prevalence ratios were less than 2:1 in each age group (Fig 3). Seroprevalence rates were low among applicants younger than 21 years, regardless of race/ethnicity or gender. However, throughout the twenties, prevalence increased sharply among black applicants, more gradually among white applicants; and at an intermediate rate among Hispanics/others (Fig 4).

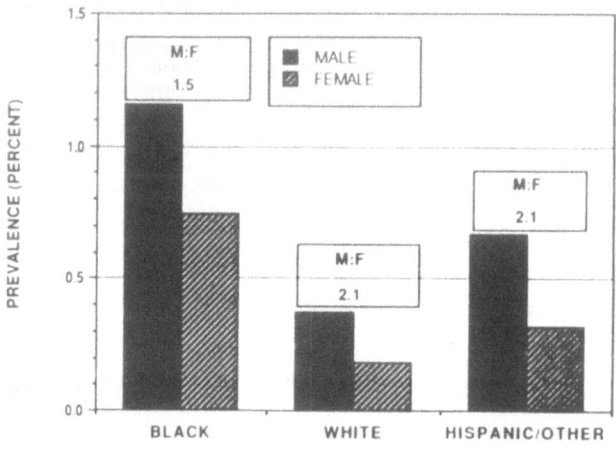

FIGURE 2. Overall seroprevalence rate among New York City metropolitan area applicants for military service, October 1985–June 1987; by sex and race/ethnicity defined subgroups.

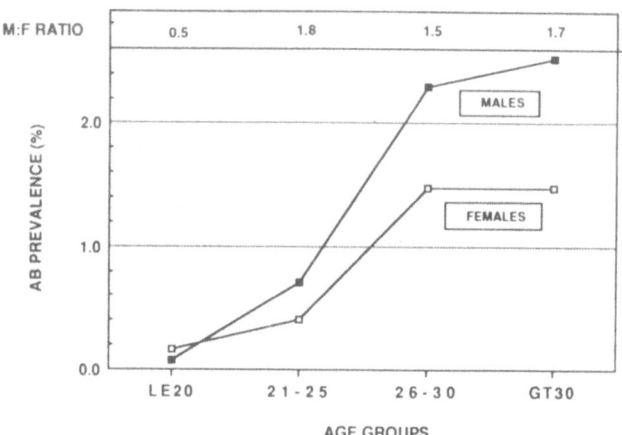

FIGURE 3. Relationship of seroprevalence with age, for male and female military applicants from the New York City-New Jersey metropolitan area. Male-to-female prevalence ratios are also indicated.

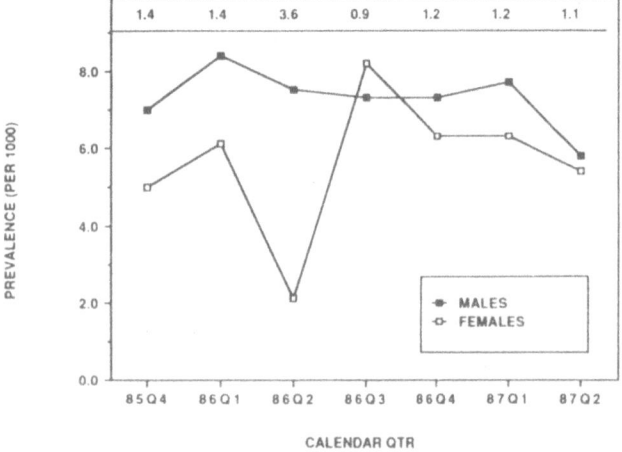

FIGURE 1. Overall seroprevalence rates among male and female applicants from the New York City metropolitan area, October 1985–June 1987, by calendar quarters. Male-to-female prevalence ratios are also indicated.

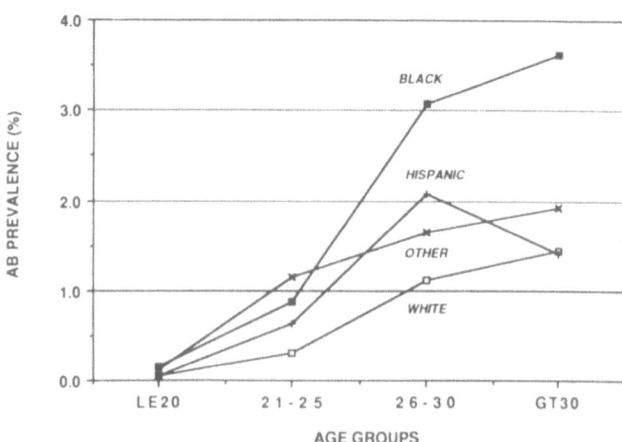

FIGURE 4. Relationship of seroprevalence with age, for race/ethnicity defined subgroups from the New York City area.

TABLE I.   Results of HIV Antibody Screening Among Male and Female Applicants for Military Service from 15 New York and New Jersey Counties in the New York City Metropolitan Region, October 1985–June 1987

	Males (per 1,000)	Females (per 1,000)
Bronx	52/4,124 (12.6)	6/ 790 (7.6)
Kings	66/6,091 (10.8)	7/1,198 (5.8)
Nassau	13/2,854 (4.6)	4/ 419 (9.5)
New York	47/2,733 (17.2)	5/ 445 (11.2)
Queens	22/4,606 (4.8)	4/ 784 (5.1)
Richmond	0/ 730 (0.0)	0/ 102 (0.0)
Suffolk	4/3,882 (1.0)	0/ 517 (0.0)
Westchester	5/1,641 (3.0)	0/ 277 (0.0)
Bergen	3/1,508 (2.0)	0/ 152 (0.0)
Essex	18/2,457 (7.3)	6/ 583 (10.3)
Hudson	16/1,507 (10.6)	0/ 223 (0.0)
Middlesex	8/1,423 (5.6)	0/ 160 (0.0)
Monmouth	10/1,581 (6.3)	0/ 229 (0.0)
Passaic	7/1,260 (5.6)	2/ 204 (9.8)
Union	9/1,441 (6.2)	0/ 218 (0.0)

Geographic Distribution (by County).   Table I shows county-specific prevalence rates among male and female applicants. In Manhattan (New York County), prevalence rates exceeded 1% among both males and females. In the Bronx and Brooklyn (Kings County), prevalence rates exceeded 1% among males and 0.5% among females. In Essex and Passaic counties in New Jersey, prevalence rates exceeded 0.5% among both male and female applicants. Overall, male-specific prevalence rates exceeded 0.5% in nine of the 15 counties, and female-specific prevalences exceeded 0.5% in seven of the 15 counties.

Location (by Zip Codes):   The New York City Health Department recently reported zip codes in Manhattan, Bronx, and Brooklyn that were associated with increased AIDS incidence during the period 1981–1984.[3] We assumed that areas defined by these zip codes had been affected by the HIV infection epidemic relatively longer than other areas of the city. The prevalence rate among applicants from AIDS-associated zip codes significantly exceeded the prevalence rate among applicants from other zip codes in the same high prevalence counties (1.52% [118/7,768] versus 0.85% [65/7,613]; χ^2 = 14.47; one degree of freedom; $p < 0.001$).

Infection Rate Estimates

Prevalence-Age Regression Method: Since antibody to HIV is a persistent marker of HIV infection, the seroprevalence rate in a sample of a population provides an estimate of the cumulative HIV infection incidence in that population. Since seroprevalence rates among applicants increase almost linearly with age in the applicant age range, the regression slope approximates the average increase in cumulative infection incidence with each additional year of age. Therefore, the slopes of prevalence-age regression lines provide estimates of annual HIV infection rates among the young adults in the region who are represented by military applicants.

Figure 5 shows age-specific prevalences for black, Hispanic/other, and white male applicants (for birth year defined groups, approximately aged 18 to 25 years). For each race/ethnicity group, regression lines were fitted to two sets of data collected during two equivalent periods exactly one year apart: October 1985–August 1986 and October 1986–August 1987. The slope of the regression line estimates the average number of new HIV infections per 1,000 persons per year (an incidence rate).

Within each racial/ethnic group, the slopes of age-prevalence regression lines from the two sampling periods were comparable. For black males, the prevalence rates by age regression slopes were 2.65/1,000/year and 2.84/1,000/year. In addition, among black males, birth-year-specific prevalence rates clearly increased between the 1985/86 and the 1986/87 sampling periods (demonstrated by the increase on the prevalence scale of the 1986/87 regression line compared with the 1985/86 line; Fig 5). For Hispanic/other males, the regression slopes were 1.53/1,000/year and 1.68/1,000/year. For white males, the regression slopes were 0.97/1,000/year and 0.78/1,000/year.

Estimated incidence of infection rates based on prevalence by age regression differed markedly among different racial/ethnic groups. Using the estimated rate among white males as the referent, infection rates were approximately 1.8 times higher among Hispanic/other males and 3.1 times higher among black males.

DISCUSSION

Applicants for military service are not randomly selected from the young adults in the New York area, so interpretations of data require consideration of the potential effects of selection bias. Young adults apply for military service subject to institutional and personal criteria. In general, selection factors that are constant over the period of screening and consistent for all age groups (eg, eligibility criteria for military enlistment) define a subgroup of the general population. Parameter estimates based on screening this subgroup provide biased estimates of general population parameters, depending on the strength of the associations of the selection factors and HIV infection risk. In addition, selection factors that change over time or that differ by age (eg, self-selection criteria) additionally bias estimates of time-dependent parameters such as incidence rates and temporal/age trends, even within the subpopulation of military applicants.

Since applicants for military service are self-selected, the consistency of selection criteria is difficult to assess. However, it is presumed that young adults are relatively unlikely to apply for military service if they know of the

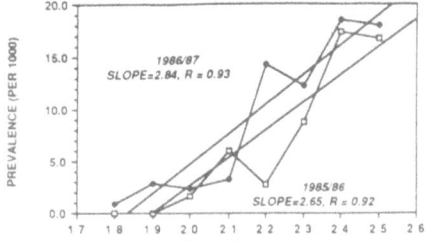
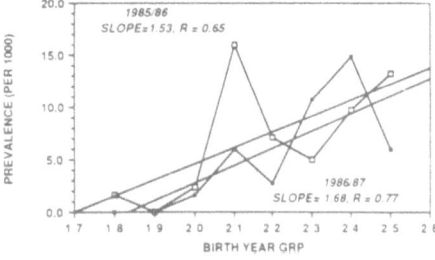
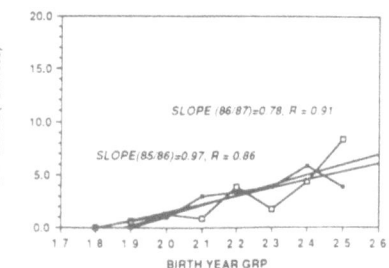

FIGURE 5.   Relationships of seroprevalences and age (defined by birth year) are shown for data collected during two screening periods a year apart in time: October 1985–August 1986 and October 1986–August 1987. Slopes and regression coefficients (R) are indicated for prevalence by age regressions for each of the sampling periods. Slopes estimate the average number of new infections per 1,000 persons per year of increasing age. Slopes are consistent within, but significantly vary among, race/ethnicity defined groups from the New York City metropolitan area. Left, black males; center, Hispanic and other males; right, white males.

Department of Defense's applicant screening program and either know or suspect that they are antibody positive.

During the two-year period of applicant screening, awareness of the Department of Defense screening program has almost surely increased among young adults living in urban epicenters of the AIDS epidemic. In addition, millions of young adults have been screened for antibody to HIV through blood donor, alternate test site, and other screening programs. Undoubtedly, many potential military applicants in the New York area were screened through such programs over the past two years. Finally, educational and mass media programs are now directed at broad segments of communities. Consequently, over the past two years, many young adults in the New York area have acquired the information necessary to accurately assess their own infection risk.

Therefore, it seems likely that self-exclusion of infected and high risk young adults has increased over the period of military applicant screening. If so, prevalence and incidence rate estimates that are based on applicant screening data will underestimate actual rates in the New York City region.

While prevalence by age regression is a simple method for estimating annual infection rates, it has at least one significant limitation. The method estimates the infection rate based on the lifelong exposure of applicants to HIV infection risk. Since the dynamics of the epidemic have evolved throughout its course, the regression method will underestimate the current infection rate if the current rate is higher than the average of the annual rates during the preceding years of the epidemic—a situation that seems likely.

In summary, potential biases based on selection factors and the changing dynamics of the epidemic probably result in estimates of prevalence and incidence rates that are lower than the actual population values.

Without question, the epidemiology of the HIV infection epidemic has changed in the period since patients now affected with end-stage HIV disease were infected with the virus. In spite of their limitations, military applicant screening data provide unique insights into the current state, as well as the recent dynamics, of the HIV infection epidemic in the New York area.

The infection epidemic has spread widely throughout the region. Yet there appear to be geographically circumscribed foci of particularly high and low infection transmission. For example, within Brooklyn, the Bronx, and Manhattan, zip codes associated with increased AIDS incidence in 1981–1984 (and therefore with HIV infection transmission for at least a decade) still define geographic areas of particularly high infection prevalence among young adults. In contrast, there are geographic areas where young adults represented by military applicants remain relatively unaffected by the epidemic (eg, Staten Island [Richmond County], New York). Identification of geographic areas with particularly high and low infection transmission rates provides opportunities to target prevention, intervention, and clinical services, and to further define sociodemographic and behavioral determinants of the current infection epidemic.

In contrast to the extreme male predominance among reported AIDS patients in the country, ratios of seroprevalence rates among male and female applicants were generally less than 2:1. While gender specific selection factors may result in underestimates of actual male-to-female infection ratios, these and other data[4] document the significant impact of the infection epidemic on young females in the region. The current involvement of young females of child bearing age in the infection epidemic has important implications regarding the futures of both the adult and the pediatric AIDS epidemics in the region.

Finally, seroprevalence rates were relatively low among teenagers, regardless of their gender or race/ethnicity, and they increased almost linearly from the late teens through the twenties, most strikingly among members of racial/ethnic minorities. These findings define opportunities and responsibilities for aggressive intervention efforts. HIV-related knowledge, attitudes, and behavioral skills that are critical during periods of greatest infection risk must be acquired by young men and women during the relatively lower risk, middle teen years, particularly in demographic subgroups in geographic areas with the highest rates of HIV infection incidence.

Acknowledgment. The authors thank Mary Goldenbaum for data management, analysis, and graphics support.

REFERENCES

1. Burke DS, Brundage JF, Herbold JR: Human immunodeficiency virus infections among civilian applicants for United States military service, October 1985 to March 1986. *N Engl J Med* 1987; 317:132–136.
2. Burke DS, Brundage JF, Bernier W, et al: Demography of HIV infections among civilian applicants for military service in four counties in New York City. *NY State J Med* 1987; 87:262–264.
3. New York City Department of Health AIDS Surveillance: The AIDS epidemic in New York City, 1981–1984. *Am J Epidemiol* 1986; 123:1013–1025.
4. Landesman S, Minkoff H, Holman S: Serosurvey of human immunodeficiency virus infection in parturients. Implications for human immunodeficiency virus testing programs for pregnant women. *JAMA* 1987; 258:2701–2703.

Chapter 9
The epidemiology of AIDS in New Jersey

RONALD ALTMAN, MD, MPH

ABSTRACT. The epidemiology of acquired immunodeficiency syndrome in New Jersey is presented for the period 1982–1986. Additional data are also presented for 1987. A total of 1,728 nonincarcerated adult AIDS cases were diagnosed in the period 1982–1986. The largest number of cases occurred in the counties that contain sizable urban populations. The proportion of cases among females is very high in New Jersey, with most of them occurring in those areas of the state near New York City. Intravenous drug abuse is the risk factor most directly associated with AIDS in the high incidence metropolitan areas of New Jersey.

New Jersey has the fifth largest number of cases of acquired immunodeficiency syndrome (AIDS) in the nation, following New York, California, Florida, and Texas. As of December 31, 1987, 3,257 cases of AIDS had been reported to the New Jersey State Department of Health. When AIDS case rates are considered, New Jersey ranks third (as of November 2, 1987), with a case rate of 346 per million population, compared to a case rate of 693 for New York and 372 for California.[1] New Jersey is unique in that the majority of AIDS patients in the state have a history of intravenous drug abuse. Probably related to this is the fact that New Jersey has the highest percentage of female AIDS cases in the nation, a large number of children with AIDS, and a large number of AIDS patients who are incarcerated.

New Jersey has always somewhat gravitated around its neighboring two large cities, New York and Philadelphia. Even the AIDS epidemic shows different patterns around New York and Philadelphia, perhaps to some extent reflecting the demographics of the AIDS epidemic in these cities. Some of these differences will be reflected in the data shown here.

METHODS

A number of years ago, the New Jersey State Department of Health administratively divided the state's 21 counties into four districts, three with five counties each and the fourth with six counties. While these administrative districts are no longer used, they provide a means of dividing the state for the purposes of analysis. Such a division gives a picture of the geographic differ-

ences of AIDS in New Jersey and eliminates the analytical problems that arise because of the relatively small number of cases in some of the counties.

As shown in Figure 1, the metropolitan district consisted of the counties immediately surrounding New York City; the northern district contained the area in northwestern New Jersey that used to be largely rural, but now is rapidly becoming suburban; the southern district consisted of all of the south of New Jersey, including rural, suburban and urban areas, much of it in the Philadelphia metropolitan area; and the central district was the region in the center of the state, with areas that can be considered in either the New York or the Philadelphia orbit. Both the central and southern districts contained the New Jersey shore.

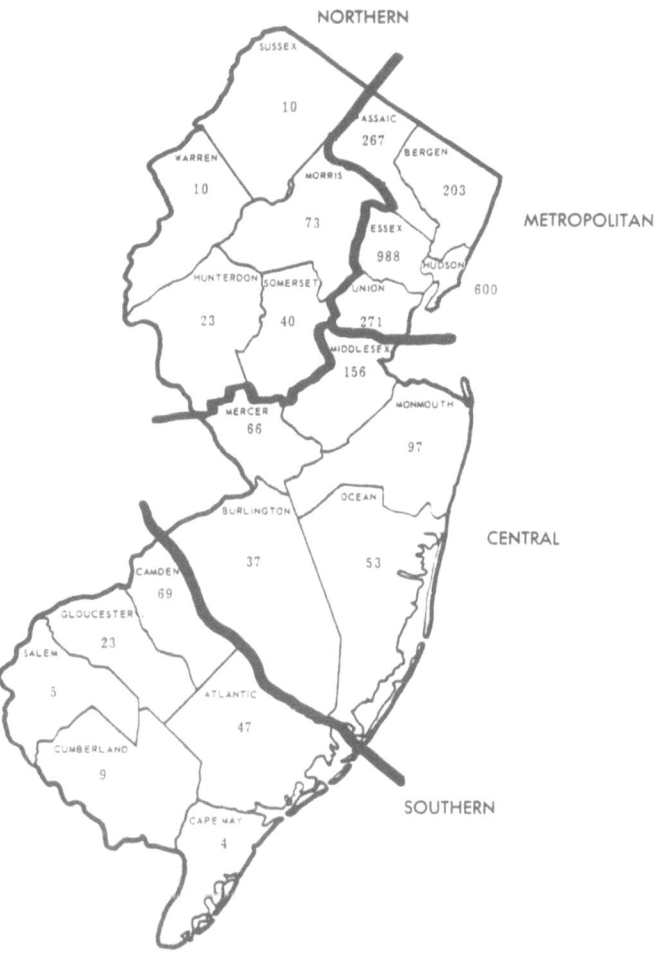

FIGURE 1. AIDS cases in the State of New Jersey as of December 31, 1987.

From the New Jersey State Department of Health, Trenton, NJ.

TABLE I. Cumulative AIDS Cases by County, New Jersey, Through December 31, 1987

County	Population	No. of Cases	Rate per 1,000,000
Atlantic	194,119	47	242
Bergen	845,385	203	240
Burlington	362,542	37	102
Camden	471,650	69	146
Cape May	82,266	4	49
Cumberland	132,866	9	68
Essex	851,304	988	1,161
Gloucester	199,917	23	115
Hudson	566,972	600	1,077
Hunterdon	87,361	23	263
Mercer	307,863	66	214
Middlesex	595,893	156	262
Monmouth	503,173	97	193
Morris	407,630	73	179
Ocean	346,038	53	153
Passaic	447,585	267	597
Salem	64,676	5	77
Somerset	203,129	40	197
Sussex	116,119	10	86
Union	504,094	271	538
Warren	84,429	10	118
Total	7,365,011	3,257	442

TABLE III. AIDS Cases by Year and Gender, New Jersey, 1982–1986

Year	Male No.	Male %	Female No.	Female %
1982	55	84.6	10	15.4
1983	146	88.0	20	12.0
1984	283	85.5	48	14.5
1985	456	82.8	95	17.2
1986	608	82.1	133	21.9

Most of the analyses presented in this paper are for the period 1982 through 1986. These data would include virtually all of the reported AIDS cases diagnosed during that period. Presenting the data for this period eliminates the problem of the small numbers of cases in the years prior to 1982, which do not give meaningful time trend data, and, since all of the cases diagnosed in 1987 would not have been reported by the time of preparation of this paper, 1987 cannot be included in time trend data. In addition, the case definition of AIDS changed during 1987, so that the case data for this year are not comparable to previous years, at least until the older data are updated to the new case definition. However, where appropriate, data are also presented which include all cases reported through 1987.

RESULTS

The largest cumulative numbers of AIDS cases reported through 1987 were reported from the counties near New York City (Fig 1). The numbers in each county do not include the people with AIDS who were incarcerated at the time of the case report, many of whom were from the counties with large numbers of AIDS cases. Epidemiologically, it is more meaningful to look at incidence rates (Table I). Essex and Hudson counties, which contain the cities of Newark and Jersey City, respectively, each had a cumulative incidence rate of over 1,000 per million population, while Passaic and Union counties, which contain the cities of Paterson and Elizabeth, respectively, each had a cumulative incidence rate of over 500 per million. There was not much difference in incidence among the 17 other New Jer-

sey counties, although a few of the counties had relatively low rates.

Of the 1,728 nonincarcerated adults with AIDS diagnosed in the period 1982–1986, 77.0% came from the metropolitan district (Table II). Overall, 16.5% of the adults with AIDS were female. There was a marked difference in the percentage of female cases in the various districts, with the largest percentage in the metropolitan district, the lowest percentages in the northern and southern districts, with the central district being intermediate, a trend generally present in the cumulative case rates. The cumulative case rates in males were essentially the same in the northern, central and southern districts, which is similar to the lack of difference in case rates among the counties noted above, except for four counties in the metropolitan district. There was an increase in the number and percentage of female cases in the later years (Table III). It should be noted that in the cumulative case data through 1987, the percentage of female patients is up to 20%, which is further evidence that the percentage of female AIDS cases in New Jersey is continuing to rise.

The northern and southern districts tended to follow the national pattern of risk group distribution of AIDS cases, with approximately three-quarters of the cases occurring in homosexual or bisexual men (Table IV). On the other hand, the metropolitan district showed slightly more cases among intravenous drug abusers compared to homosexual-bisexual men, with the central district showing an intermediate pattern between the two types of risk group distribution. The overwhelmingly larger number of AIDS cases in the metropolitan district, compared to the other three districts, resulted in a high percentage of AIDS cases in intravenous drug abusers in the state as a whole. A similar analysis by district is not presented for adult females because of the very small number of female AIDS cases in the northern and southern districts.

Tables V and VI present the risk group percentages by year for adult males and females respectively. Among adult males, there was very little change in the percentage of cases in the different risk groups over the years, the exception being a marked decline in the percentage reporting both homosexual activity and intravenous drug abuse (Table V). Among adult females, there was a marked increase in the percentage of cases reporting heterosexual contact with a person at high risk for HIV infection. Some of this increase came about because of a drop in the cases classified as undetermined, so there is some question as to whether or not all of the increase in heterosexual contact cases represented a real change.

Looking at AIDS case data only gives information about HIV infection that largely occurred several years ago. More up-to-date information on the current status of HIV infection is provided by serosurveys for HIV infection performed in various populations, al-

TABLE II. AIDS Cases by District and Gender, New Jersey, 1982–1986

District	Number of Cases Male	Female	Total	Percent by Gender Male	Female	Total	Rate per 1,000,000 Population Male	Female	Total
Metropolitan	1,075	255	1,330	80.8	19.2	100.0	708	151	415
Northern	77	8	85	90.6	9.4	100.0	175	17	95
Central	182	29	211	86.3	13.7	100.0	177	27	100
Southern	93	9	102	91.2	8.8	100.0	170	15	110
Incarcerated population	121	5	126	96.0	4.0	100.0	—	—	—
Total	1,548	306	1,854	83.5	16.5	100.0	438	80	252

TABLE IV.   AIDS Cases (%) by Risk Group and District, Adult Males, New Jersey, 1982–1986

Risk Group	Metropolitan District	Northern District	Central District	Southern District	Incarcerated Population
Homosexual/ bisexual	40.0	80.5	49.5	67.7	1.7
Intravenous drug user, heterosexual	43.5	11.7	30.8	14.0	88.4
Intravenous drug user, homosexual	7.5	0	7.7	8.6	7.4
Hemophiliac	0.7	2.6	4.4	4.3	0
Heterosexual contact	3.2	0	1.6	0	0.8
Transfusion	1.3	3.9	2.2	2.2	0
Undetermined	3.0	1.3	3.8	3.2	1.75
Total number of cases	1,075	77	182	93	121

though one-time serosurveys do not give information about the incidence of HIV infection. The New Jersey State Department of Health is currently involved in doing or planning a variety of HIV serosurveys. One of these surveys is nearing completion, a survey of specimens submitted to the State Health Department's laboratory for syphilis testing from sexually transmitted disease clinics throughout New Jersey. As might be anticipated, preliminary results are showing high HIV prevalence in specimens from those counties where there is a high incidence of AIDS cases, with lower seroprevalence rates from the remainder of the counties.

DISCUSSION

The New Jersey AIDS cases show different patterns of occurrence even within the confines of a physically small state. The largest numbers of AIDS cases are occurring in the counties that both contain sizable urban areas and are near New York City. These counties also have the highest cumulative AIDS incidence rates, with much lower case rates in most of the remaining counties in the state. The percentage of female cases is very high in New Jersey, a percentage that appears to be growing. Again, most of the female AIDS cases are also occurring in the portion of New Jersey near New York City.

In most of New Jersey, the risk group distribution of AIDS cases among men is similar to the national distribution, with about three-quarters of the cases occurring in homosexual or bisexual men. However, in the area of the

state with by far the largest number of cases, the male cases are almost equally divided between homosexual-bisexual men and intravenous drug abusers. Among women, most of the cases are occurring in intravenous drug abusers, making intravenous drug abuse the single most important AIDS risk behavior in New Jersey. In addition, a growing percentage of the AIDS cases in women in New Jersey is related to heterosexual contact with a person at high risk for HIV infection. In most such cases, the risk behavior of the contact is intravenous drug abuse.

Thus, the key to much of the AIDS problem in New Jersey is intravenous drug abuse. Intravenous drug abuse is the risk behavior most directly associated with AIDS in the high incidence metropolitan area of New Jersey. It is responsible for the very high incidence of AIDS in women in the state, both directly in drug-abusing women, and indirectly in women who are sexual partners of drug-abusing men, and is also responsible for the high incidence of AIDS in children born to HIV-infected women. It is also almost the only behavior responsible for the very large number of incarcerated persons with AIDS in the state.

Clearly, the surveillance data on the AIDS cases point to prevention of the spread of HIV through prevention of intravenous drug abuse as the primary means to slow the spread of the AIDS epidemic in New Jersey. This is necessary to diminish the already present epidemic of AIDS in the cities of the metropolitan area of the state, to do something about the increasing numbers of cases in women and children, and perhaps to prevent the areas of the state not currently as badly affected by the epidemic from soon resembling the metropolitan district. The group we need to

TABLE V.   AIDS Cases (%) by Risk Group and Year, Adult Males, New Jersey, 1982–1986

Risk Group	1982	1983	1984	1985	1986
Homosexual/ bisexual	36.4	37.0	40.3	43.6	43.2
Intravenous drug user, heterosexual	38.2	43.8	39.9	43.6	42.5
Intravenous drug user, homosexual	16.4	11.0	10.2	4.8	5.9
Hemophiliac	0	0.7	1.4	2.2	1.2
Heterosexual contact	7.2	1.4	2.8	2.0	2.7
Transfusion	0	1.4	0.7	1.5	2.0
Undetermined	1.8	4.8	4.6	2.2	2.5
Total number of cases	55	146	283	456	608

TABLE VI.   AIDS Cases (%) by Risk Group and Year, Adult Females, New Jersey, 1982–1986

Risk Group	1982	1983	1984	1985	1986
Intravenous drug user	90.0	65.0	62.5	63.2	60.2
Heterosexual contact	10.0	20.0	16.7	26.3	32.3
Transfusion	0	5.0	8.3	3.2	4.5
Undetermined	0	10.0	12.5	7.4	3.0
Total number of cases	10	20	48	95	133

reach most are those who have not yet become intravenous drug abusers, particularly people in their teenage years. Until such time as there is an effective vaccine or chemoprophylaxis, we must learn effective methods of preventing people from becoming intravenous drug abusers.

REFERENCE

1. Centers for Disease Control: *Human Immunodeficiency Virus Infections in the United States. A Review of Current Knowledge and Plans for Expansion of HIV Surveillance Activities. A Report to the Domestic Policy Council.* Department of Health and Human Services, Public Health Service, November 30, 1987.

Chapter 10

Effectiveness of distribution of information on AIDS
A national study of six media in Australia

Michael W. Ross, PhD, James A. Carson, MD

ABSTRACT. Differential use of media for providing AIDS information and attitudes toward AIDS were assessed in a geographically stratified proportional sample of 2,601 adults in all states and territories in Australia. Data indicated that exposure to media information, regardless of type, was associated with lower levels of fear of homosexual persons and less fear of death, as well as lower levels of social conservatism. Those who obtained AIDS information from health care workers were found to have fewer unrealistic concerns. Individuals who were more homosexual in expressed sexual identity and those with other at-risk behaviors tended to get information more frequently from friends and pamphlets or posters, and those in higher occupational levels and those with high levels of personal and social concerns about AIDS tended to get their information from friends and health care workers. Electronic media were not utilized more frequently by those with at-risk behaviors. These results suggest that greater emphasis should be placed on more informal sources of information for those most at risk of HIV infection, and that the public media convey little advantage in providing information to such target groups.

The spread, or potential for spread, of acquired immunodeficiency syndrome (AIDS) has instigated major media campaigns in an attempt to modify behaviors that place individuals at risk of infection with the human immunodeficiency virus (HIV), the causative agent of AIDS. Such risk behaviors include unprotected sexual intercourse, both heterosexual and homosexual, and sharing of needles for the administration of intravenous drugs. Media campaigns have been the most common form of attempting to reach the general population,[1] while pamphlets and brochures have commonly been utilized to motivate change among homosexual and bisexual men.[2]

There is little if any published research that looks at the

attitudes toward AIDS held by those who utilize various media, and whether there is a differential use of particular media by those most at risk of HIV infection. While Temoshok, Sweet, and Zich[3] found that the level of knowledge about AIDS was negatively correlated with fear of AIDS and anti-homosexual attitudes in a three-city sample, their data were based on a small sample of convenience, and its generalizability is uncertain.

METHODS

We assessed both the attitudes toward AIDS, and the differential use of media by those whose behaviors potentially put them at risk of HIV infection, as part of a national study on AIDS knowledge, attitudes, and risk behaviors in all states and territories of Australia. We noted in a related publication utilizing these data that a higher level of knowledge about AIDS was significantly related to the use of pamphlets or posters as a media source and that in some cases obtaining information from public media lead to a *lower* level of accurate knowledge about AIDS.[4]

Three research questions were asked in order to determine which media were likely to be the most effective in reaching those individuals most in need of information about AIDS: First, do attitudes toward AIDS differ according to the media from which individuals report having received their information about AIDS? Second, what demographic variables differentiate those who report receiving their information about AIDS from the various media? And third, do those whose behavior places them at greater risk of HIV infection receive their information about AIDS from particular media in preference to others?

The study was carried out on a geographically stratified, proportional sample of 2,601 individuals aged 16 years or over in all states and territories of Australia (population, 16 million). The sampling frame was provided by the Australian Bureau of Statistics on the basis of the most recent (1981) census data and was carried out in October–November 1986. Experienced market research interviewers employed by a national market research company visited the selected dwellings and carried out a face-to-face interview on knowledge of and attitudes toward AIDS. Selected census tracts were randomly generated from the state and urban-rural stratification requirements. Every third residence in the selected tracts was visited from a random start point. Respondents in each dwelling were selected by asking for the individual whose next birthday was nearest the date of the visit. Only individuals over 16 years of age were eligible to participate.

The questions and scales measuring attitudes toward AIDS have been described elsewhere.[5] Four additional questions were

From the AIDS Programme, South Australian Health Commission, and the Departments of Psychiatry and Primary Health Care, Flinders University Medical School, Adelaide, Australia (Dr Ross), and the Office of Psychiatric Services, Health Commission of Victoria, Melbourne, Australia (Dr Carson).

scored on a six-point Likert scale (the first two questions were defined at the poles by the terms "not at all concerned" and "extremely concerned"): for example, "How concerned are you about AIDS as a social issue in Australia (personally)?" A further two questions—"Do you personally know any homosexual people (intravenous drug users)?"—were scored "yes, unsure, no." Demographic data included age, state or territory, occupation, place of residence (city, town, rural), position on the Kinsey scale of sexual identity,[6] and marital status. Media sources of AIDS information (scored "yes," "no") were television, radio, newspapers and magazines, posters and pamphlets, friends, and health professionals.

At the conclusion of the 15-minute interview, an anonymous questionnaire with a reply-paid envelope was left with the respondent. The questionnaire requested yes/no responses for the following items (separate items for "ever" and "in the past 12 months"): homosexual contact, heterosexual contact, use of intravenous drugs, contact with prostitutes, and blood transfusion from 1980 to 1985. The surveyors made one return visit to interview respondents who were not at home at the time of the initial call.

The anonymous risk behavior questionnaire was matched by code number with the data from the face-to-face interview. Data analysis consisted of computing t-tests (two-tailed) and χ^2 tests (for interval/ratio and ordinal data, respectively) between those who responded "yes" and "no" to the six sources of information, with significance set at the 0.05 level.

RESULTS

Risk behavior questionnaires were returned by 60.2% of the interview subjects. Twenty-one individuals had not heard of AIDS, and their face-to-face interviews were terminated after the demographic data were collected. Results of the sampling appear in Table I. In comparison with the census data, the sample appeared to be weighted toward females, and to slightly underrepresent those younger than 24 years of age and slightly overrepresent those aged 25 to 44 years. Unmarried females also appeared to be slightly underrepresented. The marginal additional weighting given to South Australia is a result of the study's having been piloted in that state.

Comparison between the face-to-face interview results of those who did return the risk behavior forms and those who did not revealed only three significant differences at $p < 0.05$ (mean ± standard error given). Those who returned the forms were older (age 43.3 ± 0.05 vs 40.7 ± 0.05; $t = 3.9$, $p < 0.01$); had lower personal concern about AIDS on a six-point scale with the poles labelled "not at all concerned" and "extremely concerned" (3.1 ± 0.05 vs 3.4 ± 0.05; $t = 3.8$, $p < 0.01$); and were more likely to come from a lower occupational classification (classed on the Congalton[7] seven-point status ranking list of occupations in Australia (1 = highest status); $\chi^2 = 52.3$, degrees of freedom = 6, $p < 0.01$).

Results of the data analysis are summarized in Table II. The data reveal a number of differences among those who obtained their knowledge of AIDS from the six media sources (the "other" source was, without exception, the workplace). Relative importance of sources for information on AIDS was TV, 93.8%; newspapers and magazines, 89.7%; radio, 73.7%; friends, 38.3%; pamphlets and posters, 29.6%; health workers, 19.9%; and work, 9.3%.

The data in Table II illustrate that exposure to media information, regardless of type, was associated with lower levels of fear of homosexual persons and less fear of death, as well as lower levels of social conservatism. Those who obtained information from health care workers had a lower level of unrealistic concerns about AIDS, and those with who indicated higher levels of pity for people with AIDS tended to have received their information from radio and newspapers and magazines more frequently.

Individuals who were more homosexual in expressed sexual identity tended to get their information significantly more often from sources that are likely to include the homosexual subculture (friends and pamphlets/posters), and those in higher occupational classes tended to get their information from personal sources (friends and health care workers). Those with higher levels of personal and social

TABLE I. Sample Characteristics by Comparison with the General Australian Population (%)

Variable	Census	Sample
State		
New South Wales	34.8	35.7
Victoria	26.2	24.8
South Australia	8.7	12.1
Queensland	16.1	14.7
West Australia	8.9	7.8
Australian Capital Territory	1.6	1.8
Northern Territory	1.0	0.8
Tasmania	2.8	2.3
Age (yr)		
15–19	10.9	6.6
20–24	11.4	9.0
25–29	10.9	12.3
30–34	10.7	13.7
35–39	10.0	10.6
40–44	7.8	8.7
45–49	6.7	6.7
50–54	6.3	6.3
55–59	6.3	5.8
60–64	5.8	7.0
65–69	4.6	5.2
≥70	8.6	8.3
Sex		
Male	49.8	40.6
Female	50.2	59.4
Marital Status		
Male		
Single	31.4	30.4
Married	62.7	62.0
Separated, widowed, divorced	5.9	7.6
Female		
Single	23.2	17.2
Married	61.7	64.7
Separated, widowed, divorced	15.1	18.1

concerns about AIDS also tended to get information from personal sources (friends and health care workers). For those engaged in behaviors that may be associated with increased risk of HIV infection, personal sources and specific informational sources such as pamphlets and posters were more frequently used for information. The electronic media (TV and radio) were not utilized more frequently by those engaging in risk-related behaviors than by those who were not.

DISCUSSION

It is difficult to see how the differences between those who did return the risk questionnaires and those who did not might systematically bias the data. Kinsey, Pomeroy and Martin[6] have noted, however, that sexual contact occurs consistently earlier in lower socioeconomic strata. Thus, the data on those engaging in risk-related behaviors must be interpreted cautiously, as the prevalence of risk-related behavior is estimated from an incomplete sample.

Nevertheless, these data provide some useful information on the importance of various sources of information about AIDS. First, those who obtain information from a number of media sources appear to have more positive and less conservative attitudes toward AIDS, although socially conservative individuals appear to use television more frequently. Second, those with a history of engaging in risk-related behaviors generally tend to seek information from more specific sources such as pamphlets and posters

TABLE II.   Characteristics Differentiating Those Utilizing Various Media Sources for Information about AIDS

Variable	TV	Radio	Newspapers	Media Source Pamphlets/ Posters	Friends	Health Care Workers
Attitudes						
Fear of homosexuals	−*	−		−	−	−
Fear of death		−		−	−	−
Lack of unreal concerns						+
Pity for people with AIDS		+*	+			
Fear of unknown	−					
Social conservatism	+	−		−	−	−
Demographics						
Kinsey scale				+a	+a	
Occupational class					+b	+b
Marital status			−c	+d	+d	−c
Sex (more males)	−	+				
Personal concern about AIDS			+	+	+	+
Social concern about AIDS					+	+
Know more homosexuals		+	+	+	+	+
Know more intravenous drug users	−		+	+	+	+
Risk behaviors						
Transfusion 1980–1985		−		−		+
Intravenous drug use						
Male homosexual sex				+	+	+
Male heterosexual sex						
Female homosexual sex	−					
Female heterosexual sex	+			+	+	+
Male prostitute contact						

* The notation "+" indicates that those scoring higher on the variable reported use of that particular source or medium significantly more often. The notation "−" indicates that those scoring lower on the variable reported use of that particular source or medium significantly more often.
a Those more homosexual higher than those more heterosexual.
b Those in classes 1–3 higher.
c Those separated lower than those married or single.
d Those single higher than those married or separated.

on AIDS, and from friends and health care workers. This suggests that these less public and more informal sources should be emphasized to provide information to those most at risk, and that the public media convey little advantage in reaching such target groups, though they do serve to alert the general public to the issue. Third, such personal sources as health care practitioners (as well as friends) are more commonly utilized by those in the higher occupational levels. These data are consistent with the finding of Sherr[1] that information in the public media is unlikely to alter significantly attitudes or knowledge in the desired direction, even after major public information campaigns about AIDS. Sherr[1] also reported that 57.2% of high risk and 65.2% of low risk individuals would turn to doctors or clinics for information on AIDS. However, the lack of significant differences among the various public media in the present study does not imply lower rates of use of these media; rather, their use appears to be equally common across all population groups. Nevertheless, Sherr[1] found that fewer than half of the respondents in his sample had read AIDS advertisements in the UK national campaign, and that there was no significant increase in knowledge following reading of such advertisements.

These data from a large, stratified sample of adults provide useful information on the sources for information on AIDS. They suggest that the public media (radio and TV) are significantly associated with attitudes toward AIDS, but that the more intimate and personal sources of information are selectively sought by those whose behaviors may place them at risk of HIV infection. Information campaigns should concentrate on educating health care workers and providing pamphlets and posters on AIDS for those who do not wish to raise questions personally. The public media (TV, radio, newspapers, and magazines) may be of more use in directing individuals toward sources of information than in actually conveying such information.

REFERENCES

1. Sherr L: An evaluation of the UK government health education campaign on AIDS. *Psychol Health* 1987; 1:61–72.
2. Siegel K, Grodsky PB, Herman A: AIDS risk reduction guidelines: A review and analysis. *J Community Health* 1986; 11:233–243.
3. Temoshok L, Sweet DM, Zich J: A three-city comparison of the public's knowledge and attitudes about AIDS. *Psychol Health* 1987; 1:43–60.
4. Ross MW, Carson JA, Cass VC, et al: Knowledge of AIDS in Australia: A national study. *Health Educ Res* (in press).
5. Ross MW: Measuring attitudes toward AIDS: Their structure and interactions. *Hosp Community Psychiatry* (in press).
6. Kinsey AC, Pomeroy WD, Martin CM: *Sexual Behavior in the Human Male*. Philadelphia, WB Saunders, 1948.
7. Congalton AA: *Status and Prestige in Australia*. Melbourne, FW Cheshire, 1969.

Chapter 11

A seroepidemiologic profile of persons seeking anonymous HIV testing at alternate sites in upstate New York

JOHN C. GRABAU, PHD, MPH; BENEDICT I. TRUMAN, MD, MPH; DALE L. MORSE, MD

ABSTRACT. Alternate sites for human immunodeficiency virus (HIV) counseling and testing were established in New York State in the late summer of 1985. In a six-month period at the beginning of 1986, 14.4% of individuals who received HIV test results were seropositive. Questionnaire data were obtained from 1,635 persons for development of an epidemiologic profile of attendees: most were white (83%), males (72%), born in the United States (94%), well (80%), who sought testing because they had risk factors (73%) or had had sex with persons at risk (26%). Higher rates of HIV seropositivity were found among blacks (26%), Hispanics (30%), males (16%), and those with a known risk factor (18%), and among those with symptoms (21%), than among those without these characteristics. Factors associated with HIV seropositivity are described.

In his report to the nation, Surgeon General C. Everett Koop stated that "AIDS is a life-threatening disease and a major public health issue. Its impact on our society is and will continue to be devastating. By the end of 1991, an estimated 270,000 cases of AIDS will have occurred with 179,000 deaths within the decade since the disease was first recognized."[1] In that same report, Dr Koop also said that in some cases, it may be appropriate for individuals with histories of high-risk behavior to obtain a blood test for antibodies to the AIDS virus.

In April 1985, the Centers for Disease Control (CDC) established 55 cooperative agreements with state and local health departments to defray start-up costs of alternate testing sites. The purpose of the alternate sites is to make HIV antibody testing available (outside the blood banking system) to individuals wishing to learn their antibody status. Further, the nation's blood supply would benefit as the potential for false-negative donations would be reduced. By the end of 1985, 874 sites had been established in 53 project areas. During the first eight months, 17.3% of 55,500 individuals tested across the country were repeatedly reactive on enzyme-linked immunoassay (ELISA) tests for HIV.[2] While there has been a substan-

tial commitment to the alternate site effort across the country, only a limited number of published reports are available documenting the activities at the sites.

The state of West Virginia established 11 alternate test sites at local health departments throughout the state. As of mid-July 1986, 414 persons had been tested for HIV at one of the sites. The positivity rate for the state sites was 8.5%. Men were twice as likely as women to test positive, with 8.5% of the men and 4.1% of the women being positive.[3]

Through March 1986, alternate sites in the Minneapolis-St Paul areas tested 2,812 blood samples for HIV—13.2% were positive.[4] For a six-month period ending in November 1986, the state of Alabama reported 18% positive of 729 people tested at alternate sites.[5]

During the early years of the AIDS epidemic, New York State accounted for half of all cases recorded nationally. As the disease has spread across the country, New York State has contributed a decreasing proportion of the cases reported to the Centers for Disease Control. As of October 12, 1987, New York State had 28.5% of the cumulative national AIDS incidence, reporting 12,012 cases since the beginning of the epidemic.[6]

This chapter describes epidemiologic variables and the HIV serologic status of those who attended alternate sites in New York State exclusive of New York City for the first six months of 1986.

METHODS

Shortly after the Food and Drug Administration approved an ELISA test for antibodies to HTLV-III, and with the assistance of a CDC cooperative agreement, the New York State Department of Health began developing a program to establish alternate testing sites throughout upstate New York (ie, New York State exclusive of New York City). Anonymous testing for AIDS antibodies became available to those wishing to know if they had been exposed to the human immunodeficiency virus (HIV). Protocols for counseling individuals at pre- and post-test sessions were developed, staff hired and trained, locations established, and announcement of the availability of the testing sites completed in a matter of months. The first counseling site opened in late summer 1985. To obtain testing, potential clients called a hotline number, spoke with a staff member, and scheduled a pre-test counseling appointment. If, based on the discussion at the pre-test counseling session, the client elected to have the test, a blood sample was obtained and a post-test appointment was scheduled a few weeks later.

From the AIDS Institute (Dr Grabau) and the Bureau of Communicable Disease Control (Drs Truman and Morse), New York State Department of Health, Albany, NY.

In upstate New York, for a six-month period starting in January 1986, a ten-item self-administered questionnaire was utilized at all the counseling sites (seven main alternate sites and seven satellite clinics). The main sites were located in Buffalo, Rochester, Syracuse, Albany, New Rochelle, Mineola, and Farmingdale. The satellite clinics were in outlying areas surrounding the cities or towns listed above. Clients who received antibody testing were asked to complete the voluntary and anonymous questionnaire. Questions focused on basic demographics, as well as risk-group status, reasons for wanting to be tested, self-perceived health status, and sexual contacts with males and/or females since 1978. Questionnaires were completed and forwarded to the central office at the time the blood sample was drawn. All blood samples were examined initially using an ELISA test marketed by Electronucleonics; those specimens that were repeatedly reactive were confirmed using a Western Blot kit manufactured by Organo Biotechnika. Laboratory results were available two to four weeks after the specimen was submitted. As a result it was necessary to link, via computer, the questionnaire data file with the laboratory result file.

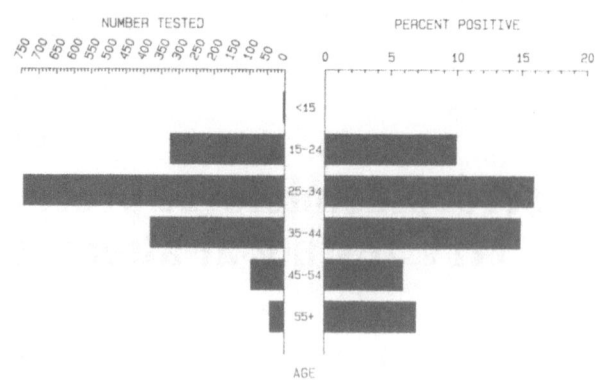

FIGURE 1. Number tested and seropositivity by age, upstate New York, January–June 1986 (42 respondents did not report their age; 19% were positive).

RESULTS

During the first six months of 1986, more than 3,100 people scheduled appointments at alternate testing sites. During that same time period, 2,127 clients electing to have the test completed the two-step counseling process and received their antibody test results. Of these, 14.4% were seropositive. Questionnaires were completed by 1,754 (82.6%) of those receiving test results. Of these, 1,635 (93.2%) were linked to laboratory report forms. A comparison of the 120 forms without laboratory data and the 1,635 complete records revealed no statistical differences except on place of birth (5% more of the group without laboratory data were born in the US) and perceived risk group membership (9% more of the incomplete records were self-classified as risk group members).

Information on the 1,635 individuals attending the alternate sites for whom complete information was available showed attendees to be primarily native-born Americans (94%). Among those born outside the continental United States, Puerto Rico and West Germany were the most frequently mentioned locations, each with 0.6% of the total. Figure 1 presents the age distribution and seropositivity data on the client group. The age distribution of persons attending alternate sites is approximately the same as persons meeting the AIDS case definition. Seropositivity varied by age, with the 25–44-year-old group having the highest rates of seropositivity.

Seropositivity rates by race and gender are presented in Table I. Eighty-three percent of those seeking testing were white, 10% were black, and 4% were Hispanic. The positivity rates for blacks and Hispanics were more than double the rate for whites ($p < 0.001$). Each minority group differed significantly from whites but not from

each other. Independent of race, males were 2.4 times more likely to be positive than females ($p < 0.001$). The differences in positivity rates by gender were most pronounced among whites, where the rate was more than four times greater in males than females ($p < 0.001$). Among blacks and Hispanics the rate among males was only about 1.5 times greater than that of females (the difference was not statistically significant). As of March 1986 (the mid-point of the study period), cumulative AIDS incidence figures for the state excluding New York City were 90.7% male and 9.3% female; 45.5% were white, 30.4% black, and 23.1% Hispanic.[7]

Seventy-three percent of clients reported having a risk factor for AIDS, and 17.5% of these were seropositive. Among the clients who did not believe they had a risk factor, 3.3% were positive. Among those indicating a risk factor, the factors cited in order of frequency were homosexuality (40.0%), intravenous drug use (21.8%), bisexuality (20.2%), blood transfusions (5.0%), and hemophilia (0.3%). Among males not reporting themselves as either homosexual or bisexual, 3.3% admitted to having had sex with a male since January 1978.

With regard to the reason for wanting to be tested, the most frequently cited reasons for testing for both men and women were risk-group membership (54.8%) or sexual contact with a risk-group member (39.1%). Family planning was listed as a reason for being tested among 6.4% of males and 8.3% of females. There were 23 women who indicated that they were pregnant at the time of testing. Two (8.7%) of them were seropositive. In response to the question concerning risk-group status, 11 of these women reported intravenous drug abuse and seven indicated a past history of sexual contact with a person who had AIDS. The racial distribution of pregnant females approximated the racial distribution of the population of alternate site attendees.

TABLE I. HIV Seropositivity by Race and Gender, Upstate New York, January–June 1986

Race	Male Tested	% Pos	Female Tested	% Pos	Gender Unknown Tested	% Pos	Total	% Pos
White (Non-Hispanic)	1,022	13.5	303	3.0	36	25.0	1,361	11.5
Black (Non-Hispanic)	84	28.6	63	20.6	12	41.7	159	26.4
	(RR = 2.1, $p < 0.001$)		(RR = 6.9, $p < 0.001$)		(RR = 1.7, p, NS†)		(RR = 2.3, $p < 0.001$)	
Hispanic	51	33.3	18	22.2	1	0	70	30.0
	(RR = 2.5, $p < 0.001$)		(RR = 7.4, $p < 0.001$)		(NA‡)		(RR = 2.6, $p < 0.001$)	
Other/unknown	27	18.5	13	0	5	40.0	45	15.6
	(RR = 1.4, p, NS)		(NA)		(RR = 1.6, p, NS)		(RR = 1.4, p, NS)	
Total	1,184	15.5	397	6.5	54	29.6	1,635	13.8

* RR = relative risks—are gender specific using whites as the standard.
† NS = not significant ($p > 0.05$).
‡ NA = not applicable.
Note: *P* values for the chi-square test are with continuity correction or Fisher's Exact Test. *P* values are not adjusted for multiple testing.

The overwhelming majority of clients attending the alternate sites reported their health status as "well" (80%). The seropositivity rate among those reported as "well" was 11.9%. One person indicated a diagnosis of AIDS, two a diagnosis of AIDS-related complex (ARC), and 38 did not report their health status. Two hundred ninety-four reported that they had one or more symptoms consistent with HIV infection, and their overall seropositivity rate was 20.7%. The reported symptoms, in order of frequency of report, were swollen glands (41.2%), cough (35.2%), sweats (34.7%), weight loss (27.6%), diarrhea (24.5%), and fever (19.7%). Seropositivity was highest in those reporting swollen glands (30.6%) and lowest among persons reporting diarrhea (11.1%).

Respondents were given the opportunity to report membership in as many risk groups as they felt appropriate. Table II lists seropositivity rates for males who listed a single risk behavior as well as some dual risk categories. Among those listing a single factor, intravenous drug abuse was associated with the highest rate of seropositivity (30.6%), followed by homosexuality (22.5%). The numbers of individuals indicating multiple risk groups were notably lower; the combination of homosexual contact and intravenous drug abuse produced a seropositivity rate in excess of 33%, but the absolute number of individuals was only six.

Analysis of the question concerning the reason for testing was performed for those respondents who listed a single risk behavior of either homosexuality, bisexuality, or intravenous drug use. Among the 383 males who listed only homosexuality as a risk group, 46.8% indicated risk-group membership as their only reason for pursuing testing. An additional 26.4% indicated risk-group membership plus sexual contact with a risk-group member. The response pattern for persons listing their only risk behavior as bisexuality was 46.4% for risk-group membership and 19% for sexual contact with a risk-group member (N = 179). Individuals listing only intravenous drug abuse as their risk behavior (N = 219) noted membership in a risk group as the reason for seeking testing 63% of the time, with risk-group membership and at least one other reason given by 26% of the respondents. Approximately 10% of both homosexual men and intravenous drug users failed to list risk-group membership as one of their reasons for seeking testing, while more than 24% of the bisexual men omitted risk-group membership as a reason for testing. It appears that intravenous drug users and homosexual men had learned of and recognized the risk behavior in which they participate. Bisexuals had not achieved the same level of awareness. At the mid-point of the study period, just under 60% of the cumulative male incidence was associated with homosexual or bisexual activity, and slightly more than 20% was related to intravenous drug use.[7]

DISCUSSION

For the period January to June 1986, the Alternate Site HIV Testing Program in New York State, exclusive of New York City, identified 306 individuals with antibodies to the human immunodeficiency virus. All persons receiving post-test results were given a similar message about safe sex and how to prevent further spread of the infection. Given the anonymous nature of the testing sites, the impact of the knowledge of HIV antibody status on future behavior cannot be assessed in the population tested.

Based on the substantial proportion of individuals identifying themselves as having engaged in high-risk behavior, it would appear that the alternate site program was attracting a substantial number of individuals at potential risk of HIV infection. This observation is reinforced by the similarity of demographic characteristics between persons attending alternate sites with those of persons with AIDS, and by the identification of a significant proportion of those tested as positive. It is important to note that in addition to identifying those who are HIV positive, the program also provided a large number of HIV-negative individuals with information on how to avoid/minimize the risk of coming in contact with the human immunodeficiency virus. Until effective prophylactic or chemotherapeutic agents are developed, education and encouragement of responsible sexual behavior remain the only tools available to control the spread of the disease.

On a programmatic level, data from the first six months' experience were useful in targeting services. For example, in March 1986 minorities and intravenous drug users made up a disproportionately high percentage of AIDS cases in upstate New York (54.5% and 53.1%, respectively),[7] but were contributing only 14% and 22% of the alternate site visits. This finding helped lead to the establishment of testing sites and increased education efforts in areas where these groups could be better served. In addition, the fact that 18% of persons seeking testing already had clinical symptoms reinforced the need to provide adequate clinical referral.

Blood donor studies have shown that some donors may acknowledge risk behavior, but may not believe they belong to a group at increased risk for infection.[8] Specifically, some seropositive males were found who did not consider themselves homosexual, but who had engaged in homosexual activity. This type of data lead to CDC's recommendation that all males with a single homosexual relationship since 1977 should self-defer donating blood.[9] As noted above, we found a similar phenomenon at the alternate sites, in that 3.3% of males not listing themselves as homosexual or bisexual admitted to having had sex

TABLE II.   HIV Seropositivity by Self-Reported Risk Groups (Males Only), Upstate New York, January–June 1986

	Total Number Tested	Number Positive	Percent Positive	Relative Risks*	p Value
Not a risk-group member	242	8	3.3		
Homosexual	383	86	22.5	6.8	<.001
Bisexual	179	23	12.8	3.9	<.001
Intravenous drug abuser (IVDA)	219	67	30.6	9.3	<.001
Hemophiliac	2	0	0		
Blood transfusion	38	5	13.3	4.0	.02
Homosexual/bisexual	22	2	9.1	2.8	NS†
Homosexual/IVDA	6	2	33.3	10.1	.02
Bisexual/IVDA	6	1	16.7	5.1	NS

* Relative risks uses "not a risk-group member" as the standard.
† NS = not significant ($p > 0.05$).
Note: P values are for the chi-square test with continuity correction or Fisher's Exact Test. P values are not adjusted for multiple testing.

with a male since January of 1978. This reinforces the need for educational efforts to emphasize individual behavior rather than only risk-group membership.

Attention has been given to the role of intravenous drug users in heterosexual transmission. Within New York City, a high proportion of the cases of heterosexual transmission are thought to be associated with intravenous drug users.[10] However, among the upstate New York sample population, the observation that one quarter or more of the self-classified homosexuals had had heterosexual relationships since 1977 indicates that this group may also be responsible for spreading the virus, via sexual contact, into the female population. This reinforces the need to emphasize the safe sex message to the population at large and not just to those in high-risk groups.

As the demand for HIV testing grows, and the need to provide timely counseling continues, the New York State Department of Health is moving toward making counseling services available at many locations throughout the state. Family planning and sexually transmitted disease clinics will be offering the HIV test on a confidential basis, or referring individuals to settings such as physicians' offices and alternate sites where counseling and testing can be obtained. Physicians in private practice have been able to conduct confidential HIV testing since the ELISA test became available, and the number of tests has increased as the spectrum of diseases associated with HIV infection has been recognized. Education, counseling, informed consent, and confidentiality will remain integral parts of this expanded testing program.

Acknowledgments. The authors thank Dr Gerald Kaufman and Mr Robert Kelly for their assistance in the computer linkage of the questionnaire and laboratory reports, Mr Forrest Mance for his programming for data analysis, and the Laboratories for Diagnostic Immunology of the Wadsworth Center for Laboratories and Research for conducting the tests.

REFERENCES

1. Koop CE: *Surgeon General's Report on Acquired Immune Deficiency Syndrome.* Washington DC, Public Health Service, US Department of Health and Human Services, October 1986.
2. Division of Sexually Transmitted Diseases, Center for Preventive Services, Centers for Disease Control: Human T-lymphotrophic virus type III/lymphadenopathy-associated virus antibody testing at alternate sites. *MMWR* 1986; 35:284–287.
3. Hopkins RS: Results of antibody testing at community-based AIDS prevention centers. *West Virginia EPI-LOG* 1986; 7:1–3.
4. Henry K, Brown RJ, Polesky HF, et al: Nondonor HIV antibody testing in Minnesota. *N Engl J Med* 1986; 315:581–582.
5. Holston JL: Testing for HTLV-III/LAV antibody. *Ala J Med Sci* 1986; 23:269–271.
6. AIDS Weekly Surveillance Report—United States, Public Health Service, Centers for Disease Control, Department of Health and Human Services, October 15, 1987.
7. New York State Department of Health, AIDS Surveillance Monthly Update, March 1986.
8. Zuck TF: Greetings—with comments on lessons learned this past year from HIV antibody testing and from counseling blood donors [editorial]. *Transfusion* 1986; 26:493.
9. Center for Drugs and Biologics, US Food and Drug Administration; AIDS Branch, Division of Viral Diseases, Center for Infectious Diseases, Centers for Disease Control: Update: Revised Public Health Service definition of persons who should refrain from donating blood and plasma—United States. *MMWR* 1985; 34:547–548.
10. Des Jarlais DC, Wish E, Friedman SR. et al: Intravenous drug use and the heterosexual transmission of the human immunodeficiency virus: Current trends in New York City. *NY State J Med* 1987; 87:283–286.

Chapter 12

Teaching about AIDS in public schools: Characteristics of early adopter communities in Massachusetts

JONATHAN HOWLAND, PhD; DIANE BAKER, BA; JULIE JOHNSON, BA; JAMES SCARAMUCCI, BA

ABSTRACT. Many teenagers are at risk for contracting AIDS because of their sexual activity and intravenous (IV) drug use. It is important that they be given information about the disease and its prevention. Some communities have taken early initiatives with respect to teaching about AIDS in their public schools. To determine whether or not there are attributes that would predict the likelihood of a community's integrating AIDS information into the public school curriculum, we explored 25 variables in a sample of 63 Massachusetts communities. None of the variables was found to be significant. We conclude that there are obviously other factors as yet unidentified, that explain why some towns teach about AIDS while others do not. Further research is necessary.

Since October 1985 the US Department of Defense has routinely screened civilian applicants for serologic evidence of infection with human immunodeficiency virus (HIV), the virus that causes acquired immunodeficiency syndrome (AIDS). Results from the first 15 months of testing indicated an overall seropositive prevalence rate of 1.5/1,000 among a population consisting predominately of young adults in their late teens and early 20s.[1] Given a delay of up to several years between exposure and seropositivity, these data provide evidence of HIV infection among the US teenage population. Because applicants for military service may underrepresent those groups at highest risk for the infection (homosexual men and IV drug users), it is possible that the actual prevalence among teens is higher.[2]

Dr Howland is Assistant Professor at the School of Public Health, Boston University School of Medicine. Ms Baker is Family Life Coordinator, Somerville Hospital, Somerville, Mass, and Ms Johnson and Mr Scaramucci are data analysts at the School of Public Health, Boston University School of Medicine, Boston, Mass.

A 1985 survey of San Francisco students (14–18 years) assessing knowledge and beliefs about AIDS showed that 8% were unaware that sexual intercourse was one mode of contracting AIDS and that 40% were unaware that the use of condoms during intercourse may lower the risk of exposure to the disease.[3] A subsequent 1986 random digit dial survey of 860 Massachusetts adolescents 16 to 19 years of age indicated that 70% were sexually active, but only 15% of these reported changing their behaviors in order to reduce exposure to AIDS. Of the teens reporting behavior change, only 20% used methods currently considered effective for preventing AIDS transmission. Of all the respondents in this survey, 8% did not know that AIDS can be transmitted by heterosexual intercourse.[4] In the absence of a vaccine or medical intervention, the US surgeon general and the National Academy of Sciences have identified public education in schools as the primary means of containing the AIDS epidemic.[5,6] In response, many states are in the process of developing model curricula for AIDS education. In Massachusetts this activity has been undertaken by the state's Department of Public Health in conjunction with the Department of Education. This curriculum was presented to local school districts during the summer of 1987. Implementation is scheduled for the following school year.

Many local school districts have taken initiatives on their own with respect to incorporating AIDS education into their curricula. These programs range from one-time lectures to students by visiting health educators to more extensive course materials developed by local district staff. With the introduction of the state's model AIDS education program it is probable that within the next few years most Massachusetts middle and high schools will to varying degrees routinely teach about AIDS. Since AIDS is a relatively new phenomenon, observation of behaviors associated with the prevention of the disease provides the opportunity to study the diffusion of innovation throughout the population and institutions.

The objective of this study was to locate those school districts which were "early adopters" of AIDS education programs and to attempt to identify characteristics distinguishing them from school districts that had delayed teaching about the disease ("late adopters").

METHODS

Community Sample. We drew a sample of 63 Massachusetts communities weighted by population size and stratified by region of the state. In December 1986 the superintendent of public schools for each of the selected communities was contacted by either one of three of the authors (JH,JJ,JS). Superintendents, or school district personnel identified by superintendents, were queried about their schools' current AIDS education activities.

Variables. The dependent variable (AIDSED) for the analysis was whether or not a community's schools had, as of the date of the survey, incorporated information about AIDS into their curricula. This dichotomous variable (yes/no) was operationalized as follows:

- Formal instruction about AIDS including information on means of transmission was taught at at least one grade level (K–12) in a course that was required for at least 80% of the students.
- AIDS instruction was imbedded in school curricula as opposed to being delivered as a special, one-time presentation.

For the purposes of this inquiry, intermittent lectures, film showings, or the distribution of literature about AIDS were not counted as AIDS education measures unless they were part of a broader program of classroom instruction.

Twenty-five independent variables representing community characteristics categorized into six domains were explored to determine which if any were associated with towns that had opted to teach about AIDS. These domains were established arbitrarily by the authors to reduce the number of redundant variables for multivariate analysis. The reduction was required because of the large number of variables relative to sample size.

Data about the political characteristics of the community were derived from 1986 voter registration data and included the percent of registered Republican voters (REPUB), the percent of registered Democratic voters (DEMO), the percent of registered uncommitted voters (UNCOM), and the ratio of Democratic to Republican registered voters (RATIO). Geographic variables included State Department of Public Works districts (DIST), a measure of geographic location, and 1980 US census population size (POP). Economic variables consisted of median family income, 1980 percent of workforce in manufacturing (MANU), and 1985 per capita school expenditures (EXPEN). The demographic variables were all derived from 1980 US census data and included the percent foreign born, the percent having changed residence in the previous five years, the percent speaking a language other than English at home, the percent black, the percent with Hispanic surnames, the percent Asian, and the percent white. Health variables were intended to measure several dimensions reflecting community health behaviors or status. These included fluoridation of town water supply as of 1986, the percent of voters voting in 1986 to maintain the state's seatbelt law, the percent of voters voting in 1986 not to limit Medicaid funding for abortion, cumulative incidence rates for AIDS as of November 1986 in the county in which the town was located, and the teenage birthrate for 1985. Education variables consisted of 1980 census measures for the percent of 3–5-year-olds enrolled in kindergarten, the percent of 18–24-year-olds enrolled in college, the percent of residents over 25 years of age who were high school graduates, and the percent of residents over age 25 who were college graduates.

Analysis. Analysis of the association between early adoption of AIDS education and community characteristics involved several steps. First, univariate analyses of variables were performed. T-tests were used for continuous variables and chi-square was used for dichotomous variables to determine the significance of differences between towns that did and did not teach about AIDS in public schools. Second, on the basis of the results of the univariate analysis, variables were selected from each of the community characteristic domains for inclusion in a multivariate logistic regression model. A stepwise logistic procedure was used with the p value for variable entrance and exit from the model set at $p = 0.15$.

RESULTS

All of the 63 school districts contacted were willing to provide information on their AIDS education activities. Thirty-five (56%) were teaching about AIDS to an extent sufficient to meet our criteria as early adopters. School districts that had had one or more special presentations on AIDS, distributed literature about AIDS, or were planning AIDS curricula were not included in the early adopter category. It should be noted, however, that among school districts that were categorized as teaching about AIDS, there was a great deal of variation with respect to the amount of material and the grade levels taught.

Results of the univariate analyses are presented in Table I. Of the 16 political, economic, and demographic variables explored, only one (% ASIAN) attained significance at the $p \leq 0.05$ level. Several other demographic variables were suggestive, with p values of 0.10 (% BLACK and % changing residency in previous five years). All three of these variables were positively correlated with AIDSED.

Among the health variables, only the percentage of voters sup-

TABLE I. Association Between Community Characteristics and Early Adoption of AIDS Education Measures: Univariate Analysis (N = 63 communities)

Domain/Variable	t-test (p value)	chi-square (p value)
Political		
% Uncommited	.70	—
% Republican	.66	—
% Democratic	.97	—
Ratio	.93	—
Geographic		
Population	.22	—
District	.32	—
Economic		
% Manufacturing	.54	—
Median family income	.78	—
Expenditures	.16	—
Demographic		
% Foreign born	.30	—
% Moved 5 years	.10	—
% Speak other languages	.72	—
% Black	.10	—
% Hispanic	.97	—
% Asian	.05	—
% White	.43	—
Health		
Fluoride	—	.21
Seatbelt	.46	—
Abortion	.08	—
AIDS cases	.83	—
Teen births	.47	—
Education		
% In kindergarten	.78	—
% In college	.41	—
% High school graduates	.44	—
% College graduates	.32	—

porting Medicaid funding for abortion (ABYES) approached significance ($p = 0.08$). AIDS education was more likely to be done in those communities that had voted not to limit Medicaid abortion funding.

None of the variables measuring community education levels were significantly associated with AIDS education.

Ten variables were selected for stepwise logistic regression on AIDSED. These were selected from each of the variable domains on the basis of univariate analysis. The only variable retained by the stepwise process was percent voting to support Medicaid abortion funding, using an entrance p value of ≤ 0.15. The p value for this variable was 0.08. The overall chi-square for the regression model (3.39, 1 df) was not significant ($p = 0.07$).

DISCUSSION

There are several reasons why it might be useful to be able to predict early adopter communities with respect to policies related to the AIDS epidemic. Foremost among them is the targeting of public health resources to encourage communities to institute AIDS prevention measures. At present state governments are focusing on AIDS education in the public schools. However, as the incidence of AIDS increases, other local institutions (eg, emergency medical squads and police departments) will be called upon to adopt new preventive policies. Knowing in advance which towns will adopt early and which will resist these changes could be valuable in allocating education and training resources.

Although this study was primarily exploratory, we proceeded with several assumptions. We supposed that communities with higher levels of education and/or family income would be more likely to be early adopters of AIDS education. In so doing we applied observations derived from behavior at the individual level (eg, income and education are positively correlated with personal health behaviors) to aggregate level characteristics. We also assumed that a community's fiscal capacity, as measured by per capita school expenditure, would be a factor in early adoption. We supposed that a town's concern with health issues generally, as measured by fluoridation status and voting in support of seatbelt legislation and abortion funding, would be reflected in the propensity to adopt AIDS education measures early. Finally, we supposed that exposure to the need for AIDS education, as measured by the regional AIDS incidence rate, might influence adoption.

None of these hypotheses was confirmed by this investigation. This result has several possible interpretations. As a cross-sectional study, the behavior of school districts was measured at one random moment in time. It is possible that the study was conducted too late in the adoption process; that early adopters could have been differentiated had we identified them at a point when only 10–20% rather than 56% of the communities had initiated AIDS education activities.

More than half of the school districts we surveyed had already adopted AIDS education programs. Others were planning to do so. Thus, it may be that all schools were in fact in the process of adopting AIDS education programs and their particular point of progress was due to a variety of random factors. This interpretation would suggest that within the context of AIDS education in the public schools, the concept of early adoption is irrelevant.

Our sample was small. Accordingly, it is also possible that the failure to detect significant differences between communities was due to lack of statistical power.

It is possible that in this context early adoption is due to the efforts and concerns of a small number of individuals who are themselves early adopters and are in a position to influence policy. In other words, whether or not a community adopts AIDS education early is not the result of consensus in the aggregate community. This would suggest that characteristics of individuals rather than populations would predict the behavior of towns. If such individuals were randomly distributed, ecological community data would not be predictive of local policies. This interpretation would be consistent with the findings of early studies on the dissemination and adoption of agricultural techniques in the American West.[7]

For the foreseeable future, behavior on both the individual and community levels is the single key to the prevention and control of the AIDS epidemic. It is likely that local communities will be encouraged to adopt an increasing number of AIDS-related policies. By understanding the dynamics of the adoption process we can hope to accelerate required change. This study is inconclusive, but our results suggest that ecological data do not predict the behavior of communities with respect to early adoption of AIDS education measures. If this result can be generalized to other AIDS policies, the implication is that efforts to bring about change in communities should focus on identifying and encouraging community leaders. Further research focusing on case studies of AIDS-related policy adoption is required to confirm this interpretation.

REFERENCES

1. Office of the Assistant Secretary of Defense (Health Affairs): Human T-lymphotropic virus type III/lymphadenopathy-associated virus antibody prevalence in U.S. military recruit applicants. *MMWR* 1986; 35:421–429.

2. Office of the Assistant Secretary of Defense (Health Affairs): Trends in human immunodeficiency virus infection among civilian applicants for military service—United States, October 1985–December 1986. *MMWR* 1987; 36:273–281.

3. DiClemente RJ, Zorn J, Temoshok L: Adolescents and AIDS: A survey of knowledge, attitudes and beliefs about AIDS in San Francisco. *Am J Public Health* 1986; 76:1443–1445.

4. Strunin L, Hingson R: Acquired immunodeficiency syndrome and adolescents: Knowledge, beliefs, attitudes and behaviors. *Pediatrics* 1987; 79:825–828.

5. Koop CE: *Surgeon General's Report on Acquired Immune Deficiency Syndrome*. US Department of Health and Human Services, 1987.

6. Institute of Medicine, National Academy of Sciences: *Confronting AIDS: Directions for Public Health, Health Care, and Research*. Washington, DC, National Academy Press, 1986.

7. Ryan B, Gross NC: The diffusion of hybrid seed corn in two Iowa communities. *Rural Sociol* 1948; 8:15–24.

Part II
Overviews

Chapter 13

Intravenous drug use and the heterosexual transmission of the human immunodeficiency virus

Current trends in New York City

DON C. DES JARLAIS, PhD; ERIC WISH, PhD; SAMUEL R. FRIEDMAN, PhD; RAND STONEBURNER, MD, MPH;
STANLEY R. YANCOVITZ, MD; DONNA MILDVAN, MD; WAFAA EL-SADR, MD;
ELIZABETH BRADY, MA; MARY CUADRADO, MA

Women, and men who deny homosexual activity, account for slightly more than one third (3,929/7,696) of the cases of acquired immunodeficiency syndrome (AIDS) in New York City through September 1986.[1] This percentage has been rising during the course of the epidemic. Intravenous (IV) drug users account for more than half (2,261/3,929) of these heterosexual cases, and an additional 134 cases have occurred in persons known to be heterosexual partners of IV drug users. The connections between AIDS, IV drug use, and the heterosexual transmission of the human immunodeficiency virus (HIV) pose one of the more difficult public health challenges facing the city and the country. In this paper we review data relevant to two questions: potential heterosexual transmission among IV drug users, and potential transmission from IV drug users to heterosexual partners who do not inject drugs.

Before reviewing data on these two questions, however, it is useful to note the history of AIDS among IV drug users in New York City. The first cases of AIDS among IV drug users were retrospectively diagnosed as having occurred in 1980.[2] Retrospective studies of sera of IV drug users revealed that the first HIV antibody positive sample was collected in 1978.[3] The trends in IV drug use and heterosexual transmission of HIV in New York City are based on at least an eight-year history of infection among IV drug users who were also active heterosexuals. While attention to heterosexual transmission in the United States is relatively new, there is actually almost a decade of experience with opportunities for heterosexual trans-

mission. This length of time allows some relatively firm conclusions to be drawn about the dynamics of transmission related to IV drug use and heterosexual behavior.

HETEROSEXUAL TRANSMISSION AMONG IV DRUG USERS

The national system used for classifying cases of AIDS tends to obscure both IV-drug-related and heterosexual transmission of HIV. Male IV drug users who also engage in homosexual behavior are often simply classified into the "homosexual/bisexual male" category, and heterosexuals who inject drugs are classified in the "IV drug use" category. This classification system tends to miss cases of IV-drug-related transmission among homosexual/bisexual men and cases of heterosexual transmission between persons who inject drugs. To study the question of potential heterosexual transmission among IV drug users, we examined the relationships between drug injection and sexual behavior in a cohort of IV drug users from the borough of Manhattan. This cohort has been previously described.[4]

A slightly higher rate of HIV infection was found among females compared to males—58% of the females were seropositive compared to 48% of the males. Since male-to-female sexual transmission of HIV may be more efficient than female-to-male transmission, these rates would be consistent with the existence of an added risk for heterosexual transmission above the risk of drug injection transmission. The difference, however, was not significant after controlling for the frequency of drug injection. Parallel findings were also obtained by Weiss et al[5] in New Jersey. They also found a slightly higher seroprevalence rate among females that was not statistically significant after controlling for drug injection frequency.

We examined a variety of sexual behaviors as possible predictors of HIV exposure among this cohort of IV drug users, including male homosexuality and, for the females, the number of IV-drug-using sexual partners. None of these sexual behaviors was significantly associated with HIV infection when drug injection behavior was con-

From the New York State Division of Substance Abuse Services (Dr Des Jarlais), Narcotic and Drug Research, Inc (Drs Wish and Friedman, Ms Brady, and Ms Cuadrado), the New York City Department of Health (Dr Stoneburner), Beth Israel Medical Center (Drs Yancovitz and Mildvan), and Manhattan Veterans Administration Medical Center (Dr El-Sadr).

The research presented in this paper was supported primarily through grant R01 DA 03574 from the National Institute on Drug Abuse. Additional support was provided by grant 85-IJ-CX-0025 from the National Institute of Justice.

trolled for. Twelve females reported engaging in prostitution in the year prior to the interview. Ten of these were
HIV seropositive. While the women who reported engaging in prostitution did have a higher seroprevalence rate
than those who denied engaging in prostitution, this was
also not statistically significant when the frequency of
drug injection was entered into the analysis. The probability level associated with prostitution in the multivariate
analysis was 0.21, however, which does not lead one to
completely reject a hypothesis that engaging in prostitution is associated with higher rates of seropositivity among
female IV drug users. Schoenbaum and colleagues[6] did
find that engaging in prostitution was a significant predictor of HIV exposure in their sample of IV drug users from
the Bronx, though not as strong a predictor as the drug
injection variables.

One conclusion from the available data is that, to date,
heterosexual transmission among IV drug users is at most
a slight added risk compared to the risk of HIV infection
from the sharing of equipment for drug injection. This
added risk would seem to be greater for female IV drug
users who engage in prostitution. Even in this instance,
extreme care must be used in drawing any conclusion
about the sources of this potential added risk. Many IV-
drug-using females who engage in prostitution have customers who inject drugs (D. Strug, personal communication, 1985). They also frequently have boyfriends who
inject drugs, and the use of condoms and other forms of
"safer sex" are particularly unlikely with these boyfriends
(J. Cohen, personal communication, 1986). It is also possible that the female prostitutes have slightly different
patterns of drug injection behavior that were not identified in the interviews but were the underlying reason for
higher rates of seropositivity, or that the effects of frequent infection with sexually transmitted diseases make
them more susceptible to heterosexual transmission.

The hierarchical risk classification system may result in
the misclassification of some AIDS cases as being related
to IV drug use when transmission actually occurred
through heterosexual activity. Comparisons of sexual behavior and IV drug use behavior as predictors of HIV exposure, however, indicate that such misclassifications are
currently infrequent in New York City.

HETEROSEXUAL TRANSMISSION FROM MALE IV DRUG USERS TO WOMEN WHO DO NOT INJECT DRUGS

Comparisons of the relative risk of developing AIDS
among females who inject drugs versus females who do
not inject drugs but are the heterosexual partners of male
IV drug users also suggest that, to date, the risk of heterosexual transmission is relatively small compared to the
risk of transmission through sharing equipment for IV
drug use.

Such a comparison was first made in September 1984,
at which time there had been 132 cases of AIDS among
female IV drug users and 25 cases among females who did
not inject drugs but were heterosexual partners of IV drug
users.[7] In calculating the relative risks, one must first estimate the sex ratio among IV drug users and the ratio of
male IV drug users to their heterosexual partners who do
not inject drugs. Based on studies of more than 10,000

persons entering treatment for heroin abuse in New York
City in 1983, the percentage of male IV drug users was
estimated as 73%, giving a male-to-female ratio of 2.70:1.
This high male-to-female ratio indicates that the majority
of male IV drug users must be having sexual relationships
with females who do not inject drugs. A survey of 50 male
IV drug users admitted to detoxification treatment programs showed a total of 53 regular heterosexual partners,
of whom 40 were reported not to inject drugs. This gave a
ratio of 1:0.80 male IV drug users to female heterosexual
partners, and a ratio of 1:2.16 female IV drug users to
females who are heterosexual partners of IV drug users
but do not inject drugs themselves.

The relative risk of AIDS among female IV drug users
compared to female heterosexual partners was estimated
as 11 to 1 in September 1984. Through September 1986,
472 cases of AIDS among female IV drug users and 134
cases among female heterosexual partners had been reported to the New York City Department of Health.[8] Using the same ratio of 1:2.16 of female IV drug users to
female heterosexual partners gives a relative risk of 7.8:1
for female IV drug users compared to female heterosexual
partners of male IV drug users. Both of these ratios suggest that, to date, the risk of developing AIDS from heterosexual contact is relatively small compared to the risk
from IV drug use.

Both the data on sexual behavior as a predictor of seropositivity and the data on the relative risk of AIDS among
female IV drug users compared to female heterosexual
partners indicate that, to date, heterosexual transmission
has been relatively infrequent compared to IV-drug-use
transmission.

An examination of the available data on AIDS and
prostitution in New York City also leads to the same conclusion.

As a first step in this argument, evidence suggests that
many "street-worker" prostitutes are IV drug users. Interviews were conducted with 95 female prostitutes who
had been arrested in New York City.[9] (These street-work-
ers should not be considered representative of call girls or
prostitutes working through escort services.) Intravenous
drug use was common in this sample of arrested prostitutes, 40 (42%) reported histories of drug injection, and
urinalysis revealed that 28% were positive for opiates and
69% for cocaine.

Second, many prostitutes who use IV drugs are HIV
seropositive. Because the women referred to above were
interviewed in a jail facility, it was not possible to obtain
blood samples. Wallace and colleagues[10] have conducted
a serosurvey of street-working prostitutes and found that
half of those who injected drugs were HIV antibody positive. This is consistent with the above-noted findings of
high seropositivity among female IV drug users who engaged in prostitution.[2,6]

In spite of this, however, there have been few AIDS
cases in New York City among men who lack other risk
factors. Given the length of time that HIV has been
present among IV drug users in New York City, and the
substantial proportion of street prostitutes who inject
drugs and are seropositive, there has been very little apparent transmission from prostitutes to their customers.
More than 8,000 cases of AIDS have been reported to the

New York City Department of Health; only 39 occurred in men in whom no risk factor is identified, and in fewer than half of these is contact with prostitutes claimed as a risk factor.[11]

Further evidence for the infrequency of prostitute-to-customer transmission comes from a study by Rabkin and colleagues.[12] They examined HIV seropositivity in a sample of men attending a clinic for sexually transmitted diseases in New York City. They specifically examined contact with prostitutes as a potential risk factor, but it was not a statistically significant predictor of HIV exposure.

One possible explanation for the apparently low rate of transmission of HIV from prostitutes to customers in New York is the use of "safe sex" procedures. The great majority—62/67 (92%)—of the female prostitutes interviewed in jail reported that they usually required their customers to use condoms. (Questions about safe sex procedures were added to the interview after the first 28 subjects were interviewed.) When the customer did not want to use a condom, the prostitute would charge extra and/or deceive him by substituting manual masturbation. These subjects also reported that oral sex was the predominant activity with their customers, and while HIV has been found in saliva, infection from saliva appears to be very rare if it occurs at all.[13]

Our interviews with key informant ex-prostitutes indicate that these safe-sex practices were adopted in the early 1970s, certainly before HIV was widely spread among IV drug users in New York City. General concern about sexually transmitted diseases, including herpes, was the main stated reason for the increase in the use of condoms at that time. It should also be noted that sexually transmitted diseases pose a significant economic threat to prostitutes, particularly those with regular customers.

DISCUSSION

It is likely that HIV was first introduced into the intravenous drug user group in New York City during the middle to late 1970s. Since then the virus has spread among this group through the sharing of equipment for injecting drugs and through homosexual and heterosexual contact. We have examined sets of data that compared drug-injection-related transmission to heterosexual transmission in seroprevalence studies of IV drug users and that compared the relative risk of developing AIDS among females who inject drugs and females who do not inject drugs but are sexual partners of men who do inject drugs. These comparisons suggest that, to date in New York City, transmission related to IV drug use has been approximately an order of magnitude more frequent than male-to-female heterosexual transmission. The available data on prostitution indicate that prostitutes who inject drugs are relatively likely to have been exposed to HIV, but to date there has been relatively little transmission to customers.

There are several possible reasons why there has been relatively little transmission through heterosexual activity compared to the sharing of drug injection equipment to date in New York City. First, the efficiency of transmission through sharing of drug equipment may simply be much greater than that for unprotected vaginal intercourse. Second, even if the relative efficiencies of transmission were approximately equal, the observed differences might also be explained in terms of two variables that are key to rapid transmission during the early stages of an epidemic: the frequency with which an individual performs acts likely to transmit the virus, and the number of different persons with whom the individual practices those acts. At least prior to the awareness of AIDS, many IV drug users injected several times per day at so-called "shooting galleries"—where rented equipment permitted sharing with large numbers of anonymous partners. In New York, these IV drug users engaging in high-frequency sharing of equipment were also likely to be sharing with each other, regardless of sex or sexual orientation. One would thus expect a relatively rapid transmission of HIV among those persons frequently engaging in high-risk behavior with multiple partners.

Regarding heterosexual transmission, there are certainly some persons who average several different partners per day, but most of these are likely to be prostitutes, who generally seem to have been using "safer sex" procedures since before the AIDS epidemic began. While there are few data available on the levels of male heterosexual activity in New York, it is doubtful that there are large numbers of men who average several different heterosexual partners per day over long periods of time. Thus, women with high numbers of heterosexual partners are relatively likely to be taking precautions against sexual transmission, and there are probably relatively few men with high numbers of heterosexual partners. Heterosexual transmission is therefore likely to occur at a much slower rate.

Given that an HIV-infected person may be infectious for an indefinite period of time, the slower initial spread of HIV through heterosexual transmission compared to drug equipment transmission tells us little about whether heterosexual transmission will eventually become more frequent. Most heterosexual transmission that is currently occurring in New York is probably between IV drug users and their partners. Efforts are urgently needed to prevent more IV drug users from being infected with HIV. Prevention of further HIV infection among IV drug users will also prevent heterosexual transmission. Indeed, prevention of HIV transmission from shared drug injection equipment may be critical for the eventual control of heterosexual transmission in New York City. Effective means of preventing transmission to persons who are current or potential sexual partners of IV drug users are also urgently needed.

A number of such projects for preventing drug injection transmission and heterosexual transmission from IV drug users are currently under way. These include expanded drug treatment programs to help drug users stop using drugs, and education within these programs so that clients who continue to use drugs will be able to reduce their risks. Street outreach education and antibody-testing and counseling projects are targeting IV drug users and their sex partners. There are also attempts to organize drug users to help each other make it less likely that they will share injection equipment.[14,15] The newness of these projects does not permit any systematic assessment of their relative or absolute effectiveness. Research will be needed not only to evaluate specific programs, but also to develop a concep-

tual understanding of the behavior changes needed to interrupt HIV transmission through both drug injection
equipment and heterosexual activity.

In addition to these prevention projects oriented towards drug users and their sexual partners, education of
the entire population with respect to preventing heterosexual transmission will also be needed on a long-term basis.

REFERENCES

1. New York City Department of Health AIDS Surveillance, September 1986.
2. Des Jarlais DC, Friedman SR, Hopkins W: Risk reduction for the acquired immunodeficiency syndrome among intravenous drug users. *Ann Intern Med* 1985; 103:755–759.
3. Novick DM, Kreek MJ, Des Jarlais DC, et al: Antibody to LAV among intravenous drug users: Historical, therapeutic and ethical aspects, in Harris L (ed): *Problems of Drug Dependence 1985: Proceedings of the 47th Annual Scientific Meeting.* NIDA Research Monograph 67. Washington, DC, The Committee on Problems of Drug Dependence, Inc, 1985, pp 318–320.
4. Cohen H, Marmor M, Des Jarlais DC, et al: Risk factors for HTLV-III/LAV seropositivity among intravenous drug users. Presented at the International Conference on the Acquired Immunodeficiency Syndrome (AIDS), Atlanta, Ga, April 14–17, 1985.
5. Weiss SH, Ginzburg HM, Goedert JJ, et al: Risk for HTLV-III exposure and AIDS among parenteral drug abusers in New Jersey. Presented at the International Conference on the Acquired Immunodeficiency Syndrome (AIDS), Atlanta, Ga, April 14–17, 1985.
6. Schoenbaum EE, Selwyn PA, Klein RS, et al: Prevalence of and risk factors associated with HTLV-III/LAV antibodies among intravenous drug abusers in a methadone program in New York City. Presented at the International Conference on AIDS, Paris, France, June 23–25, 1986.
7. Des Jarlais DC, Chamberland ME, Yancovitz SR, et al: Heterosexual partners: A large risk group for AIDS [letter]. *Lancet* 1984; 2:1346–1347.
8. New York City Department of Health Bureau of Health Statistics, 1986.
9. Wish ED, Johnson BD: The impact of substance abuse on criminal careers, in Blumstein A, Cohen J, Visher CA (eds): *Criminal Careers and Career Criminals.* Washington, DC, National Academy Press, 1986, vol 2, pp 52–58.
10. Wallace JI, Christonikos N, Merlink R, et al: HTLV-III/LAV exposure in New York City prostitutes. Presented at the International Conference on AIDS, Paris, France, June 23–25, 1986.
11. New York City Department of Health AIDS Surveillance, 1986.
12. Rabkin CS, Thomas PA, Jaffe H, et al: Prevalence of antibody to HTLV-III/LAV in a population attending a sexually transmitted disease clinic. *Sex Transm Dis* 1986; 13:80–83.
13. Friedland G, Saltzman B, Rogers M, et al: Lack of transmission of HTLV-III/LAV infection to household contacts of patients with AIDS or AIDS-related complex with oral candidiasis. *N Engl J Med* 1986; 314:344–349.
14. Friedman SR, Des Jarlais DC, Goldsmith DS: An overview of current AIDS prevention efforts aimed at intravenous drug users. *J Drug Issues* (in press).
15. Friedman SR, Des Jarlais DC, Sotheran JL, et al: AIDS and self-organization among intravenous drug users. *Int J Addict* (in press).

Chapter 14

AIDS in Africa: Evidence for heterosexual transmission of the human immunodeficiency virus

THOMAS C. QUINN, MD

Since its initial recognition in 1981, acquired immunodeficiency syndrome (AIDS) has become a global epidemic.
Nearly 40,000 cases have been reported from over 85
countries on five different continents. Presently, an estimated 5–10 million people worldwide have been infected
with the causative agent, referred to as the human immunodeficiency virus (HIV).[1,2] From natural history studies,
it can be expected that at least 10–30% of these HIV-infected individuals may develop AIDS within the next
three years,[3–6] resulting in a cumulative number of more
than one million cases of AIDS worldwide by 1990. With
the present lack of effective curative therapy or a vaccine,
this disease now represents one of the most serious epidemics of the century.

SURVEILLANCE FOR AIDS IN AFRICA

Shortly after the recognition of AIDS in the United
States, cases were identified among Africans residing in
Europe.[7,8] In contrast to European cases, with a male-to-
female ratio of 16:1, African cases had a male-to-female
ratio of 1.7:1, and 90% of affected individuals had no identifiable risk factors.[9] This recognition of African AIDS
cases with unusual epidemiologic features prompted a series of investigations in Africa.[10,11] Initially limited to urban areas of Central Africa, recent reports have documented the spread of AIDS to nearly all countries of
Africa, with major foci primarily in Central and East African countries.[12–15] Unfortunately, accurate statistics regarding the number of AIDS cases are not available, since
surveillance has only been instituted within the past six
months in several African countries and remains nonexis-
tent in other countries. Presently, 19 African countries
have officially reported over 2,000 cases of AIDS to the
World Health Organization. In 1985, in Kigali, Rwanda,
and Kinshasa, Zaire, it was estimated that the annual incidence of AIDS for adult residents was approximately
500–1,000 cases/million adults.[11,14] Unlike in the United
States, where the sex ratio is 13:1 men to women, the sex
ratio of AIDS cases in Africa is now 1:1.[14] As in developed
countries, AIDS in Africa primarily affects young and
middle-aged persons. The mean age of AIDS patients in
Kinshasa was 33.6 years (mean, 32 years; range, 1.5–64
years), and men were significantly older than women—
mean ages, 37.4 years and 30.0 years, respectively. Peak
age-specific incidence rates of 786/million and 601/mil-
lion were present among 30–39-year-old men and women,

Dr Quinn is Senior Investigator, Laboratory of Immunoregulation, National Institutes of Allergy and Infectious Diseases, National Institutes of Health, Bethesda, Md, and Associate Professor of Medicine, Johns Hopkins University School of Medicine, Baltimore, Md.

respectively.[14] These sex and age distributions of AIDS cases reflect patterns seen with other sexually transmitted diseases, both in developed and developing countries, in which the incidence and morbidity rates are higher among younger women and older men.[12]

In addition to the equal sex distribution of cases, other evidence that suggested heterosexual transmission was the fact that women with AIDS were more likely than men to be unmarried (61% versus 36%), and nearly one third of the married AIDS patients had had at least one previous marriage or "union libre" (persistent cohabitation without formal marriage).[14] One third of AIDS patients reported having had at least one sexually transmitted disease during the three years preceding their illness. In many areas of Africa, a large proportion of the AIDS cases comprise female prostitutes, or men and women with a history of multiple sexual partners within the previous five years.[10,11,13,17-19] However, additional factors that may influence transmission of HIV include frequent exposure to unsterilized needles (80% of AIDS cases), and a history of blood transfusion within the previous three-year period prior to the onset of illness (9%).[14] More recent case-control studies have further demonstrated that AIDS is primarily transmitted in Africa by heterosexual activity, blood transfusions, exposure to blood-contaminated needles and syringes for medical or ritual purposes, and via perinatal transmission from mother to infant.[12,18-23]

Seroprevalence data on HIV infection suggest that of these different modes of transmission, heterosexual transmission appears to be the predominant mode of infection in Africa. In a recent study of HIV infection among 6,000 healthy persons residing in Kinshasa, Zaire, a bimodal distribution of infection was evident with a peak prevalence under one year of age and among young adults aged 16-29 years (Fig 1).[12] The first peak in seroprevalence among children under one year of age represented a combination of passive antibody transfer and transmission of virus from mother to infant. The low prevalence rate between ages 2 and 14 argues strongly against arthropod transmission, since arthropod-transmitted diseases usually

have peak infection rates among these age groups.[24] As sexual activity increased during adolescence, the rate of HIV infection increased dramatically, particularly among women aged 15-29 years. This increase was followed by a rise in HIV infection among men between the ages of 20 and 39 years. This pattern, in conjunction with the distribution of AIDS cases, is consistent with that of a sexually transmitted disease with higher prevalence rates among younger, sexually active women having sexual relations with older men.[12,16]

RISK FACTORS FOR HETEROSEXUAL TRANSMISSION

Risk factors associated with HIV infection among heterosexuals residing in Africa include the number of sexual partners, having sex with prostitutes, being a prostitute, and being a sexual partner of an infected person.[12] In Africa, prostitutes show the highest rate of infection (27-88%),[13,18] and they may have played an important role in the dissemination of HIV in areas such as Nairobi, where HIV antibody prevalence was initially higher in prostitutes than in men with sexually transmitted diseases who frequented the prostitutes.[13] In a recent study by Piot et al,[26] HIV seroprevalence rates among prostitutes in Nairobi, Kenya, rose from 4% to 59% between 1980 and 1986. This rapid dissemination of HIV infection in a high-risk group in Africa was similar to that observed among homosexually active men in San Francisco during the same time period.[3,5] This rise in infection among the prostitutes was subsequently followed by a steady increase in seroprevalence rates, from 1% to 18%, among men attending clinics for treatment of sexually transmitted diseases (STD) in Nairobi during the same time period.[26]

HIV infection among female prostitutes correlated with socioeconomic status and mean number of sexual encounters per year. For example, a seroprevalence rate of 66% was present among prostitutes of low socioeconomic status who averaged 963 sexual encounters per year, compared to a prevalence rate of 31% among prostitutes of higher socioeconomic status who averaged 124 sexual encounters per year.[13] In this same study, sexual exposure to men from Central Africa was significantly associated with HIV infection among these female prostitutes, suggesting transcontinental spread of the epidemic into East Africa. Similarly, the history of sexual exposure to these female prostitutes correlated with infection in Kenyan men attending the STD clinics, suggesting initially male-to-female followed by female-to-male bidirectional transmission.[13]

In further studies of HIV infection among the Nairobi prostitutes and the men attending the STD clinics, HIV seropositivity was significantly associated with current infection with sexually transmitted diseases such as gonorrhea, genital ulcers, and syphilis.[13,26] In a study in Zambia, seropositivity in men also correlated with the presence of genital ulcers.[15] These observations suggest that the disruption of genital epithelial integrity caused by sexually transmitted diseases that are common in Africa may facilitate transmission of HIV during vaginal intercourse. Alternatively, the presence of these sexually transmitted diseases may be indicative of high-risk activities for HIV infection or of exposure to unsterilized needles for the

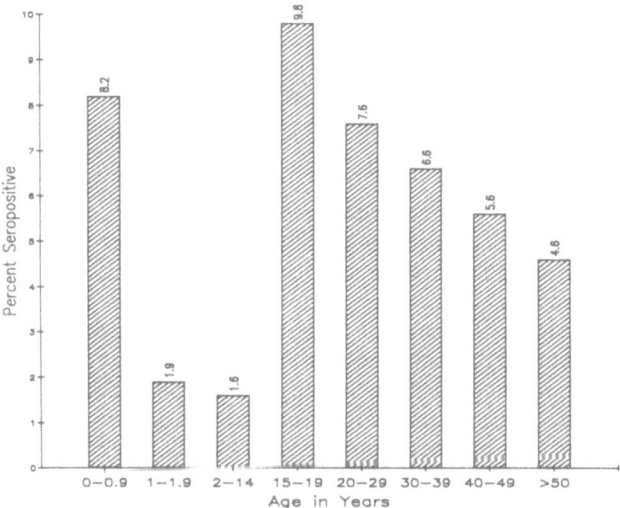

FIGURE 1.   HIV seroprevalence rates among 6,000 healthy persons by age in Kinshasa, Zaire, 1984–1986.

treatment of sexually transmitted diseases, and may not be causally related to HIV transmissability. However, in two studies of female prostitutes and of men attending STD clinics in Africa, HIV seropositivity was directly associated with the number of sexual exposures independent of the frequency of needle exposures—which was not associated with HIV seropositivity.[13,25]

Further evidence for heterosexual transmission comes from a household study of AIDS patients in Zaire, in which HIV antibody was significantly higher among spouses than among other household members or controls. In this study by Mann et al,[27] 20 (9.8%) of 204 case household members and three (1.9%) of 155 control household members were HIV seropositive (relative risk = 5.1; 95% confidence interval, 1.7-15.2). Eleven (three men and eight women) (61%) of 18 spouses of three women and fifteen men with AIDS were HIV antibody positive compared to only one (3.7%) of 27 spouses of seronegative control patients (relative risk = 16.5; 95% confidence interval, 3.7-75.0). Except for spouses, the rate of HIV seropositivity did not differ significantly between case and control households. Furthermore, of adults in case households who were not spouses, the number who were seropositive for HIV was identical to that predicted from sex- and age-specific HIV seroprevalence rates. These data document the potential for heterosexual transmission among sexual partners of HIV-infected individuals, and that bidirectional transmission is possible. In addition to this study, several clusters of AIDS cases in Africa have been identified in the chronology of events suggesting both female-to-male and male-to-female transmission of HIV.[10,28]

Unlike HIV infection among homosexual men in the United States and Europe, specific sexual activities other than vaginal intercourse do not appear to play a significant role in heterosexual transmission. Anal intercourse, reported by only 4-8% of female AIDS patients, was not associated with HIV infection in surveys in Kenya, Zaire, and Rwanda.[13,17-19,25] Clearly, the most important variable for heterosexual transmission is the number of sexual exposures within a given time period. In a recent study of female prostitutes in Zaire by Mann et al,[25] HIV seroprevalence rates were 19% for those women with fewer than 200 sexual partners per lifetime, which increased steadily to a high of 34% for those women with a history of more than 1,000 lifetime sexual partners (Fig 2). The only variable that had a negative effect on seropositivity was a history of condom use. Although the numbers are small, none of eight female prostitutes who insisted their partners use condoms were seropositive, compared to an infection rate of 33.8% among female prostitutes whose partners used condoms less than half of the time. These data provide indirect evidence that even with promiscuity, barrier contraceptives such as the condom may effectively prevent transmission of HIV.

OTHER MODES OF HIV TRANSMISSION

Heterosexual transmission of HIV in Africa is amplified by further dissemination of the AIDS virus into the general heterosexual population via blood transfusions and injections with blood-contaminated needles for medicinal purposes. In some areas of Africa, such as Uganda,

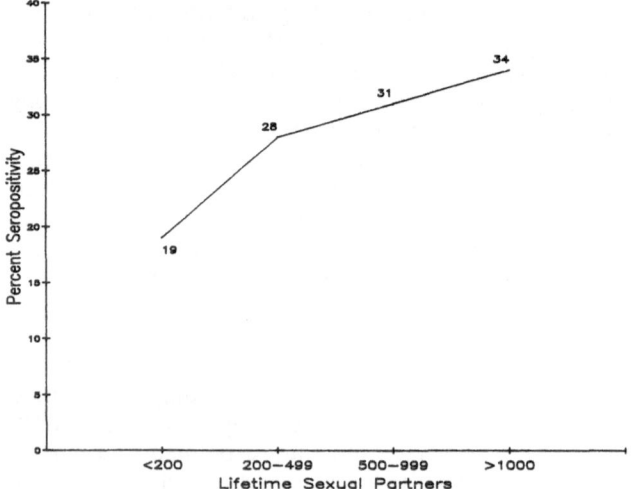

FIGURE 2. HIV seroprevalence rates in 377 female prostitutes according to mean number of lifetime sexual partners, Zaire, 1986.

Rwanda, and Zaire, seroprevalence rates among blood donors range from 8% to 18%, suggesting that the risk to transfusion recipients in these areas is very high. In Kinshasa, 9% of 295 AIDS patients reported receiving at least one blood transfusion during the three to five years prior to onset of illness.[22] Among 2,384 hospital workers in Kinshasa, 9.3% of seropositive workers and 4.8% of seronegative workers reported transfusions within the past ten years ($p < 0.05$).[21] Even among children in Central Africa, 60% of 40 seropositive children compared to 32.7% of 328 seronegative children and 14.3% of 92 healthy outpatient control children had a history of prior blood transfusions ($p < 0.001$).[20]

Similarly, in the same seroprevalence study of hospital workers in Kinshasa,[21] significantly more HIV seropositive than seronegative workers reported receiving medical injections during the previous three years. Among those reporting injections, seroprevalence was nearly twice as high for those who received five or more injections as for those receiving fewer than five injections. Together, these two additional factors, blood transfusions and exposure to blood contaminated needles and syringes, contribute significantly to the dissemination of HIV among the general population. With increasing prevalence of HIV infection in the general population, heterosexual transmission becomes more efficient, and promiscuity becomes a less important variable.

CONCLUSIONS

The present available data in Africa demonstrate that heterosexual transmission exists, and that it can, given the right circumstances, sustain an epidemic of HIV infection in the general population. The rate at which HIV infection will spread by heterosexual contact outside Africa depends on many factors, such as the prevalence of HIV in the heterosexual population, its introduction and amplification in a highly promiscuous subpopulation of heterosexuals, the degree of sexual promiscuity, the efficiency of heterosexual transmission, and the prevalence of genital infections and use of barrier contraceptives.[29] Most importantly, the long latency period between viral exposure and the development of clinical disease harbors the delayed recognition of the epidemic in a heterosexual population. Thus, it is appropriate to institute studies to determine the occurrence of HIV infection in heterosexual populations in the United States known to be at high risk, such as sexual partners of individuals with AIDS or at risk for AIDS, heterosexual prostitutes, and patients with sexually transmitted diseases. Educational programs on AIDS prevention should be instituted immediately and should be directed at heterosexuals as well as at other high-risk groups. The major emphasis of these programs should be on reducing risk factors and on safer sexual practices, including condom use. For Africa, the obstacles to AIDS control are even greater and include cultural, sociologic, and economic factors. To be successful, these programs will have to be integrated into the existing health and educational programs and will require full support by appropriate government agencies. Controlling the spread of HIV worldwide will require a major international commitment, not only in terms of providing financial help, but also in providing scientific, educational, and technical assistance.

REFERENCES

1. Mahler H, Assad F: The World Health Organization's programme on AIDS. *Abstracts of the Second International Conference on AIDS*, Paris, France, June 23–25, 1986, p 5.

2. Coffin J, Haase A, Levy JA, et al: Human immunodeficiency viruses [letter]. *Science* 1986; 232:697.

3. Curran JW, Morgan WM, Hardy AM, et al: The epidemiology of AIDS: Current status and future prospects. *Science* 1985; 229:1352–1357.

4. Melbye M: The natural history of human T lymphotropic virus-III infection: The cause of AIDS. *Br Med J* 1986; 292:5–12.

5. Jaffe HW, Darrow WW, Echenberg DF, et al: The acquired immunodeficiency syndrome in a cohort of homosexual men: A six-year follow-up study. *Ann Intern Med* 1985; 103:210–214.

6. Goedert JJ, Biggar RJ, Weiss SH, et al: Three-year incidence of AIDS in five cohorts of HTLV-III infected risk group members. *Science* 1986; 231:922–995.

7. Clumeck N, Sonnet J, Taelman H, et al: Acquired immunodeficiency syndrome in African patients. *N Engl J Med* 1984; 210:492–497.

8. Brunet JB, Ancelle R: Update: Acquired immunodeficiency syndrome—Europe. *MMWR* 1985; 34:583–589.

9. World Health Organization: Acquired immunodeficiency syndrome (AIDS): Situation in Europe as of 31 December 1985. *Wkly Epidemiol Rec* 1986; 61:125–128.

10. Piot P, Quinn TC, Taelman H, et al: Acquired immunodeficiency syndrome in a heterosexual population in Zaire. *Lancet* 1984; 2:65–69.

11. Van de Perre P, Rouvroy D, Lepage P, et al: Acquired immunodeficiency syndrome in Rwanda. *Lancet* 1984; 2:62–65.

12. Quinn TC, Mann JM, Curran JW, et al: AIDS in Africa: An epidemiological paradigm. *Science* 1986; 234:955–963.

13. Kreiss JK, Koech D, Plummer FA, et al: AIDS virus infection in Nairobi prostitutes: Spread of the epidemic to East Africa. *N Engl J Med* 1986; 314:414–418.

14. Mann JM, Francis H, Quinn T, et al: Surveillance for AIDS in a Central African city: Kinshasa, Zaire. *JAMA* 1986; 255:3255–3259.

15. Melbye M, Njelesani EK, Bayley A, et al: Evidence for heterosexual transmission and clinical manifestations of human immunodeficiency virus infection and related conditions in Lusaka, Zambia. *Lancet* 1986; 2:1113–1115.

16. Aral SO, Holmes KK: Epidemiology of sexually transmitted diseases, in Holmes KK, Mardh PA, Sparling PF, et al (eds): *Sexually Transmitted Diseases.* New York, McGraw-Hill, pp 127–141.

17. Clumeck N, Robert-Guroff M, Van de Perre P, et al: Seroepidemiological studies of HTLV-III antibody prevalence among selected groups of heterosexual Africans. *JAMA* 1985; 254:2599–2602.

18. Clumeck N, Van de Perre P, Carael M, et al: Heterosexual promiscuity among African patients with AIDS. *N Engl J Med* 1985; 313:182.

19. Van de Perre P, Clumeck N, Carael M, et al: Female prostitutes: A risk group for infection with human T-cell lymphotropic virus type III. *Lancet* 1985; 2:524–527.

20. Mann JM, Francis H, Davachi F, et al: HTLV-III/LAV seroprevalence in pediatric in-patients 2–14 years old in Kinshasa, Zaire. *J Pediatrics* 1986; 78:673–677.

21. Mann JM, Francis H, Quinn TC, et al: HTLV-III/LAV seroprevalence among hospital workers in Kinshasa, Zaire: Lack of association with occupational exposure. *JAMA* 1986; 256:3099–3102.

22. Mann JM, Francis H, Quinn TC, et al: Role of blood transfusions in transmission of HTLV-III infection in Zaire. *JAMA* 1986; 256:721–724.

23. Mann JM, Francis H, Davachi F, et al: Risk factors for human immunodeficiency virus seropositivity among children 1–24 months old in Kinshasa, Zaire. *Lancet* 1986; 2:654–657.

24. Zuckerman AJ: AIDS and insects. *Br Med J* 1986; 292:1094–1095.

25. Mann JM, Quinn TC, Francis H: Sexual practices associated with LAV/HTLV-III seropositivity among female prostitutes in Kinshasa, Zaire. Presented at the International Conference on AIDS, Paris, France, June 23–25, 1986.

26. Piot P, Plummer FA, Rey M, et al: Retrospective seroepidemiology of AIDS virus infection in Nairobi populations. *J Infect Dis* (in press).

27. Mann JM, Quinn TC, Francis H, et al: Prevalence of HTLV-III/LAV in household contacts of patients with confirmed AIDS and controls in Kinshasa, Zaire. *JAMA* 1986; 256:721–724.

28. Jonckheer T, Dab I, Van de Perre P, et al: Cluster of HTLV-III/LAV infection in an African family. *Lancet* 1985; 1:400–401.

29. Piot P, Mann JM: Bidirectional heterosexual transmission of human immunodeficiency virus (HIV). Presented at the International Conference on AIDS, Paris, France, June 23–25, 1986.

Chapter 15

AIDS in adolescents: A rationale for concern

KAREN HEIN, MD

Adolescents between the ages of 13 and 19 years comprise approximately 10% of the American population, accounting for approximately 25 million individuals.[1] Adolescents are not currently identified as a high-risk group for the acquisition or spread of the human immunodeficiency virus (HIV) infection, although the definition of risk has been changing to encompass the notion of risk behavior rather than risk groups. Based on current knowledge of adolescent behavior and development, this age group has been targeted as a "bridging" group to those currently infected.

Although only a few hundred adolescents were diagnosed as having acquired immunodeficiency syndrome (AIDS) in 1986 (Centers for Disease Control, AIDS Surveillance Unit, Atlanta, Ga, personal communication, December 1986), many aspects of the life styles of American adolescents, especially those in the inner cities, seem to place them directly in the path of this epidemic. The youngest members of each of the groups known to be at highest risk for contracting and transmitting AIDS are themselves adolescents (ie, young bisexual and homosexual men, and intravenous drug abusers). But, more critically, it is the chain of heterosexual partners of both of these groups who may form a bridge to a much larger adolescent population whose patterns of sexual behavior may expose them to the virus. As we come to understand more about the heterosexual transmission of AIDS, it appears that adolescents coming into sexual contact with those already infected may face a substantial risk.

CASE HISTORIES

The following two case histories of 17-year-olds illustrate some of the reasons why adolescents should be a focus of concern.

An adolescent female presented to a comprehensive adolescent health clinic after being rejected by the military. An HIV antibody screening test had been performed as part of a recruitment requirement and was found to be positive. The young woman had previously considered herself to be in good health. In the course of a general health assessment she was found to be in the first trimester of an unintended pregnancy. She elected to terminate the

pregnancy, but within six months she became pregnant for a second time. She stated that in the past she had had intercourse with another adolescent whom she believes was an intravenous drug abuser.

A 17-year-old male presented to a general adolescent medicine clinic for health screening that was required for enrollment in a job training program. He complained of back pain and fatigue. He admitted to intravenous substance abuse ending five months prior to evaluation. On evaluation, several problems were identified, including glomerulonephritis, evidence of previous hepatitis B infection, and a positive tuberculin skin test. After eliciting the history of previous intravenous drug abuse, HIV status was assessed. Screening and confirmatory tests were positive for HIV infection. During counseling regarding HIV status, the patient revealed that he had had at least two sexual partners within the previous three months with whom he continued to have intercourse after he became aware of his HIV status. He informed only one of these partners and did not use condoms or other forms of contraception.

These case histories illustrate the basis for our current concern about adolescents. These two youngsters did not seek help because they suspected HIV infection or because they recognized themselves as being members of a known high-risk group. They were identified only because of their normal adolescent activities. In the first case, detection was made inadvertently as part of a career decision to join the military. In the second case, detection resulted from a comprehensive evaluation following a request for a routine physical examination that was required for entry into a job-related training program. Both adolescents sought medical care through the usual channels open to them, namely health services specially geared to their age group. Neither might have been appropriately cared for in health facilities for children or adults. The health services, type of counseling, and support that adolescents receive must be appropriate for their age group.

RATIONALE FOR CONCERN

Most adolescents do not seek health services on a regular basis. Thus risk status for HIV infection must be inferred from data collected for other purposes. This information can be summarized in three categories: sexual behavior and relevant consequences, physiologic considerations, and drug abuse.

Dr Hein is Associate Professor of Pediatrics, Department of Pediatrics, Albert Einstein College of Medicine, Jacobi BE-21, Pelham Pkwy and Eastchester Rd, Bronx, NY 10461.
Partial funding for this research was provided by The Carnegie Corporation of New York.

SEXUAL BEHAVIOR AND RELEVANT CONSEQUENCES

Adolescent Sexual Experience. In the United States, roughly half of all teenagers have had intercourse by the age of 19.[2] However, among the 25 million adolescents in the US, there are subgroups who either have intercourse at an early age or whose patterns of sexual behavior may put them at increased risk. Studies conducted by Zelnick and Kantner[3] in the 1970s (Fig 1) revealed changes during that decade that have profound implications for the possible spread of HIV if it were to be introduced into the adolescent population. In comparing data from 1971, 1976, and 1979, some important changes are evident. The latest survey[3] found that approximately 60% of white urban females and approximately 80% of black urban females have had intercourse by age 19. The greatest increase in the three survey years was among the adolescent white female population.

To complement the national data, regional data support the assertion that some adolescents are currently at greater risk than others for the acquisition and spread of AIDS (Fig 2). Three curves are presented that compare the age at first intercourse of young inner-city women.[4] The curve on the left represents data for young women housed in a detention center. The curve in the center is based on data for young women living in group homes in the Bronx. The curve on the right was derived from a national survey conducted by Sorenson[5] in the 1970s. The average age of first intercourse in the detention population was 12 as compared to an average age of first intercourse for the nation

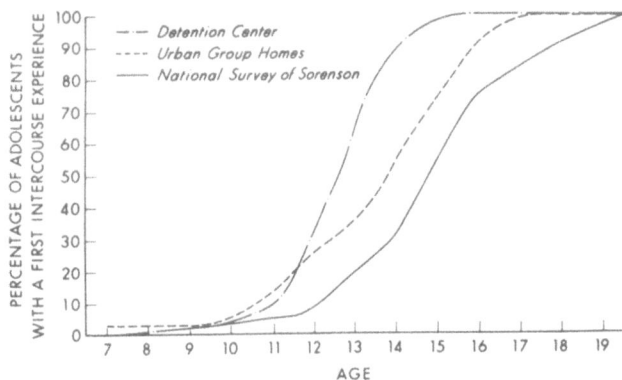

FIGURE 2. Percentage of sexually experienced adolescents aged seven to 19 years for three populations of teenaged females (from Hein, et al[4]) (courtesy of C.V. Mosby Company).

at that time of age 16. The age of sexual initiation for the group home residents was intermediate between that of the other two groups. Some of these young women were runaways. Most were having intercourse with multiple partners with whom they had no lasting relationships and little knowledge of their partners' prior sexual or drug-related behavior. These data begin to define a population of urban adolescents who may be at immediate and particular risk of HIV infection.

Knowledge of some of the patterns of sexual behavior among adolescents who have had intercourse may help identify teenagers who are at greater risk. Following the scheme of Sorenson,[5] two such patterns of sexual relationships are the "serial monogamous" pattern and that of the "sexual adventurer." According to Sorenson's[5] survey of American adolescents in the 1970s, roughly half of the nonvirginal females and only one quarter of the nonvirginal males could be described as being serially monogamous. Some serial monogamists also occasionally had intercourse with other partners besides the primary consort at that time. More than half of all sexually experienced adolescent females had intercourse with male partners who were 20 years of age or older.

The "sexual adventurer" was defined by Sorenson[5] as an adolescent who by the age of 19 had had a total of 17 sexual partners, and who, in the month preceding the interview, had had an average of 3.2 sexual partners. The sexual adventurer, therefore, becomes another subgroup of adolescents at risk for the acquisition or spread of AIDS to his/her partners, as compared to the serially monogamous adolescent. The sexual adventurer pattern describes approximately 41% of the sexually experienced adolescent males and about 13% of the sexually experienced females in the country.[5]

Contraception. Approximately half of sexually experienced adolescents use any form of contraception at first intercourse, whatever the age at initiation.[2] Oral contraceptives are used by approximately one third of teenaged females, and condoms, depending on the study and the population, are used by approximately 12%. One third to one fourth of adolescents have never used any form of contraception at all.[2]

Pregnancy. Pregnancy, another consequence of the early initiation of sexual activity among American teenagers, occurs in approximately one million teenagers ev-

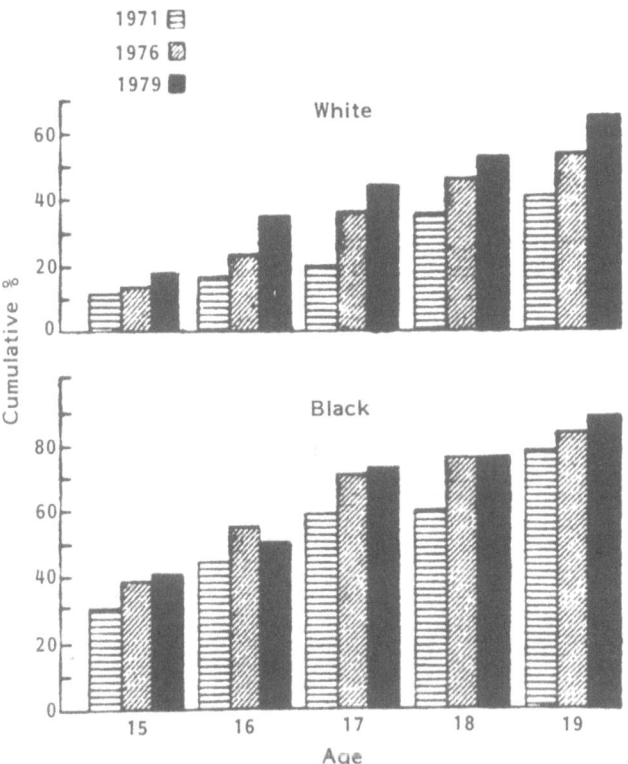

FIGURE 1. Proportion of black and white urban US females aged 15 to 19 years who were sexually experienced in 1971, 1976, and 1979 (from Bell and Hein,[9] adapted from Zelnick and Kantner[3]) (courtesy of Alan Guttmacher Institute).

ery year, and roughly 85% of these pregnancies are unintended.[2] Since adolescent females tend to have intercourse with males who are two to three years older than they, these younger females may be exposed to HIV infection and thus unintentionally expose their offspring.[5] Pregnant young teenage girls are less likely to obtain prenatal care as compared to adults; thus they and their babies currently have little opportunity to benefit from counseling or services that might inform them about possible risk to themselves or their offspring.

Issues relevant to pregnant teenagers living in New York were recently reviewed. In New York State every day roughly 180 teenagers become pregnant.[6] Minority group status appears to be associated with increased risks to both mother and child.[7] In New York City and some other urban centers, HIV infection has been disproportionately identified in black and Hispanic groups. Cumulative incidence rates of AIDS among blacks and Hispanics are more than three times the rate among whites.[8]

Venereal Disease. National data regarding the incidence and prevalence of various venereal diseases can be very misleading when applied to the adolescent age range. If data are reported per 100,000 of population at a given age, it would appear that rates for the youngest adoles-

cents (10–14-year-olds) are the lowest as compared to other age groups through young adulthood.[9] However, this is an artifact produced by using a denominator that is not relevant to the question.

In Figures 3–5, data are presented which give a more accurate portrayal of the rates of venereal disease in American youth.[9] Instead of reporting the number of cases per 100,000 of population (Fig 3), national data have been recalculated and graphed using the percent of sexually active adolescents and young adults in each age group as the denominator (Figs 4, 5). For 1971 and 1976, the 10–14-year-olds and 15–19-year-olds showed the highest rates of gonorrhea (Fig 4), not the lowest, accounting for roughly 3,500 cases per 100,000 sexually active teenagers. For syphilis, the rate was 100–200/100,000 for the youngest groups (Fig 5). Rates of hospitalization for pelvic inflammatory disease were similarly highest in the youngest age groups when the denominator was corrected for the percent of sexually active females.

Thus, the youngsters who are having intercourse at a very early age also have higher rates of venereal disease than their young adult counterparts. Similar analyses of data regarding syphilis and chlamydia reveal that the highest rates occur among the young adolescents, despite the impression that much of venereal disease resides within the young adult population.

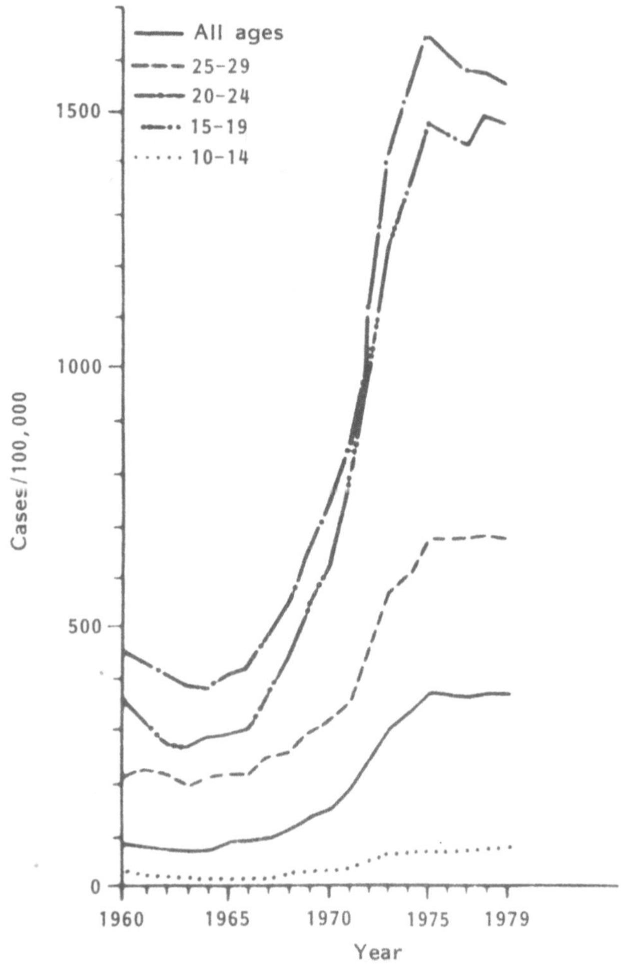

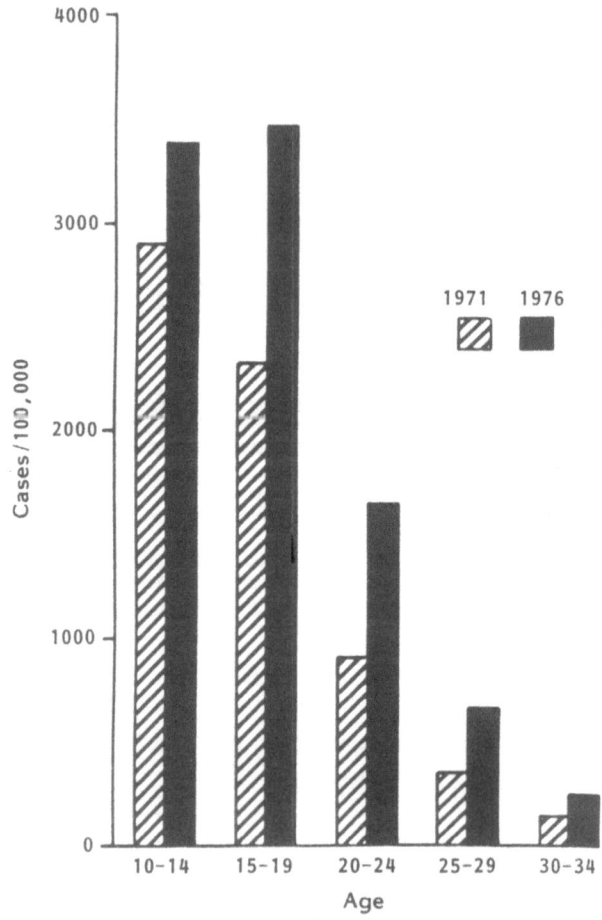

FIGURE 3. Apparent increase in the incidence of gonorrhea among females in the age groups 10 to 14, 15 to 19, 20 to 24, and 25 to 29, and in all females (from Bell and Hein[9]) (courtesy of McGraw-Hill Book Company).

FIGURE 4. Rates of gonorrhea expressed as number of cases per 100,000 of sexually experienced females aged 10 to 14, 15 to 19, 20 to 24, 25 to 29, and 30 to 34[9] (courtesy of McGraw-Hill Book Company).

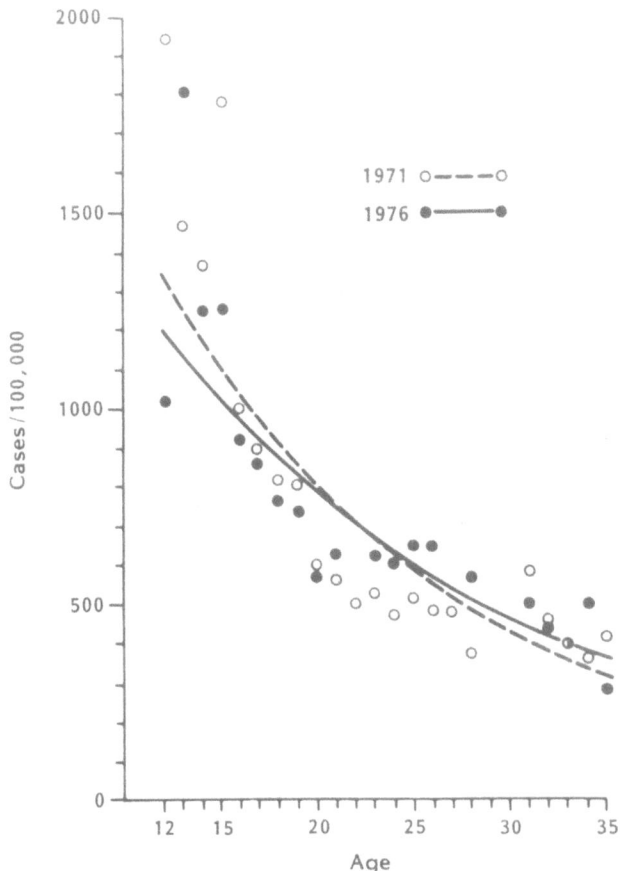

FIGURE 5. Incidence of pelvic inflammatory disease in hospitalized adolescents[9] (courtesy of McGraw-Hill Book Company).

Asymptomatic venereal disease continues to be a problem in some segments of the adolescent population. In the 1970s in the Bronx, youngsters arrested as "persons in need of supervision" or for committing acts of delinquency were screened for the presence of gonorrhea.[10] In a study in which 600 females under the age of 17 years were tested for the presence of cervical infection with gonorrhea, after eliminating all who were symptomatic for any genitourinary symptoms (including any history or any evidence of vaginal discharge or the presence of white blood cells in urine), asymptomatic gonorrheal cervical infection was detected in 7% of these young women.[10]

A similar study conducted during the 1970s involving more than 2,000 males, all under the age of 17, documented a reservoir of 1.9% who had positive urethral cultures but no symptoms of gonorrhea.[10]

Since these young people harbor venereal diseases that were prevalent prior to the introduction of HIV, such as gonorrhea, syphilis, and/or chlamydia, we might therefore expect that these youngsters may be a new reservoir of undetected AIDS virus.

PHYSIOLOGIC REASONS WHY ADOLESCENTS MAY BE AT SPECIAL RISK

There are anatomic and physiologic differences between adolescents and young adults that indicate that teenage females may be at even greater risk than young adult females for the complications of some venereal diseases, and, by analogy, possibly AIDS.

Differences in ovarian function and differences in the cervical milieu in young adolescents may facilitate entry and spread of certain organisms.[9] There are differences in properties of cervical mucous that affect the penetrability of sperm and also the ability of the motile organisms to penetrate through the cervix. As a female progresses through puberty there are changes in vaginal pH. The adult pH is more protective against the invasion of some organisms associated with venereal diseases.

The location of the squamo-columnar junction changes with age. The junction at which squamous epithelial cells that line the vagina and external portion of the cervix that protrudes into the vagina (portio vaginalis) overlaps with endometrial cells differs in the adolescent as compared to the adult woman. The location of this "transition zone" in adolescents may expose young women to organisms or other factors that may predispose them to a greater risk of developing cervical intraepithelial neoplasia.[9]

There is a high prevalence of anovulatory cycles within two years after menarche. It has been observed that the use of oral contraceptives may confer some protective effects against some venereal diseases.[9] The hypothesis is that the presence of progesterone (or the progestins present in oral contraceptives) alters characteristics of cervical mucous and the length of menses. These two factors plus other physiologic effects help prevent or alter the establishment and spread of some venereal diseases. By analogy, the adolescent who is not ovulating is also not producing progesterone. Therefore, the young adolescent female would not benefit from whatever protective effects may come from the presence of this hormone. These factors may contribute to the documented high rates of venereal disease in this population. Whether or not these factors will also be relevant to HIV infection is not known.

The association between cervical infection with human papilloma viruses and cervical cancer has been documented in recent years.[11] Factors that have been identified as being useful in predicting increased risk of developing cervical carcinoma include early age at first intercourse and a history of multiple sexual partners. Once again the adolescent female may be at particular risk. The rates of abnormal cervical cytology seen in a study of young women under the age of 17 years housed at the Spofford Juvenile Detention Center were very high.[12] Pap smear screening revealed rates of dysplasia and early forms of cervical intraepithelial neoplasia (CIN) of 35 per 1,000. This rate is comparable to that of the highest risk groups in the adult population. Whether or not young adolescent females with early age at first intercourse are also at increased risk for HIV infection and consequent alterations in immune status is unknown at this time.

DRUG ABUSE

Past experience in the 1960s and 1970s regarding drug abuse patterns may have relevance for the current AIDS epidemic. We have much to learn from the past regarding adolescents. Figure 6 shows data collected at the Spofford Juvenile Detention Center from the late 1960s through 1977 (just prior to the documentation of AIDS).[13] Usage patterns for various drugs are shown for the adolescent

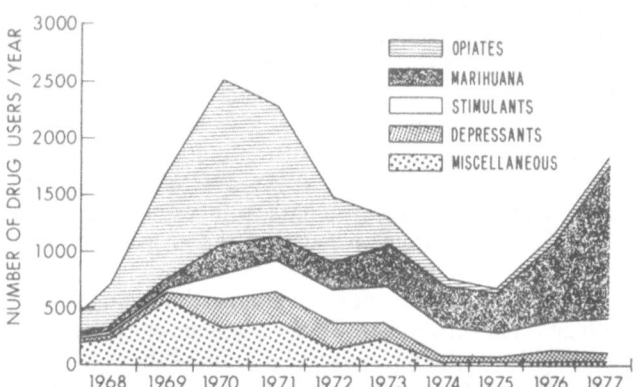

FIGURE 6. Analysis of types of drugs used by 14,810 of 66,000 adolescents admitted to a youth detention center between 1968 and 1977[13] (courtesy of the American Medical Association).

population arrested for status offenses or acts of delinquency. All youngsters were 17 years of age or younger. During the late 1960s and early 1970s, considerable publicity was given to the young adult drug abuser. Heroin was not thought to be a problem among adolescents. The medical consequences of heroin use in adolescents were not documented in the medical literature until the epidemic was long established in the adult population. Medi-

cal correlates of heroin use were noted and published in 1979.[13,14] Medical sequelae that followed increased use of heroin were then reported; these included increased admissions to in-patient units and increased cases of hepatitis and drug-related deaths. The pattern of these sequelae followed the heroin usage pattern, as shown in Figures 7 and 8.

The problem in the teenage population was not appreciated because adolescents are traditionally grouped statistically with children or adults, not studied as a unique population. Services were organized for young adults long before an appropriate response was mounted by public health and educational agencies serving youth. We should learn from previous errors. In this case, we have an opportunity to intervene before large numbers of adolescents are infected and before the obvious medical sequelae of HIV infection have become apparent.

The opportunity now presents itself to focus attention on the adolescent population as distinct from young adults or children. They are not big children and they are not small adults. They have a unique set of sociologic, epidemiologic, and physiologic circumstances that require special attention now, before wider spread of HIV infection is documented in this segment of the population.

In the Bronx, drug addiction is currently the major risk factor for AIDS. Two thirds of all AIDS cases are associated with intravenous (IV) drug abuse and about 50% of

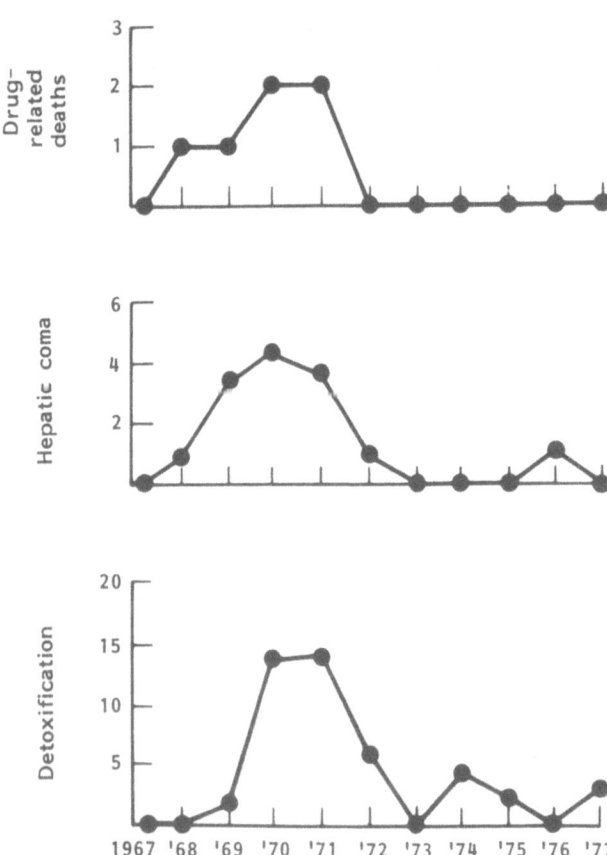

FIGURE 7. Ten-year experience from an in-patient unit for adolescents describing the number of teenagers admitted who died of drug-related causes or hepatic coma or who were admitted for drug detoxification[13] (courtesy of the American Medical Association).

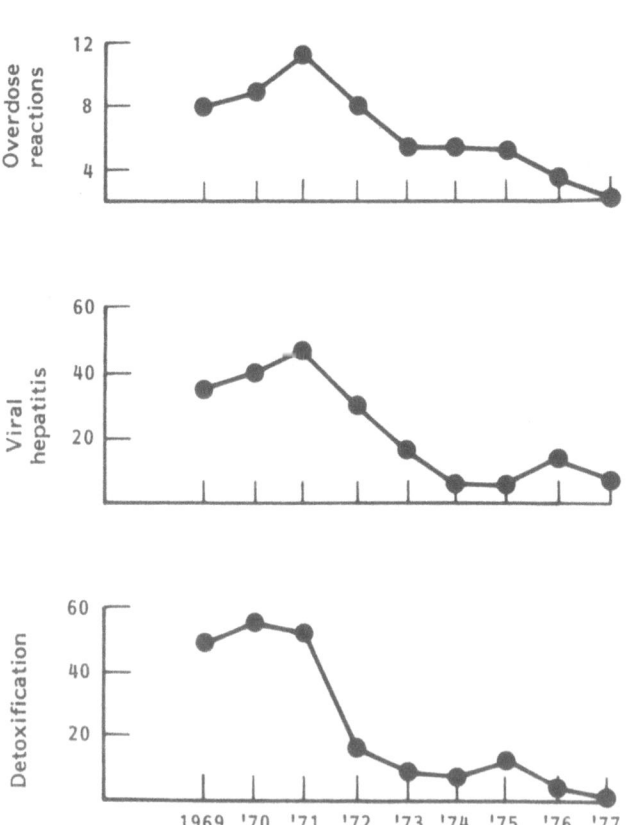

FIGURE 8. Nine-year experience with juvenile detention facility describing number of cases of overdose reactions, hepatitis, and heroin detoxification[13] (courtesy of the American Medical Association).

the borough's 60,000–70,000 IV drug users are believed to be positive for HIV antibodies.[15] This group is mostly composed of young adults (aged 20–40 years) who are black and Hispanic and who are sexually active with multiple partners, making large scale heterosexual transmission a genuine possibility.[16]

One indication of the emerging problem of HIV infection in a young heterosexually active population can be found in the results of the blood testing program for new military recruits. While the national rate of HIV infection is still low (1.6/1,000), the figure for the Bronx (and for Manhattan; Newark; Washington, DC; and Puerto Rico) appears to be about ten times this rate, or 1.6%.[17,18] The ratio of males to females in this sample is 3:1 as compared to 13:1 nationally for AIDS cases. This pattern is more characteristic of that observed among IV drug abusers and may also implicate heterosexual transmission. Further, these rates must represent an underestimation since the military does not attract those adolescents who are the most marginal, and who would be expected to have the highest rates of sexually transmitted diseases, drug abuse, promiscuity, and pregnancy.

IMPLICATIONS FOR EDUCATIONAL INTERVENTIONS

In the absence of an effective treatment or vaccine against HIV infection, risk reduction programs must be developed to restrict the introduction and spread of AIDS to the adolescent population.[19] Sampling adolescents themselves to learn about their specific concerns, attitudes, and beliefs regarding AIDS should be the basis for designing interventions for teenagers. Educational materials prepared for teenagers should be based on their own questions, perceptions, fears, and convictions.

It appears that there are two groups within the adolescent population, though we do not currently know the dimensions of each group. They include those young people who may be currently infected or at risk, and those whom we might call the "worried well" (adolescents who are very concerned or anxious, but who do not have reason to be concerned at present). Neither group has adequate age-appropriate services or support. We should begin to separate the "worried well" from the smaller group of teenagers for whom concern is warranted. A major goal of risk reduction programs for the latter must be to try to alter current patterns of sexual behavior, including attitudes toward use of contraceptives.

CONCLUSION

Because of contemporary American adolescent life styles, teenagers are an important group for targeted interventions to prevent further spread of HIV infection. The factors that support our current concern are prevailing patterns of adolescent sexual activity, the age of initiation of first intercourse, current contraceptive practices, the choice of sexual partners, rates of venereal diseases, and anatomic and physiologic considerations.

It is hypothesized that the "sexual adventurers," in particular, form a subpopulation of adolescents who are most likely to be the entree of HIV infection into the adolescent population, just as this group has been a reservoir for other sexually transmitted diseases. While more effective treatments and possibly primary preventive methods are being developed for all age groups, special attention should be paid to adolescents. They are a proximal group that may become rapidly infected in the near future. Therefore, they require the immediate attention of health policy and health care agencies.

Acknowledgments. I wish to acknowledge a group of individuals with whom I have been working over the past year. Together we have considered the implications of AIDS in adolescents and are jointly planning new programs to address the issues raised in this paper. Key members include Ernest Drucker, PhD, Nancy Reuben, MD, Sten Vermund, MD, and Sandra Shephard, MD. Special acknowledgment is made to Sharon Lockett and Carol Ruffo for their assistance in preparing this manuscript.

REFERENCES

1. Projections of the population of the United States. *Current Population Reports.* Series 25, No. 952. Bureau of the Census, 1986.
2. *Teenage Pregnancy: The Problem That Hasn't Gone Away.* New York, The Alan Guttmacher Institute, 1981.
3. Zelnick M, Kantner JF: Sexual activity, contraceptive use and pregnancy among metropolitan-area teenagers: 1971–1979. *Fam Plann Perspect* 1980, 12:230–231, 233–237.
4. Hein K, Cohen MI, Marks A, et al: Age at first intercourse among homeless adolescent females. *J Pediatr* 1978; 93:147–148.
5. Sorensen RE: *Adolescent Sexuality in Contemporary America.* New York, World Publishing Co, 1973, pp 180–280.
6. Randolph LA, Gesche M: Black adolescent pregnancy: Prevention and management. *J Community Health* 1986; 11:10–18.
7. Clarke MI: Black teenage pregnancy: An obstetrician's viewpoint. *J Community Health* 1986; 11:23–30.
8. AIDS among Blacks and Hispanics—United States. *MMWR* 1986; 35:655–666.
9. Bell T, Hein K: The adolescent and sexually transmitted disease, in Holmes K, et al (eds): *Sexually Transmitted Diseases.* New York, McGraw-Hill, 1984, pp 73–84.
10. Hein K, Marks A, Cohen MI: Asymptomatic gonorrhea: Prevalence in a population of urban adolescents. *J Pediatr* 1977; 90:634–635.
11. Howley P: On human papillomaviruses. *N Engl J Med* 1986; 315:1089–1090.
12. Hein K, Schreiber K, Cohen MI, et al: Cervical cytology. The need for routine screening in the sexually active adolescent. *J Pediatr* 1977; 91:123–126.
13. Hein K, Cohen MI, Litt IF: Illicit drug use among urban adolescents. A decade of retrospect. *Am J Dis Child* 1979; 133:38–40.
14. Hein K, Cohen M, Litt I, et al: Juvenile detention. Another boundary issue for physicians. *Pediatrics* 1980; 66:239–245.
15. Drucker E: AIDS and addiction in New York City. *Am J Drug Alcohol Abuse* 1986; 12:165–181.
16. Schoenbaum EE, Selwyn PA, Klein RS, et al: Prevalence of and risk factors associated with HTLV-III/LAV antibodies among intravenous drug abusers in a methadone program in New York City. Presented at the International Conference on AIDS, Paris, France, June 23–25, 1986.
17. *Human T-lymphotropic Virus Type III/Lymphadenopathy-Associated Virus Antibody Prevalence in U.S. Military Recruit Applicants.* US Dept of Health and Human Services. Atlanta, Centers for Disease Control, 1986.
18. Burke D, Brundage JF, Bernier W, et al: Infections among prospective U.S. military recruits. Presented at the International Conference on AIDS, Paris, France (Poster 676), June 23–25, 1986.
19. Koop E: *Surgeon General's Report on Acquired Immune Deficiency Syndrome.* US Dept of Health and Human Services, Public Health Service, October 1986.

Chapter 16

Education and contact notification for AIDS prevention

DEAN F. ECHENBERG, MD, PHD

Epidemics are dynamic phenomena. The strategies used to deal with epidemics generally evolve as knowledge increases. These strategies must be evaluated continually to insure success. This paper discusses how disease control strategies evolved in San Francisco as the prevalence of acquired immunodeficiency syndrome (AIDS) in different groups changed.

The goal of an AIDS prevention program is to prevent transmission of the human immunodeficiency virus (HIV). A broad range of intervention programs is required to attain this goal. These programs must be appropriate to the particular circumstances of each community where they are to be implemented, and, even though no one approach will be successful everywhere, education must be the cornerstone of every effort. This education must focus on the appropriate groups of individuals—that is, those who are either infected or at risk of becoming infected.

PREVALENCE OF DISEASE

One factor that determines how this education will be applied in any population group is the prevalence of the disease in that population. When many people are infected, mass education directed to the entire population is one of the most important methods. When very few people are infected, then attempts must be made to locate these individuals and individually educate them, because of the potential health consequences of a sexually active and uninformed infected individual.

If one looks at the epidemiology of AIDS in San Francisco one can understand how the city's different strategies evolved. A cohort of homosexual men in San Francisco, recruited from the Department of Public Health's sexually transmitted disease clinics, has been followed since 1978.[1,2] Originally, these men volunteered for hepatitis B studies. In 1984 it was realized that many of these men were infected with the AIDS virus. Consequently, they were asked to participate in AIDS studies, and blood specimens which had been drawn from them between 1979 and 1980 and saved were examined.

One of the saddest statistics in the AIDS tragedy is that by the time the first publication on AIDS appeared in the medical literature in July 1981, 30–40% of the men in this cohort were already infected.[3] It was another six months to a year before the mode of transmission was understood, at which time 40–50% of the cohort was infected.

The strategies that evolved at that time to deal with this situation in San Francisco are obviously different from those that are applied where the prevalence of the disease is much lower. In addition, today there is a blood test for potential infectivity which was not available then.

In the initial stages of the epidemic, a strategy was evolved that said in effect that all people in the classic high-risk group should consider themselves to be infectious through sexual contact. This included not only gay men but also individuals with hemophilia and intravenous (IV) drug users. This strategy of mass education has been relatively effective. It has had a great impact in decreasing the level of unsafe sexual activities that facilitate transmission of the virus.[4] In 1982, an average of 382 cases of rectal gonorrhea were seen each month in San Francisco at a sexually transmitted disease clinic. This number has now decreased to fewer than 30 per month.[5] However, it subsequently became apparent that cases could occur outside of the classic high-risk groups. This then called for the use of additional strategies.

Fifty percent of the gay men in San Francisco are infected with the AIDS virus.[6] In the general heterosexual population, the prevalence of HIV infection is less than a fraction of one percent. In this latter group, the progress of the epidemic might be even more insidious because heterosexual individuals often may not know they are infected. The incubation period for AIDS can be up to seven years and possibly longer.[2] An infected individual might be able to carry the virus and unknowingly infect others during this time. Even with mass education campaigns applied to the general population, one cannot assume an overall decrease in unsafe sexual activity. The immediacy of the epidemic is very different among heterosexuals than it has been among homosexual men.

The approach in San Francisco has been to find individuals in the heterosexual community who have been exposed and do not know it and to offer them risk-reduction education and serological testing.[7] If this is not done one will see rivulets of AIDS extending unchecked into the general heterosexual population, resulting in a much larger problem in the future.

Dr Echenberg is Director, Bureau of Communicable Disease Control, San Francisco Department of Public Health, San Francisco, CA.

INTERVENTION STRATEGY

Two strategies have been developed in San Francisco to deal with both high- and low-prevalence groups. In both groups a mass education campaign is being used and in the latter, a contact notification program has been started in addition. An active surveillance program seeks out all AIDS cases in San Francisco and each case is investigated. Anyone who has been diagnosed as having AIDS is asked for the names of their heterosexual partners so that they can be contacted and the situation explained to them. Once the program is explained (we use very sensitive investigators who have had long experience in dealing with sexually transmitted diseases in the community in San Francisco), a very high degree of cooperation is obtained. The identity of the index case is never revealed and the program is completely voluntary. It is permissible for individuals to tell their partners themselves. If in some cases they would rather not participate, that is their prerogative, although that has been rare.

The same techniques have been used in San Francisco during the past few years for over 6,000 cases of syphilis and gonorrhea. Although there is no treatment for AIDS as there is for syphilis and gonorrhea, an intervention is still available. It is possible to tell people who would not otherwise know it that they might be infected. A major assumption of the program is that an individual would not want to infect others unknowingly. The program has located quite a number of women who were infectious and did not know it. In fact most of the individuals named as heterosexual partners are women of childbearing age, so a contact tracing program is especially important in preventing perinatal transmission of HIV.

RESULTS

Twenty-seven heterosexual contacts have been investigated since the beginning of the program. Seven of them were HIV antibody positive. Almost all of them were women of childbearing age. It is interesting that about half of the women had concerns about being infected even before they were contacted by our investigators. They thought they were at risk because of their sexual activities and were greatly relieved when the blood tests proved to be negative. Those who were positive did not know they were infected.

It is extremely important for anyone who is contemplating these kinds of programs to understand that confidentiality is essential. There must be very strong legal protections to safeguard this information from all subpoenas. In addition, there is a need for a precise technical approach based on current knowledge of HIV transmission, as well as a need for very sensitive and informed investigators.

In addition to contact tracing of the heterosexual partners of AIDS patients, we have begun a similar program of contact tracing among individuals who have become infected after having received contaminated blood, and among mothers of pediatric AIDS cases. Partner referral is also encouraged among all HIV-infected cases.

CONCLUSIONS

Each geographic region will have to examine its own AIDS epidemiology. In some situations where the prevalence is extremely high, contact tracing is inefficient and inappropriate. On the other hand, where the number of cases is still small, where there are confidentiality safeguards, and where there are sensitive case counselors, contact tracing and partner referral can play an important role in dealing with the AIDS epidemic by identifying individuals who are unknowingly infected with the AIDS virus.

This technique will be especially useful in dealing with what may be the next phase of the AIDS epidemic, the spread via heterosexual contact into those groups where one now sees the highest rates of syphilis and gonorrhea. These are the same groups among which there is a high level of intravenous drug use. They include adolescents and young adults, especially in minority groups in low-income socioeconomic areas.

In addition, it will become extremely important that all health care providers understand the consequences of their being the first to diagnose HIV infection in a particular individual from a low-prevalence group. These individuals must be advised to refer other sexual partners who might have become unknowingly infected. If this is not done the result will be an unending chain of infections extending further into the community.

REFERENCES

1. Jaffe HW, Feorino PM, Darrow WW, et al: Persistent infection with human T-lymphotropic virus type III/lymphadenopathy-associated virus in apparently healthy homosexual men. *Ann Intern Med* 1985; 102:627–628.

2. Jaffee HW, Darrow WW, Echenberg DF, et al: The acquired immunodeficiency syndrome in a cohort of homosexual men. A six-year follow-up study. *Ann Intern Med* 1985; 103:210–214.

3. Echenberg DF, Rutherford GW, O'Malley P, et al: Update—Acquired immunodeficiency syndrome in the San Francisco cohort study 1978–1985. *MMWR* 1985; 34:573–575.

4. McKusick L, Wiley JA, Coates TJ, et al: Reported changes in the sexual behavior of men at risk for AIDS, San Francisco 1982–1984—the AIDS behavioral research project. *Public Health Rep* 1985; 100:622–629.

5. Rectal gonorrhea in San Francisco, October 1984–September 1986. *San Francisco Epidemiologic Bulletin*, vol 2, no. 12, December 1986.

6. Winkelstein W Jr, Lyman DM, Padian N, et al: Sexual practices and risk of infection by the human immunodeficiency virus. The San Francisco Men's Health Study. *JAMA* 1987; 257:321–325.

7. Echenberg DF: A new strategy to prevent the spread of AIDS among heterosexuals [editorial]. *JAMA* 1985; 254:2129–2130.

Chapter 17
AIDS care in New York City: The comprehensive care alternative

JACK A. DEHOVITZ, MD, MPH, VIRGINIA PELLEGRINO, MSC, MPH

In Chapter 2, Arno and Hughes[1] critically examined the differences in the policy responses of San Francisco and New York City to the epidemic of acquired immunodeficiency syndrome (AIDS). They note that while both cities have devoted an enormous amount of financial support to fighting the epidemic, the timing of the development of specific services varied. For example, the first outpatient program for AIDS patients in San Francisco was opened in September 1981, with the first inpatient unit being established there in July 1983. In contrast, a dedicated AIDS outpatient clinic did not begin in New York until 1984, with the first discrete inpatient unit following in November 1985.[1] Although the San Francisco experience provides an important foundation on which to build, the unique risk-factor and case mix of New York's population of AIDS patients requires the development of innovative programs to deal with these diverse populations.

New York State has embarked on a program to designate comprehensive AIDS centers at various hospitals both in New York City and upstate. The first center was designated at St Clare's Hospital and Health Center in May 1986. From our experience in developing this program, we have developed a framework that addresses the needs of patients with AIDS and other manifestations of HIV infection.

The initial impetus for the development of comprehensive AIDS programs stemmed from the unique medical problems of AIDS patients. While some of the problems resemble those of patients with other catastrophic diseases such as cancer, there are some differences that require unique medical interventions. Perhaps the most obvious is the fact that the clinical spectrum of AIDS and severe human immunodeficiency virus (HIV) infection is extremely variable. Although some patients with Kaposi's

sarcoma (KS) have an excellent prognosis for survival for three to five years, many patients present with an opportunistic infection which leads to rapid deterioration and death. Other patients present with severe dementia without any of the opportunistic infections or cancer that fulfill the current diagnostic criteria for AIDS. In addition to the various acuity levels, the conditions of those who have symptomatic HIV infection are subject to rapid fluctuation. These individuals may be fully ambulatory and feeling relatively well one day, and be acutely ill the next.

Although the opportunistic infections that appear with this disease are not new, the conventional therapies often cause unexpectedly frequent or severe toxicities. Treatment of the various malignancies that accompany HIV-induced immunosuppression is also difficult. Often the use of conventional chemotherapeutic regimens results in severe myelosuppression, or increased risk of opportunistic infection. Finally, the introduction of new antiviral regimens such as azidothymidine (AZT) may be accompanied by toxicities not revealed in comparatively brief initial clinical trials.

As health care professionals have become more experienced in caring for those with HIV infection, several other unique characteristics have emerged which support a comprehensive approach to care. In addition to their complex medical problems, persons with symptomatic HIV infection or asymptomatic seropositivity face intense psychosocial problems. These range from the isolation and stigmatization they encounter from friends, family, and society, to learning to cope with having a terminal illness at an early age.[2]

A majority of AIDS patients develop neurological and psychiatric complications as a result of HIV infection.[3] In addition to recurrent episodes of acute opportunistic infections, many patients will have some clinical manifestation of neurologic disease which can leave them permanently debilitated and unable to live outside of an institutional setting.

The supervision of the care of AIDS patients requires a dedicated team consisting of, at a minimum, infectious disease specialists, oncologists, pulmonologists, and neurologists. As the population of patients with AIDS invariably expands, more broadly trained practitioners such as internists assisted by physician assistants and/or nurse practitioners can extend the expertise of these subspecialists.[4] The availability of a dedicated medical staff will

Dr DeHovitz is Assistant Professor, Department of Preventive Medicine and Community Health, SUNY Health Science Center at Brooklyn, and Assistant Medical Director, Spellman AIDS Program, St Clare's Hospital and Health Center, New York, NY. Ms Pellegrino is Vice-President for Planning at St Clare's Hospital and Health Center.

allow rapid intervention in acute medical problems, improved communication, and increased patient compliance. In addition, the presence of dedicated AIDS practitioners will facilitate the process of clinical investigation.

DESIGNING AN INSTITUTIONAL RESPONSE

In view of the unique dimensions of HIV-related disease described above, the acute care hospital is the only resource that can deliver the range of services this population requires. A comprehensive approach to care may prevent the inappropriate utilization of resources by AIDS patients and ensures that all of the needs of patients with AIDS are addressed.

A hospital-based program for persons with AIDS should endeavor to provide a comprehensive range of services that should include at least the following: acute inpatient services, alternate level of care services, outpatient services, home care services, and access to dental services. In addition, the large number of homeless people with AIDS presents a significant problem in New York City. While housing does not fall within the normal range of services provided directly by hospitals, linkages to community-based organizations involved in this service should be established.

Acute Inpatient Care. A number of acute care hospitals have developed discrete inpatient units as the core service of their AIDS program.[5] While controlled studies have not been done, a discrete unit may be more effective in caring for AIDS patients than scattered placement from both a cost and a quality of care standpoint. In a discrete unit the staff members have chosen to care for AIDS patients, which prevents the isolation and resistance to caring for patients that exists in many hospitals. The availability of extensive psychosocial support services and other specific programs for AIDS patients, which can be readily accomplished in a discrete unit, ensures that patients receive the level and range of services they require. For example, the formation of patient support groups is facilitated in the environment of a discrete unit. A discrete unit also helps to reduce the length of acute hospitalization through focused, early interventions by discharge planning and financial resource staff.

The existence of a discrete inpatient unit alone, however, will not solve the problems of lengthy acute hospital stays. The development of alternate levels of care within institutions and community-based home care and housing services are, therefore, key components of the comprehensive care model.

Alternate Levels of Care. A significant number of AIDS patients being treated in acute care hospitals in New York City are there only because there are no alternatives for them in either an institutional or community-based setting. At St Clare's Hospital, for example, as many as 15% of the patients on any given day do not require acute care services. Within this group of hospitalized AIDS patients are a substantial number who suffer from neurologic or psychiatric conditions associated with HIV infection. These conditions, which include neuropathies and severe dementias, frequently require long-term institutional care, but not at an acute care level. The level and type of services that these patients require do not cur-

rently exist in the institutional sector and will have to be developed.

The solution to the alternate level of care needs of many of these patients cannot be achieved simply by increasing access to traditional skilled nursing facilities. The services they need may be more comparable to a general acute care service than a long term care service as traditionally defined. Hospitals should consider developing extended care units for persons with neurologic or psychiatric conditions related to HIV infection as part of the development of the comprehensive care model.

Outpatient Services. The development of a multi-faceted outpatient program is an essential component of the comprehensive care model. A full range of services should be available, from HIV screening through diagnosis and treatment.

The outpatient program should be designed with two goals in mind. First, it should result in decreased use of the emergency room by AIDS patients. Second, it should facilitate the referral of patients to the appropriate level of outpatient care. To accomplish these goals, a triage system should be implemented to assess patient needs and rapidly integrate individuals ranging from the worried well to those who are acutely ill. Using a triage system, for example, new patients are evaluated by an adult nurse practitioner and referred to the appropriate service within the outpatient program. The triage system can also facilitate the response to current outpatients who need to be seen by someone immediately rather than waiting for their scheduled appointment.

In the outpatient setting a primary care physician and/ or physician extender, ideally one who is also involved in the inpatient unit, should be assigned to each patient.[6] A full range of multispecialty services must also be available, such as neurology, gastroenterology, hematology/ oncology, and dermatology.

An important service of the outpatient program is ambulatory infusion therapy. Through this program patients can receive intravenous antibiotics and blood transfusions on an outpatient basis. This program has significant cost-saving potential since the alternative is short-term admission to the hospital. It also provides a psychological benefit for AIDS patients by allowing them to remain at home.

A comprehensive outpatient program for people with HIV infection must also include a mental health component. Persons with HIV infection—ranging from those who are seropositive to those with confirmed AIDS—face multiple psychosocial issues which are appropriately addressed on an outpatient basis. As in the inpatient program, the outpatient service should use various types of support groups as well as individual counseling.

The high number of intravenous (IV) drug abusers among the AIDS patients in New York City necessitates that linkages be established to drug treatment programs. In some instances hospitals should consider developing a methadone maintenance treatment program or other drug treatment program as a component of the outpatient service. The integration of drug treatment services with other services for persons with AIDS is essential to address the increasing problem of IV drug abusers with AIDS being admitted to the hospital for therapy for an opportunistic infection, responding appropriately to therapy, and then returning to actively using drugs after discharge.[7]

Dental Services. The provision of dental services is another important component of the comprehensive care program for persons with HIV infection. Dental professionals should be an integral part of the medical and support team caring for persons with HIV infection.

There are several diseases associated with HIV infection which manifest themselves in the head and neck region. These diseases include discrete oral lesions which can be detected and treated early by trained dental professionals. Also, many patients with AIDS experience excessive weight loss, a condition which is often exacerbated by dental problems that can be effectively treated.

In addition to treating dental problems, a considerable amount of clinical research can be done by the dentists involved in a comprehensive care setting. These dentists can also design and conduct educational programs for the dental community at large regarding the treatment of patients with AIDS.[8]

Home Care. Out-of-hospital management of AIDS patients requires rigorous planning and close integration with inpatient services. In addition to simple assistance with activities of daily living, AIDS patients at home often require sophisticated and specialized nursing intervention. For example, they may require IV hydration because of persistent diarrhea, IV antibiotics because of an opportunistic infection, or even simple intramuscular injection of narcotics for pain control.

Other service components of community-based care, such as home attendant care, residential facility support, and home hospice care, overlap with the needs for specialized nursing intervention. The hospital provides the ideal site for the coordination of such services. In this way management plans can be designed in consultation with both hospital-based and community-based nursing personnel prior to discharge. It will also encourage careful monitoring of the patient after discharge. This coordination between inpatient, outpatient, and community-based staff will prevent frequent and avoidable readmissions as well as provide a means of communication for the various staff members.

The Visiting Nurse Service (VNS) of New York currently provides home care for patients in New York City who are Medicaid eligible and have AIDS. In 1986 they provided care to over 1,000 patients in the five boroughs.[9] Although both the quality and breadth of services offered is exceptional, delays in instituting services, as well as communication problems, have resulted in both increased length of stay as well as avoidable readmissions. To address this problem plans are underway to staff comprehensive AIDS programs with VNS personnel to facilitate the transition from inpatient care to home care.

CONCLUSION

The scope of the AIDS epidemic in New York and the unique characteristics of the disease demand that hospitals, as the focal point of the health care system, develop an immediate response to addressing the needs of persons with HIV infection. The most appropriate and meaningful approach is one which is comprehensive and incorporates diverse levels of services.

The comprehensive care model as described represents an appropriate hospital-based response to this epidemic for the immediate future. However, in the absence of an effective vaccine or antiviral therapy to alter the course of the epidemic, we will be faced with over 10,000 severely ill individuals with HIV infection in New York City by 1991. As an outgrowth of the implementation of the comprehensive care model, presumably at multiple hospitals throughout New York City, it may become necessary, as has been suggested, to designate specialized regional hospital centers for the care of persons with HIV infection.[10] This option, however, requires careful study because of the implications it may have for further isolation of this population.

REFERENCES

1. Arno PS, Hughes RG: Local policy responses to the AIDS epidemic: New York and San Francisco. *NY State J Med* 1987; 87:264–272.
2. Morin SF, Charles KA, Malyon AK: The psychological impact of AIDS on gay men. *Am Psychol* 1984; 39:1288–1293.
3. Navia BA, Jordon BD, Price RW: The AIDS dementia complex: I. Clinical features. *Ann Neurol* 1986; 19:517–524.
4. Institute of Medicine, National Academy of Sciences: *Confronting AIDS: Directions for Public Health, Health Care and Research.* Washington, DC, National Academy Press, 1986, p 140.
5. Volberding PA: The clinical spectrum of the acquired immunodeficiency syndrome: Implications for comprehensive patient care. *Ann Intern Med* 1985; 103:729–733.
6. LaCamera DJ, Masur H, Henderson DK: Symposium on infections in the immunocompromised host. The acquired immunodeficiency syndrome. *Nurs Clin North Am* 1985; 20:241–256.
7. DeHovitz J. Planning for the AIDS epidemic: Public health control measures and the provision of patient care. *J Community Health* 1986; 11:215–218.
8. Andriolo M, Rosenberg J, Wolf J: AIDS and AIDS-related complex: Oral manifestations and treatment. *J Am Dental Assoc* 1986; 113:586–589.
9. *AIDS Program Summary.* New York, Visiting Nurse Service, 1986.
10. Barnes D: AIDS stresses health care in San Francisco. *Science* 1987; 253:964.

Chapter 18
The epidemiology of HIV in New York State

Lloyd F. Novick, MD, MPH; Benedict I. Truman, MD; J. Stan Lehman, MPH

This examination of the epidemiology of acquired immunodeficiency syndrome (AIDS) by the New York State Department of Health (NYSDOH) in 1987 takes into account three factors. First, New York State has the largest number of reported AIDS cases of any state. As of October 28, 1987, there were 12,790 cases reported among New York State residents.[1] However, the prevalence of AIDS is not uniform throughout New York State communities and displays marked variation by age, sex, race, and geography. Further, the dominance of risk factors and the phase of the epidemic vary between regions within the state. New York State, excluding New York City, has approximately 10% of the total cases. However, this proportion still accounts for 1,181 cases, with an additional 432 cases occurring among prisoners housed in New York State Department of Correction facilities. If New York City cases were excluded, New York State would have the sixth highest number of cases among the 50 states.

The second critical factor in any consideration of AIDS epidemiology in New York State is that most of the information describing the epidemic has relied on reported AIDS cases. Reporting of AIDS cases may not in fact reflect the true number of cases, as described in a recent report by New York City Department of Health staff members on deaths of intravenous (IV) drug users.[2] Further, reported cases of AIDS represent only one part of the spectrum of disorders related to human immunodeficiency virus (HIV) infection. The lag time between HIV infection and the appearance of reportable cases, compounded by the largely unknown natural history of this infection, limits the value of relying on reports of disease to understand the distribution and extent of the epidemic. However, reliance on case reports alone will soon no longer be necessary. The capability now exists to determine the extent of HIV infection in the New York State population, particularly in a number of subgroups.

Another critical issue in regard to AIDS epidemiology in New York State is the validity of projections that forecast the future course of the epidemic. At NYSDOH, projections have been developed that rely on the past experience with AIDS as described by surveillance. This projection forecasts 46,000 cumulative cases in 1991.[3] The problem with this type of projection is that it is based on a static mathematical model reflecting past experience. It does not take into account the current or future dynamics of the epidemic, such as changes in the size of the pool of susceptible individuals or in the frequency or types of contacts between individuals.

ACQUIRED IMMUNODEFICIENCY SYNDROME IN NEW YORK STATE

At the beginning of the epidemic in 1982, the majority of AIDS cases in the United States were reported from New York State. By 1987, the proportion of national AIDS cases reported by New York State had declined to 30% (Fig 1), and this rate is projected to decrease to 17% by 1991. The rate of increase for the United States as a whole is now greater than that for New York State.

Figure 2 shows the number of reported cases of AIDS in adults in New York State and in the United States by month of diagnosis. Approximately 370 cases of AIDS are reported each month in New York State. Some 325 cases per month are reported by New York City and 45 are reported by upstate New York (Fig 3).[1] The ratio of cases reported by upstate New York in relation to New York City has remained constant (Fig 4). The increasing number of upstate counties with confirmed AIDS cases demonstrates the spread of this epidemic. By the end of 1986,

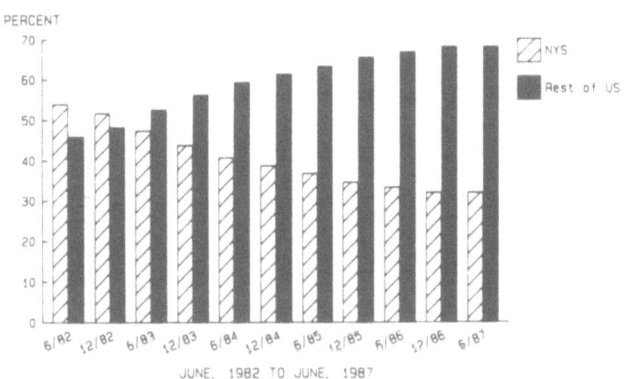

FIGURE 1. Percent of cumulative AIDS cases in the United States reported from New York State at six-month intervals, June 1982 through June 1987.[1]

Dr Novick is Director of the Center for Community Health, Dr Truman is Director of the AIDS Epidemiology Program, and Mr Lehman is a research scientist for the AIDS Epidemiology Program of the New York State Department of Health.

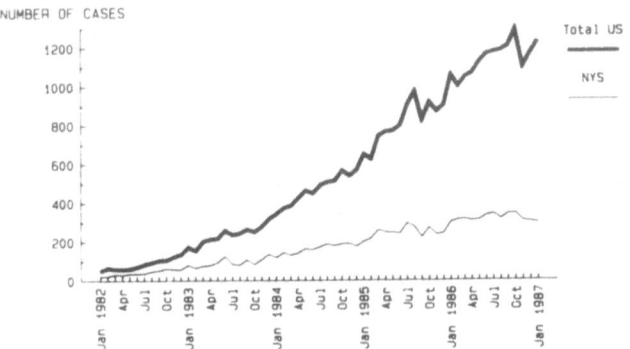

FIGURE 2. Reported cases of AIDS in adults among New York State residents and total in United States by month of diagnosis, January 1982 to January 1987.[1]

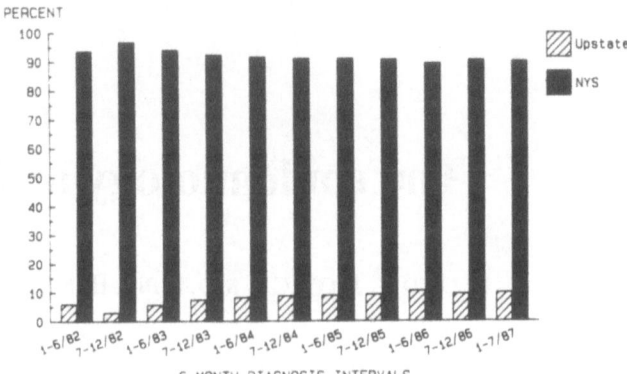

FIGURE 4. Percent of reported New York State adult AIDS cases from upstate general population, by six-month intervals of diagnosis, as of July 17, 1987.[1]

52 out of 57 upstate New York counties had reported AIDS cases (Fig 5). In New York City, the largest number of reported cases as of June 1987 was in Manhattan (5,914), followed by Brooklyn (2,269) and the Bronx (1,634).[4]

Adult AIDS cases in the 57 upstate counties were grouped into four regions on the basis of the degree of urbanization, physical proximity to New York City, and cumulative burden of AIDS to date. Region 1 (New York City vicinity) includes Nassau, Suffolk, and Westchester counties. Together they account for 61% of the AIDS morbidity outside of New York City. They are highly urbanized areas and closest to the New York epicenter. Region 2 (Mid-Hudson Valley) includes the counties of Dutchess, Orange, Putnam, Rockland, Sullivan, and Ulster. Further away from New York City and less urbanized, these counties account for 11.5% of cumulative AIDS morbidity upstate. Region 3 (urban upstate) includes the counties of Albany, Schenectady, Onondaga, Erie, and Monroe. These highly urbanized counties include the cities of Albany, Schenectady, Syracuse, Rochester, and Buffalo. They are physically distant from New York City, yet the factors that contribute to the spread of AIDS in New York City may also be operating in these communities. Region 3 accounts for 18% of the upstate AIDS morbidity. Region 4 (upstate rural) includes the remaining 43 counties outside of New York City. These counties are as far away from New York City as those of region 3, but only one has reported more than ten cases of AIDS. Nine have reported no cases. Region 4 is composed mainly of

small towns and rural communities, and accounts for 9.5% of the upstate morbidity.

AGE, SEX, RACE, AND RISK FACTORS

The percentage distribution of adult AIDS cases is shown in Figure 6 by age group and by place of residence at time of diagnosis. In New York City, New York State, and the United States, the age group 20-39 years accounts for the majority of cases.[3,4] For both New York City and upstate, about 10% of the reported cases are among women (Fig 7). This is approximately twice the proportion observed in the United States as a whole and can be related to the prominence of IV drug use as a risk factor in New York State.

Distribution of adult AIDS cases by race and place of residence at time of diagnosis is shown in Figure 8. In New York City approximately 25% of the AIDS patients are Hispanic and 30% are black. Thus, the majority of the reported AIDS cases occurred in minority groups. Conversely, whites account for 67% and 68% of the cases reported from upstate New York and from the United States, respectively.

Reported risk groups for New York State AIDS cases are shown in Figure 9. Of these risk groups, homosexual or bisexual behaviors can be related to approximately 50% of the cases, and IV drug use is a factor in approximately 35% of the cases.

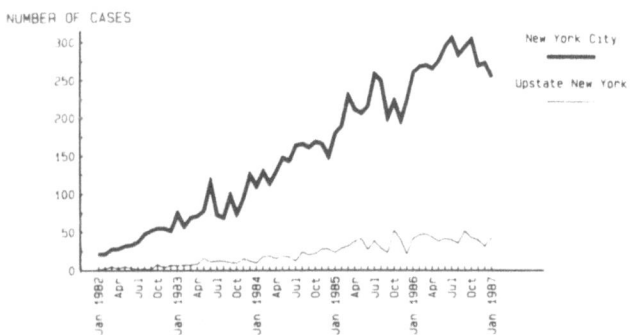

FIGURE 3. Reported cases of AIDS in adults among residents of New York City and upstate New York, by month of diagnosis, January 1982 to January 1987.[1]

YEAR	CUMULATIVE NUMBER OF COUNTIES	CUMULATIVE NUMBER OF CASES
<1982	3	6
1982	11	46
1983	20	171
1984	29	402
1985	45	799
1986	52	1301

FIGURE 5. Upstate counties with confirmed AIDS cases (inmate or general population) by year of diagnosis.[1]

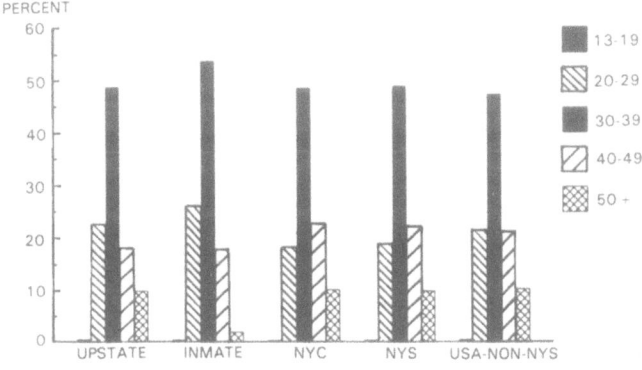

FIGURE 6. Percentage distribution of adult AIDS cases by age group and place of residence at time of diagnosis, as of July 17, 1987.[1]

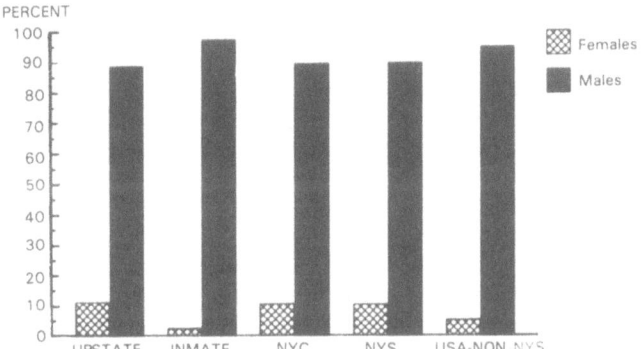

FIGURE 7. Percentage of adult AIDS cases by sex and place of residence at time of diagnosis, as of July 17, 1987.[1]

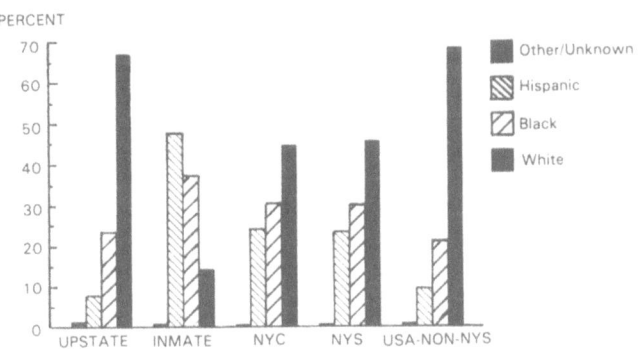

FIGURE 8. Percentage distribution of adult AIDS cases by race and place of residence at time of diagnosis, as of July 17, 1987.[1]

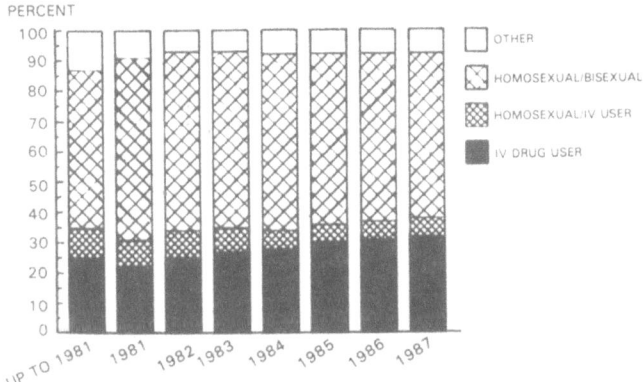

FIGURE 9. New York State AIDS risk groups, percent distribution by year, as of July 17, 1987.[1]

The distribution of adult AIDS cases by risk group varies by place of residence (Fig 10). The major difference between both upstate and New York City and the rest of the United States is the proportion of IV drug users. This proportion is approximately 35% for New York City and upstate and only 15% for the rest of the United States.

Of interest is that the upstate proportion for IV drug use as a risk factor is similar to that of New York City. Examining the IV drug use risk factor by the four regions described earlier, however, a different pattern emerges. In Region 1 (New York City vicinity) and Region 2 (Mid-Hudson Valley), the proportion of IV drug abuse as a risk factor is similar to that of New York City. However, for Region 3 (upstate urban), designated as urban and including a number of upstate cities, the proportion of drug abusers is somewhat lower (28%), and in Region 4 (upstate rural) only 15% have a drug abuse risk factor.

Risk and race distribution among New York State men with AIDS is shown in Figure 11. Among blacks and Hispanics, IV drug abuse is the leading risk factor (50% and 55%, respectively). However, among whites, IV drug abuse is reported among 15% of the cases.

A dissimilar pattern is found among women (Fig 12). IV drug use is the most common risk factor for black, Hispanic, and white women.

PROJECTIONS

In 1991, incident cases per year are projected to be approximately 8,100 for New York City and 9,600 for New York State as a whole (Fig 13).

The adult AIDS cases diagnosed each month between January 1984 and December 1986 (adjusted for reporting

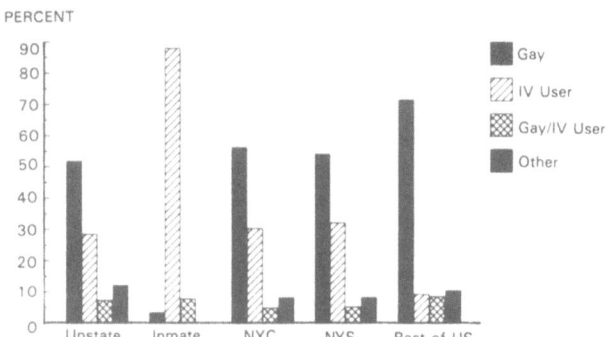

FIGURE 10. Percentage distribution of adult AIDS cases by risk group and place of residence at time of diagnosis, as of July 17, 1987.[1]

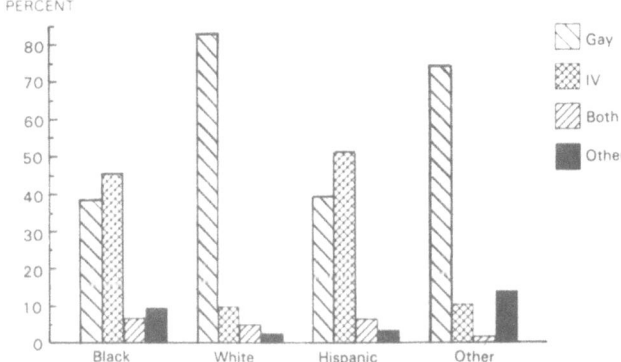

FIGURE 11. New York State men with AIDS by risk group and race/ethnicity.[1]

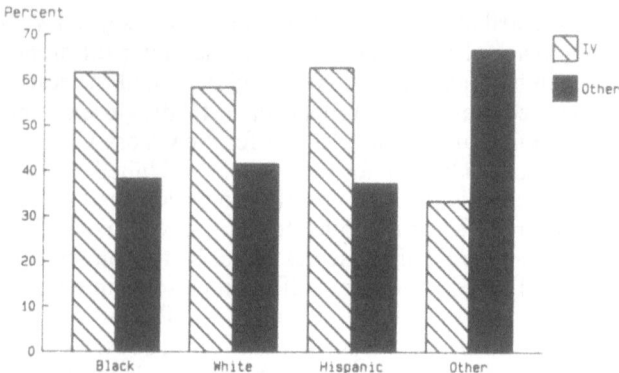

FIGURE 12. New York State women with AIDS by risk group and race/ethnicity.[1]

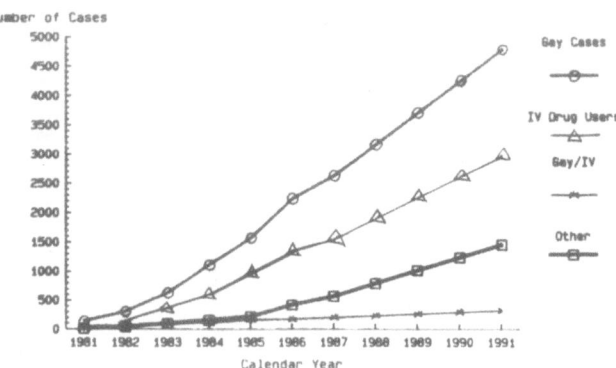

FIGURE 14. New York State AIDS cases by risk group. Cases for 1987 to 1991 are projected.

lag) were divided into five risk group categories: homosexual and bisexual males, IV drug abusers, a group reporting both homosexual and IV drug use behaviors, women of childbearing age, and a group reporting other risk factors. For each category a linear model was extrapolated forward to predict the monthly incidence of AIDS cases through 1991 (Fig 14). These predictions are simply linear extrapolations and do not take into account changes in the dynamics of the epidemic or the susceptibility of various groups. Projections of AIDS cases among women in New York State indicated a 100% increase by 1991 (Fig 15).

A revised case definition for surveillance of acquired immunodeficiency syndrome was instituted by the Centers for Disease Control in the fall of 1987.[5] The major proposed changes applied to patients with laboratory evidence of HIV infection. This new definition includes HIV encephalopathy, HIV wasting syndrome, and a broad array of specific indicator diseases. The inclusion of AIDS patients whose indicator diseases are diagnosed presumptively and the elimination of exclusions due to other causes of immunodeficiency were also important revisions to the surveillance case definition.

The change in definition is expected to increase the number of reportable cases by 13% (Fig 16). Projected prevalent and incident cases taking into account the new definition are shown in Figure 17.

NEW YORK STATE DEPARTMENT OF HEALTH SEROPREVALENCE STUDY

A seroprevalence study comprising a group of studies is

being implemented to better determine the HIV antibody prevalence in the population of New York State. This initiative is necessary because of the lack of information about HIV infection in our communities. Previous estimates of the extent of HIV infection have been speculative and not useful for planning or preventive purposes.

Seroprevalence is determined in a number of groups by utilizing blood specimens collected for other purposes. Groups undergoing testing include newborns; clients of family planning clinics, sexually transmitted disease and tuberculosis clinics, and drug treatment programs; and prison entrants. Hospital and emergency room admissions and other categories may be considered in the future for this type of study.

In the newborn study, mandatory blood specimens for detection of hereditary disorders are obtained from all newborn infants prior to discharge or within 14 days of birth and submitted to the NYSDOH Wadsworth Center for Laboratories and Research in Albany, NY. Since maternal antibodies cross the placenta, serologic testing of newborns reflects the HIV antibody status of the mother and not necessarily infection of the infant.

Testing of all specimens is completely blind. The absence of identifying information will protect the anonymity of the individual. Efforts are made to provide the women with information about HIV and to assure the availability of testing and counseling where this is elected.

As of February 5, 1988, 40,259 blood specimens of new-

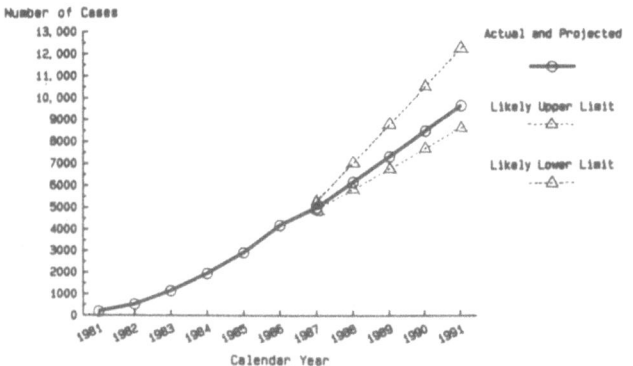

FIGURE 13. New York State AIDS cases with upper and lower limits. Cases for 1987 to 1991 are projected.

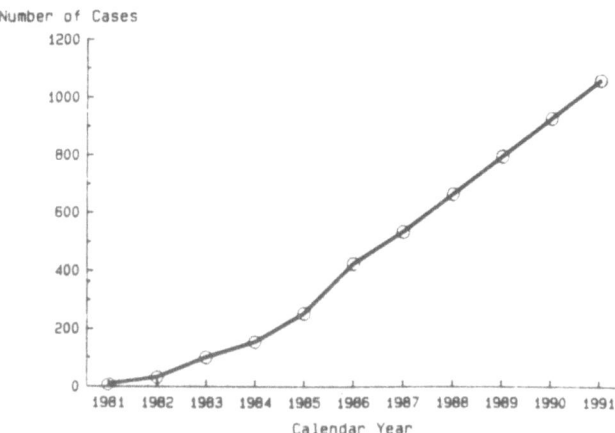

FIGURE 15. New York State AIDS cases in women aged 15 to 44. Cases for 1987 to 1991 are projected.

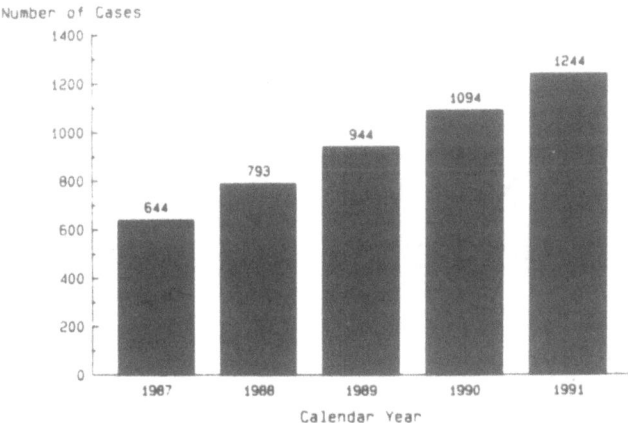

FIGURE 16.   Potential added New York State AIDS cases from 1987 to 1991. New case definition increases incident cases by 13%. Mortality experience will remain constant.

borns had been submitted and analyzed for HIV serologic status. The overall seroprevalence rate was 0.84 percent. These seroprevalence rates were 293/18,718 births (1.57%) for New York City and 36/20,809 births (0.18%) for upstate New York. Substantial rates of infection in New York City are linked to areas where intravenous drug abuse is predominant.

Information gained from this type of study can be utilized to develop programs for preventive recommendations and activities. These include educational programs

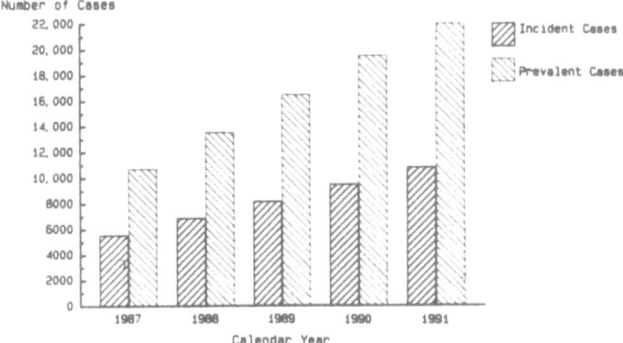

FIGURE 17.   New definition projected prevalent and incident New York State AIDS cases, 1987 to 1991.

and expanded counseling and testing. A similar seroprevalence testing effort has been initiated by the Centers for Disease Control. A "family of studies" is being implemented in 30 cities across the country, including 20 high prevalence areas and ten low prevalence areas. New York State is the site of two of these studies, with New York City designated as a high prevalence and Rochester as a low prevalence area.

Seroprevalence studies in New York State have already increased our knowledge of the extent of infection with human immunodeficiency virus. Measurements of seroprevalence over time will lead to a better understanding of the future course of this epidemic. Relationships can now be elucidated between cases of reported AIDS and HIV seroprevalence, especially for particular groups such as infants and young children.

A blind methodology utilizing available blood specimens in the New York State seroprevalence study cannot fully access a cross section of the general population and, therefore, actual prevalence in the entire population cannot be determined. However, an estimate of the prevalence of HIV infection, heretofore unavailable, is now available for subpopulations including women at the time of childbirth. The proportion of this group that is infected has profound implications for the community at large.

These serosurveys supplement but do not supplant case report information for AIDS. In many cases, case information obtained will complement the knowledge obtained from serosurveys, but we will also undoubtedly learn in the near future from an epidemiology based on population and community rather than derived from cases of illness.

REFERENCES

1.   AIDS Epidemiology Program, Bureau of Communicable Disease Control, Division of Epidemiology, New York State Department of Health.

2.   Stoneburner RL, Des Jarlais DC, Guigli P, et al: Increasing mortality among intravenous drug users in New York City and its relationship to the AIDS epidemic: Evidence for a longevity specimen of HIV-related disease. Presented at the 115th Annual Meeting of the American Public Health Association, New Orleans, La, October 18, 1987.

3.   Bureau of Communicable Disease Control: Estimating AIDS-related morbidity and mortality in New York State through 1991. New York State Department of Health, December 5, 1986.

4.   AIDS Surveillance Unit: AIDS Surveillance Update. New York State Department of Health, November 25, 1987.

5.   Centers for Disease Control: Revision of the CDC surveillance case definition for acquired immunodeficiency syndrome. *MMWR* 1987; 36(1S).

Chapter 19

The impact of AIDS on New York's not-for-profit hospitals

KENNETH E. RASKE

Surgeon General Dr C. Everett Koop has been quoted as saying, "How many are infected? That's our whole problem—we don't know that number."[1] The numbers we do know tell the story of the ever-worsening problem of acquired immunodeficiency syndrome (AIDS) in New York City. As of October 19, 1987, the US Centers for Disease Control (CDC) reported 11,166 diagnosed cases of AIDS in New York City, placing the city at the top of the AIDS census.[2] Approximately 30% of AIDS cases nationwide have been reported from New York.

The AIDS patient profile in New York City is unique. Whereas other cities with a large AIDS population see more uniformity in the risk factors relating to the incidence of AIDS, risk factors in New York City's caseload are diverse, including intravenous drug use and transmission of AIDS through both heterosexual and homosexual activity and from mothers to babies at birth.

THE AIDS CENSUS

The Greater New York Hospital Association's (GNYHA) recent survey of not-for-profit voluntary and public hospitals, conducted in June 1987 with the Health and Hospitals Corporation (HHC), showed 1,266 AIDS and AIDS-related complex (ARC) inpatients in New York City (Fig 1). That is a full 18% over the number reported in GNYHA's first survey of AIDS and ARC inpatients in March 1987, when a total of 1,071 were counted. The results of GNYHA's latest survey revealed an average daily census of 1,335 patients with AIDS or suspected AIDS in New York City during the week of October 18, 1987. According to these figures, the number of hospitalized patients with AIDS or suspected AIDS increased overall by 24.6% between March and October 1987. However, the census increase from June to October (5.5%) was considerably less than the March to June increase.

This new demand on health care resources comes at a time when New York's hospitals are stretched to capacity. A spot check of occupancy rates of not-for-profit voluntary and municipal hospitals in October 1987 showed 34 of 46 voluntary hospitals citywide at or above 90% occupancy, as were all 11 municipal hospitals. Seventeen of the

voluntary hospitals were at or above 100% occupancy. Throughout the voluntary hospital system, 379 patients were awaiting admission in emergency rooms.

This bottleneck in the system is created by the overcrowding problem, as the capacity of New York's hospital system is pushed to its natural limit. As hospital occupancy increases and demand for beds outpaces supply, patients are forced to wait in emergency rooms for admission, making it more and more difficult for emergency rooms to accommodate additional emergency cases. Indeed, GNYHA's same spot survey showed that of 37 hospitals, 22 had either asked for and been refused or were on diversion status from 911.

While the increasing numbers of AIDS and ARC patients may be an easy explanation of the occupancy problem of hospitals in New York, it is likely not the complete explanation. The New York State Department of Health is currently undertaking an analysis of additional factors that may be affecting occupancy, including changes in the number of alternate level of care days, patterns of elective surgery, and average lengths of stay. GNYHA will be cooperating with Department of Health officials on this project and will be contributing data for analysis.

PLANNING AIDS TREATMENT FOR THE FUTURE

A major part of the challenge of coping with the AIDS crisis is literally predicting the future, and then planning

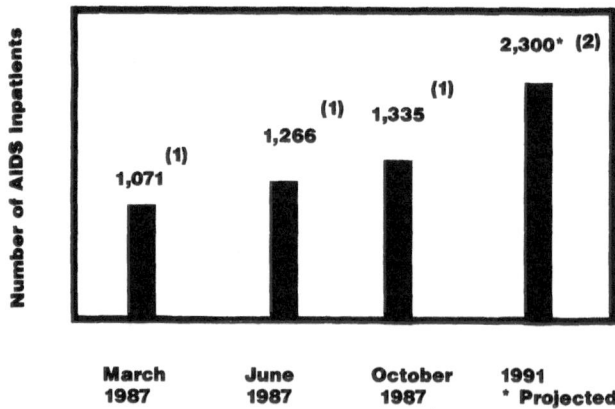

FIGURE 1. Inpatients in New York City with AIDS and AIDS-related complex (Sources: (1) GNYHA and Health and Hospitals Corporation; (2) New York State Department of Health.)

Mr Raske is President of the Greater New York Hospital Association, New York, NY.

for it. That is no easy task, as is seen from the differing numbers of AIDS cases predicted by city and state officials and other sources. According to recently released figures presented in a New York State Department of Health draft report, by 1991 New York City will have an average daily inpatient census of more than 2,300 patients with AIDS or AIDS-related illnesses.[3] The mid-point projection of these figures for 1987–1988, at 1,296, is close to GNYHA's June 1987 survey figure of 1,266 AIDS inpatients.

These new estimates reflect a substantial upward revision from previous Department of Health estimates. Since these figures corroborate GNYHA's actual count of AIDS inpatients, they may be more reliable than other predictions. But some would argue that even those figures may be too low. However, the appropriate question is not who may eventually be right and who may be wrong in estimating future numbers of AIDS patients, but rather finding a way to provide current information and to update estimates accordingly. Projection equations, therefore, should be adjusted periodically, perhaps quarterly, to reflect the most recent experience. In the final analysis, we need to be alerted to the need for a resource response to any changes in demand.

COSTS OF TREATING AIDS INPATIENTS

As the number of AIDS and ARC patients in New York City increases, so do the demands on the health care system, from nursing and social work to laundry, housekeeping, and dietary facilities. In April 1986, GNYHA commissioned a study of the differential cost increase in treating AIDS patients over the average per diem cost.[4] The following routine cost centers at the two hospital study sites were significantly affected by the AIDS caseload: general nursing service, central services, social work, housekeeping, laundry and linen services, and dietary services. The study found that the cost of treating AIDS patients was approximately 22% greater than the cost of treating an average medical/surgical patient. (The reported total health bills for AIDS patients from time of diagnosis to time of death ranged from a low of approximately $42,000 to a high of $150,000.[5])

Hospitals, it was found, assign more nursing resources to the care of AIDS patients, who require up to 28% more nursing hours per patient day than average medical/surgical patients. In addition, AIDS patients incur four times as many bed linen changes as the average medical/surgical patient. Every AIDS patient receives social work services, while cases with social work referrals, in general, are a small proportion (approximately 17.5%) of the total patient population. Hospitals follow more extensive room cleaning procedures for isolation patients, and many AIDS patients require such precautions. And as the incidence of AIDS increases, the overall costs of treating potentially infectious waste will clearly rise.

Based on this study of the routine costs of treating AIDS patients, and a state-generated analysis of SPARCS data, in which a 19.6% difference for ancillary components including laboratory, radiology, blood bank, pharmacy, and other services was identified, the New York State Department of Health agreed to adjust hospital reimbursement rates for AIDS patients. The new rates, applied to inpatient days from 1984 to 1987, provide for a 22.5% increase in the routine portion of the inpatient rate and a 19.5% increase in the ancillary component. This rate adjustment, designed to account for the costs of treating AIDS patients, is applicable to the current reimbursement methodology entitled the New York Prospective Hospital Reimbursement Methodology.

The state has also developed an initiative to designate some hospitals as AIDS Centers, a concept which GNYHA supports because of its potential to increase access and quality services and to enhance coordination of the continuum of care—all appropriate goals for the treatment of AIDS patients and all patients with chronic and terminal illnesses. AIDS Centers receive a prospective per diem reimbursement rate for treating AIDS patients with Medicaid and Blue Cross based on budgeted costs approved by the state. It will be important to monitor and evaluate the appropriateness and adequacy of this payment approach to allow each center to meet the comprehensive care requirements of AIDS patients and to comply with state standards. The performance of both the AIDS Centers and other hospitals that care for AIDS patients should also be carefully examined in terms of organizational structure, cost, and quality of care.

As we move into the case payment system in 1988, a distinct series of diagnosis related groups (DRGs) to recognize the illnesses of AIDS patients will be utilized to reflect greater accuracy in the weights assigned to AIDS cases, and therefore the resource intensity and payment on behalf of AIDS patients. While it is the providers' responsibility to deliver quality care, it is GNYHA's belief that the state has a public responsibility to continue to recognize the financial implications of delivering this care and to reimburse hospitals accordingly.

STAFFING DEMANDS: THE BURNOUT FACTOR

Use of hospital resources is not only measured in dollars, however. In addition to the medical interventions and treatments and support services required to manage the disease, hospital staff members who have contact with AIDS patients are frequently called on to provide emotional support to patients and their friends and relatives, to assist in daily living tasks, to identify appropriate community resources, and to assist in preparations for death. Unfortunately, few staff members are adequately prepared to deal with the full range of needs of AIDS patients. And this shortcoming has become more and more apparent as the number of AIDS patients grows.

Individuals who choose careers in health professions seek to cure sickness, save lives, and improve the overall quality of life. Modern medicine permits the overwhelming majority of patients to recover fully from episodes of illness and to return to productive lives. Occasionally, however, this outcome is not achieved. Such is the case with AIDS patients. Furthermore, the unique needs of these patients create problems for patients and health care workers alike. The result may be the psychological burnout of the professional and support staff. One must remember, however, that there are tens of thousands of health care workers who come face to face with AIDS patients every day and who provide them with compassionate, quality care. Their daily heroics should not be dwarfed by the isolated cases we hear so much of in news reports of health care professionals who may be reluctant to treat AIDS patients.

GNYHA is keenly aware of the demands on hospital staff and the additional stress involved in caring for patients with AIDS. In a major project, Greater New York Hospital Foundation, Inc, a subsidiary of GNYHA, in cooperation with representatives of the academic community in New York City, is developing an educational program aimed at health care personnel working primarily in hospitals and long term care facilities. It is being designed with major funding support from the W.K. Kellogg Foundation and supplemental funding from the United Hospital Fund of New York and the Health Services Improvement Fund. The pilot sessions to help health care personnel cope with the treatment of AIDS and other chronic illnesses took place in April 1988.[6]

It is still to be determined how the prevalence of AIDS affects recruitment and retention of interns and residents, a question of great concern for this city's major teaching hospitals. GNYHA is currently drafting a grant proposal and will soon be seeking funding to explore this issue.

UNIVERSAL PRECAUTIONS

Clearly, AIDS patients draw more heavily on existing resources and practices in the health care system than do patients who do not have AIDS. In addition, management of the disease is necessitating major changes in daily hospital operations. In August 1987, the CDC published revised recommendations for the prevention of transmission of the AIDS virus in the health care setting. In establishing "universal blood and body fluid precautions," this document emphasized the need for health care workers to consider all patients as potentially infected with the AIDS virus and to adhere rigorously to infection control precautions for minimizing the risk of exposure to blood and body fluids. These precautionary procedures are especially important in emergency care settings where the risk of exposure to blood is increased and the infection status of the patient is usually unknown.[7] GNYHA has asked the CDC for clarification of its universal precautions guidelines regarding the possible waste disposal implications of these procedures.

These new procedures have practical consequences. It is no surprise, for example, that GNYHA's group purchasing arm reports a 30–40% increase in orders for gloves from 1986 to 1987. Some back orders for the latex gloves preferred by hospital personnel have taken as long as two to three months to fill.

CONCLUSION

AIDS has left no component of the health care delivery system untouched. However, facing us today is not merely an assessment of a present problem and a measurement of current resources. We must confront the long term future of treating patients with AIDS and AIDS-related diseases. There are no quick, temporary solutions to the AIDS problem and, barring a medical miracle, AIDS will be a continuing health care challenge at least until the end of the century. All involved parties, including the New York State Legislature, the New York State Department of Health, the New York City Department of Health, GNYHA, Health and Hospitals Corporation, Health Systems Agency of New York City, and others must work closely together to develop and implement effective solutions.

Most importantly, bed needs in New York City must be reassessed to reflect the demands of AIDS cases and to build a reserve capacity of 10–15% into the acute care system to respond to other emergencies. Assessing the current situation, it appears that by 1991 a minimum of two to three new or refurbished hospital facilities must be added to the stock of hospitals in New York City. Public policymakers must begin examining ways to get new capital on line at the appropriate times. In the meantime, we must also find new ways to channel inpatient care into alternate delivery systems.

When an AIDS patient no longer requires the services of an acute care institution, a major stumbling block to timely and humane discharge has been the lack of appropriate community or long term care placement options. Placement options for all AIDS patients, especially the very difficult to place intravenous drug users and babies who have AIDS, need to be established. Organized home care services, hospice services, and beds in long term care facilities need to be encouraged and increased, and options for day care services and support services for children of AIDS patients need to be explored.

In addition, improvements to the present system of delivering outpatient services to AIDS patients should be examined. Since 1981, however, reimbursement for clinic services provided to Medicaid patients in New York State has been capped at an all-inclusive rate of $60 per visit. Such reimbursement constraints do not encourage creativity and innovation. AIDS Centers do receive special pricing for providing outpatient services to AIDS patients, however, the majority of hospitals caring for AIDS patients today are not designated as AIDS Centers. Reimbursement rates, therefore, need to address the resource requirements and costs for treating a significant segment of the AIDS population. We must continue to study and evaluate outpatient costs of treating AIDS patients, and consequent adjustment to the clinic rate cap relating to AIDS should be recommended.

In many instances, however, neither long-term placement options nor outpatient services will be able to provide the care AIDS patients require. In the final analysis, there may prove to be no substitute for acute inpatient care in the complete treatment of AIDS patients. How the health care community responds to the AIDS epidemic in the coming months and years will determine not only the future treatment of AIDS but the future of the health care system as well. If we are to continue to respond meaningfully to the needs of patients with AIDS and AIDS-related illnesses for quality health care, responsible and effective planning must begin immediately.

REFERENCES

1. "AIDS forecasts are grim—and disparate." *NY Times*, October 25, 1987, p 24.
2. *AIDS Weekly Surveillance Report—United States AIDS Program*. Atlanta, Centers for Disease Control, October 19, 1987.
3. *Health Care Resource Requirements for AIDS Patients in New York State, 1986–1991*. New York State Department of Health, October 1987 (draft).
4. *Study of Routine Costs of Treating Hospitalized AIDS Patients*. New

York, Peat, Marwick, Mitchell & Co, April 1986.
  5. Peyser N: AIDS—Implications for health care providers. *Amherst Q* 1987 (Fall), p 2.
  6. *Coping with Chronic and Terminal Illness: A Model Education Program*

for Hospital Staff. New York, Greater New York Hospital Foundation, Inc, November 14, 1986 (revised).
  7. Centers for Disease Control: Recommendations for prevention of HIV transmission in health-care settings. *MMWR* 1987; 36:3S–18S.

Chapter 20
AIDS in Connecticut

JAMES L. HADLER, MD, MPH; JULIA WANG MILLER, PHD; MARGE EICHLER, RN, MPH

In order to understand the epidemiology of acquired immunodeficiency syndrome (AIDS) in Connecticut, it is important to review the demographic features that underlie the manner in which the data have been analyzed.

Connecticut is by far the smallest of the three states in the tri-state (New York, New Jersey, Connecticut) area. With a population of 3.2 million, it is the 25th largest state in the US.[1] Geopolitically, it is divided into eight counties and 169 towns. Unlike in New York and New Jersey, the counties have little political significance. There are no county governments or county health departments. Rather, the relevant political and health organization is at the town level. Correspondingly, for practical epidemiologic purposes, most data analysis is done at the town level. For a disease such as AIDS, in which morbidity is measured as cumulative incidence per million population, this can pose difficulties, as the average town population is only 20,000.

The five largest towns have between 100,000 and 150,000 residents. When their metropolitan areas are taken into consideration, their populations expand to between 200,000 and 700,000. The population is most dense in the southwest corner close to New York City: nearly half the population lives in Fairfield and New Haven counties, in the urban-suburban corridor leading out of New York City (Fig 1, areas labelled 1). The rest of the state is predominantly suburban and rural with the one exception of the City of Hartford.

In terms of proximity to New York City, Connecticut can be divided up by county into four regions with decreasing commuting and public transportation potential to reach the city. These are shown in Figure 1.

Racially, Connecticut's population is mainly white: 87% white, 7% black, and 4% Hispanic, making it the state with the lowest proportion of minorities in the tri-state area.[1 (pp 220–221,225)] Most of the minority population lives in seven towns in the southwest corner of the state (Fig 1); these towns comprise 24% of the total state population, but house 70% of all black and Hispanic persons.

Finally, in spite of Connecticut's ranking as one of the wealthiest states in the US, and in spite of the small size of its urban areas, at least three of these towns have neighborhoods in which socioeconomic conditions are nearly as poor as any to be found in New York or New Jersey. These towns are Bridgeport, New Haven, and Hartford.

EPIDEMIOLOGY OF AIDS IN CONNECTICUT

Although Connecticut is small and lacks large urban centers, the epidemiology of AIDS in Connecticut is more similar to than different from the epidemiology of AIDS in New York or New Jersey.

Magnitude of the AIDS Problem. The magnitude of the AIDS problem in Connecticut is relatively large. As of October 15, 1987, 515 cases of AIDS had been reported for a cumulative incidence ratio (CIR) of 156 cases per million population. Nationally, Connecticut ranked 14th among states in number of cases reported, and ninth in per capita incidence (expressed as CIR), behind New York (first, CIR of 683) and New Jersey (third, CIR of 347) but ahead of New York State minus New York City (CIR of 129).

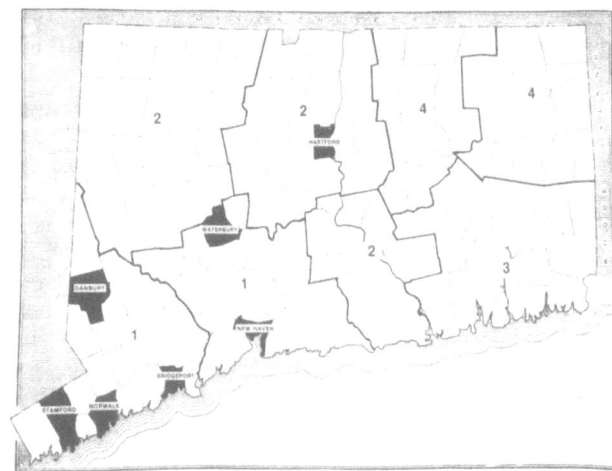

FIGURE 1. Map of Connecticut by region, counties, and major cities. Region 1, Fairchild and New Haven counties; Region 2, Litchfield, Hartford, and Middlesex counties; Region 3, New London County; Region 4, Tolland and Windham counties. Regions are numbered in decreasing proximity to New York City. Towns outlined in black include Stamford, Norwalk, Bridgeport, New Haven, Danbury, Waterbury, and Hartford.

From the Connecticut State Department of Health Services, Epidemiology Section, Hartford, Conn.

In spite of their small size, urban-metropolitan areas of Connecticut also have a relatively significant AIDS problem. Until mid-1987, the Centers for Disease Control routinely reported information ranking metropolitan areas (expressed as Standard Metropolitan Statistical Areas (SMSAs)) with ten or more AIDS cases by CIR. As of June 19, 1987, three Connecticut SMSAs ranked in the top 30 nationally, along with two from New York and five from New Jersey. These included New York City (CIR, 1,083), Jersey City (CIR, 790), Newark (CIR, 458), Patterson (CIR, 413), New Haven (CIR, 307), Poughkeepsie (CIR, 298), Trenton (CIR, 266), Norwalk (CIR, 213), Stamford (CIR, 201), and New Brunswick (CIR, 198). More focally, the City of New Haven had a CIR of 848 at that time. Thus, Connecticut has geographic foci of AIDS which would be of major concern anywhere.

Finally, projections based on Connecticut data have not yet been made. However, Connecticut has contributed a steady 1.2% to the national total of reported AIDS cases. Borrowing from the projections made by the US Public Health Service at Coolfont, West Virginia, in 1986 and assuming that the Connecticut contribution will remain stable, more than 800 new cases are expected to be reported in 1991. On the other hand, this assumption may not hold up. As the next section demonstrates, the dynamics of AIDS in Connecticut are somewhat different than those nationally.

AIDS by Transmission Category. Table I shows the relative contribution to AIDS by underlying risk behavior category and trends over time. As with New York and New Jersey, Connecticut has a much higher proportion of AIDS cases comprising intravenous (IV) drug users than is seen nationally (33% vs 16%). In addition, the relative percentage of all cases attributable to IV drug use has been increasing over time, so that IV drug use is becoming the leading AIDS risk behavior in Connecticut. The trend toward an increasing contribution to AIDS incidence from intravenous drug users has not been observed nationally.

In parallel to the increase of AIDS in IV drug users, the percentage of AIDS cases attributable to heterosexual contact has also increased (Table I). Nearly all of these cases are the sexual partners of IV drug users.

AIDS by Sex. Connecticut also has a much higher proportion of AIDS cases among women than is seen nationally (16% vs 7%). Overall, Connecticut ranks third nationally in sex- and race-specific incidence in women, behind only New York and New Jersey (Table II). Thus, women in the tri-state area have the highest AIDS risk of women anywhere in the country. The risk to women is largely related to IV drug use. More than 80% of the women with AIDS in Connecticut are either intravenous drug users (56%) or their sexual partners (25%).

Pediatric AIDS. The theme for pediatric AIDS is similar to that for AIDS in women: Connecticut has a disproportionately high representation, and most of the cases are directly or indirectly IV drug related. As of mid-October 1987, 3.1% of Connecticut's AIDS cases were in children, compared to 1.4% nationally. Eighty percent (12/15) were directly or indirectly related to IV drug use.

AIDS in Minorities. Minorities in Connecticut have been at particularly high risk of AIDS. Although only

TABLE I. Transmission Categories for AIDS Trends Over Time, Connecticut, October 30, 1987

Transmission Category	1980–1983	1984–1985	1986–1987	All Years	P-value Trend
Homosexual/bisexual*	51%	46%	40%	43%	.08
Intravenous drug user*	20%	27%	39%	33%	.002
Heterosexual†	0%	3%	6%	4%	.05
Total cases	41	173	273	487	

* Excluding those with both homosexual/bisexual and intravenous drug use exposure.
† Excluding persons whose heterosexual risk was birth in a country where heterosexual transmission is believed to be the primary mode of transmission.

11% of the population is black or Hispanic, nearly 50% of all reported AIDS cases have occurred in these two groups. Furthermore, blacks and Hispanics in Connecticut have a higher relative risk of AIDS than do their counterparts nationally. Compared to whites, blacks in Connecticut have been 8.6 times more likely to have developed AIDS; Hispanics have been 7.1 times more likely. Nationally, the comparable figures are 3.0 for each. This high relative risk has been corroborated in seroprevalence studies in Connecticut. Black and Hispanic men and women attending sexually transmitted disease (STD) clinics and counseling and testing sites, entering methadone clinics, and taking the human immunodeficiency virus (HIV) antibody test as part of military recruitment all have more than four times the probability of being seropositive than their white counterparts. This disproportionate representation among minorities is of major importance in devising and targeting prevention efforts in Connecticut.

Among minorities, intravenous drug use and sexual transmission from drug users appear to be the largest sources of HIV transmission. Altogether, 76% of AIDS cases in minorities have been drug related: 61% in drug users, 9% in heterosexual contacts of drug users, and another 6% in their offspring. Although only 21% of minority AIDS cases have been in homosexual/bisexual men, 22% of all cases in homosexual/bisexual men have been minorities, a figure that is double the minority population representation. Thus, prevention efforts targeted to minorities need to be directed at all types of risk behavior, including drug use, sexual transmission, and perinatal transmission.

AIDS by Place. AIDS in Connecticut is not equally distributed geographically. Residents of urban areas have been at considerably greater risk than residents of non-

TABLE II. Cumulative AIDS Incidence Ratios* in Women By State† and Race, July 29, 1987

State	Race		
	White	Black	Hispanic
New York	4.5	69.9	64.7
New Jersey	4.0	76.0	22.6
Connecticut	2.4	50.8	20.1
Massachusetts	1.9	30.7	7.9
California	1.7	(6.2)	(1.8)
Florida	1.5	51.0	(2.6)

* Cases per million population, 1980 census.
† Highest ranking states nationally by incidence in white women. Numbers in parentheses indicate less than top six ranking.

TABLE III. AIDS Incidence in Connecticut By Proximity to New York City and Year of Diagnosis, October 15, 1987

Region*	1980–83	1984–85	1986–87	CIR†	RR‡
1	78%	67%	66%	220	3.8
2	22%	27%	28%	129	2.2
3	—	3%	4%	71	1.2
4	—	4%	2%	58	—
Total cases	41	171	303	—	—

* Regions defined by county (Fig 1).
† Cumulative incidence ratio: no. AIDS cases/population in millions.
‡ Risk ratio of the region compared to Region 4.

urban areas. Sixty percent of AIDS cases have occurred in residents of seven towns comprising only 24% of the population (Bridgeport, Danbury, Hartford, New Haven, Norwalk, Stamford, Waterbury). Residents of these seven towns have been 4.6 times more likely to develop AIDS than nonresidents, based on comparison of CIRs. When analyzed by race-ethnicity, whites in the seven towns have had 2.7 times the risk of their nonurban counterparts, and minority groups have had 2.1 times the risk.

New York City AIDS Connection. Connecticut's geographic proximity to New York City and the ease with which the city can be reached by public transportation make it likely that much of Connecticut's AIDS problem, at least initially, represented spread from the New York "epicenter." At least four types of epidemiologic information suggest that this is what did indeed occur.

First, all initial AIDS cases in Connecticut occurred in the southwest region in the urban-surburban corridor leading out of New York City. No cases were seen east of the Connecticut River until 1984 (Table III, Regions 3 and 4). Second, as part of surveillance during 1983–1984, randomly selected incident AIDS patients, including both gay men and intravenous drug users, were interviewed as to where their risk-taking behavior had taken place. All interviewed persons had been to New York City for either shooting gallery use or sexual activity in bathhouses between 1980 and the time their disease was diagnosed.

In addition, the incidence of AIDS increases the closer one gets to New York City, at least at the county level (Table III). Finally, in the one statewide seroprevalence study, entrants to methadone clinics closer to New York have been more likely to have antibodies to HIV than those further from New York. This has been true regardless of race-ethnicity (Figure 2).

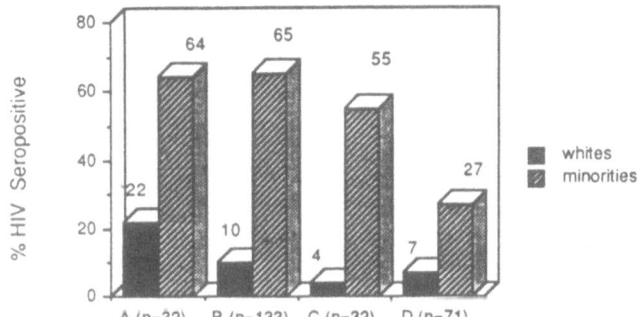

FIGURE 2. HIV seropositivity in methadone clinic entrants by proximity to New York City, for Connecticut, March 1986–March 1987. (Location A is nearest New York City, location D is furthest.)

TABLE IV. Sources of HIV Antibody Seroprevalence, Connecticut, October 30, 1987

Source	Group Tested	Number Tested	Percent Seropositive*	RR† in Minorities
Anonymous counseling and testing sites (3/86–6/87)	Total	2,200	6.9	3.5
	Intravenous drug abusers	306	18.3	—
	Homosexual men	699	10.6	—
	Heterosexuals	938	1.9	—
Methadone maintenance clinics (3/86–3/87)	Intravenous drug abusers	268	24.0	5.0
Sexually transmitted disease clinic (3/87–10/87)‡	Clients	159	3.8	
Military (10/85–9/87)	Recruits	11,287	0.14	8.3
Red Cross, Connecticut chapter (1/87–9/87)	Donors	152,124	0.005	—

* Confirmed seropositive by Western blot.
† Relative risk = probability of seropositivity for blacks and Hispanics divided by probability for whites only.
‡ Six out of 90 minority group members vs 6 out of 67 whites were seropositive.

Although these data suggest that at least some of the AIDS cases in Connecticut, especially early on, have been attributable to exposure to HIV in New York City, it is clear that there is indigenous transmission as well. Many of the seropositive intravenous drug users have not been to shooting galleries outside of Connecticut, there is an increasingly wide geographic distribution of cases within the state (Table III), and nearly all of the cases involving heterosexual contacts and children appear to have been acquired in the state.

Seroprevalence Studies. As of October 1987 there were five ongoing sources of information on HIV antibody seroprevalence in Connecticut. These are shown in Table IV. As noted previously, race-ethnicity has been the best predictor of seropositivity in each of these, thus far.

There will be an expansion of surveillance for seroprevalence in 1988. Additional multiyear seroprevalence studies that have started or will begin shortly include seroprevalence in tuberculosis cases statewide, in newborns statewide using the filter paper disc method, and in additional selected sexually transmitted disease clinics, family planning clinics, and prenatal clinics. Particular emphasis will be placed on the newborn study. It is hoped that this will become a major component of Connecticut's surveillance to monitor the extent of ongoing transmission of HIV to women and children.

REFERENCE

1. *The World Almanac and Book of Facts 1987*. New York, Pharos Books, 1987, pp 220–221.

Chapter 21
Current issues concerning AIDS in New York City

STEPHEN C. JOSEPH, MD, MPH

This is a critical period in the acquired immunodeficiency syndrome (AIDS) epidemic. Today's public policy decisions will determine the state of the epidemic, and its impact on New York City, five, seven, and even ten years hence.

As of October 1987, 12,000 people had been diagnosed with AIDS in New York City—comprising 28% of the national total—with more than 6,500 deaths. More than 300 new cases of AIDS are reported every month. AIDS is the current leading cause of death in the city among men aged 25–44 years and women aged 25–34 years.[1]

Currently, upwards of 400,000 New Yorkers are estimated to be infected with the human immunodeficiency virus (HIV), including some 250,000 homosexual and bisexual men and 120,000 intravenous (IV) drug abusers.

AIDS AMONG INTRAVENOUS DRUG ABUSERS

Dr Rand Stoneburner, Director of AIDS Research for the New York City Department of Health, presented a paper at the recent American Public Health Association meeting that received a good deal of media attention.[2] It is important to understand the relevance of Dr Stoneburner's findings. For more than three years, we have reported what we think is a compelling hypothesis that the number of HIV-related deaths is substantially undercounted in the IV drug abuser community because of shortcomings in the Centers for Disease Control (CDC) case definition. We now estimate that the number of AIDS-related deaths among IV drug abusers in New York City is more than 150% higher than previously thought.[2]

A study of all drug-related deaths in the city from 1982 through 1986 found that an additional 2,500 people died of AIDS-related conditions than we had previously counted in our surveillance. These deaths are not included because they did not meet the strict federal definition of AIDS. Investigation of death records revealed, over time, this evidence of excess mortality among IV drug abusers. When we sampled charts of people who died of nonspecific pneumonia, endocarditis, and tuberculosis, many charts exhibited evidence of HIV infection or symptoms compatible with AIDS, such as oral thrush.[2]

If the HIV mortality rate is readjusted to account for these excess deaths, AIDS-related deaths involving IV drug abusers would account for 53% of all AIDS-related deaths in New York City since the epidemic began, while deaths among homosexual men would account for 38%. Previous figures showed that homosexual men accounted for 55% of all AIDS-related deaths, and intravenous drug abusers for 31%[2] (Fig 1). These figures represent a compelling hypothesis that needs validation.

Besides increasing the number of drug abusers who are so sick with HIV-related illness that they are dying, the new data are disturbing because recent evidence suggests that people at the end stage of illness have a return of viremia, making them more infectious and a greater danger to the community than in the middle stage of the illness. The actual rates of transmission from addicts here may be underestimated.

This is particularly worrisome because IV drug abusers have been the main conduit of HIV infection to women and children (Fig 2). Of the more than 1,200 cases of AIDS in women in New York City, 80% have been IV drug abusers or their sex partners. Most of the 231 children with AIDS were infected through their mothers, 80% of whom were IV drug abusers or their sex partners (Fig 3).

Epidemiologic investigation and early results of serologic surveys have shown that HIV infection in heterosexuals is primarily linked to exposure to IV drug users or bisexual men. There is little current evidence for secondary or tertiary spread among heterosexuals. The large pool of infected people in New York City does increase the

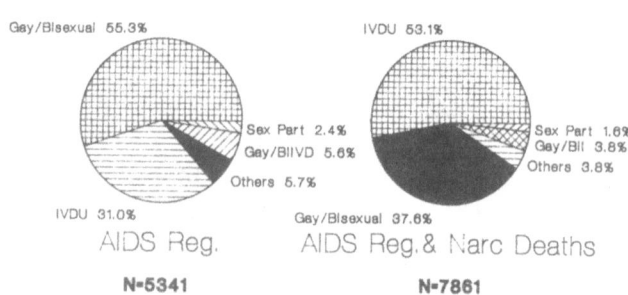

FIGURE 1.   Postulated impact of narcotic deaths on total AIDS mortality by risk group, New York City, 1982–1986.

Dr Joseph is the New York City Commissioner of Health.

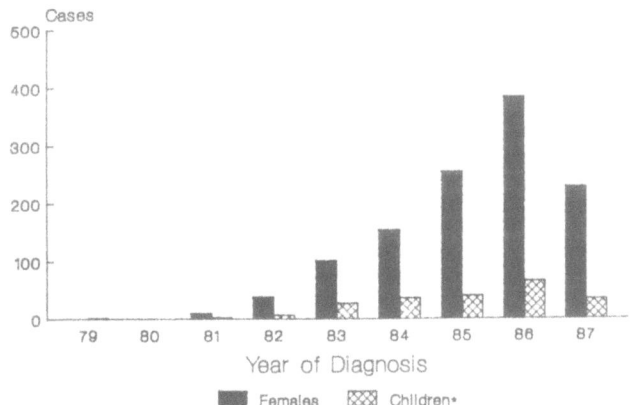

FIGURE 2. AIDS incidence among women and children in New York City, August 1987 (preliminary data). Transfusion-associated cases are excluded.

probability of HIV spread through heterosexual sex. At particular risk are sex partners of IV drug users, who are mostly minority women.

A Department of Health study is now under way to determine the rate of HIV infection among women at high risk, primarily IV drug users and sex partners of men at high risk. Early results indicate that 40% of these women are infected. Early results from Health Department studies estimate that 1.5% of all women in New York City who become pregnant may be infected with HIV.

Three-quarters of the children with AIDS in New York City have died, most by the age of three years. An estimated 600 HIV-infected children are expected to be born this year. Among teenagers aged 13 to 19 years, 35 AIDS cases have been reported. Ominously, young women represent 40% of these cases, compared to 11% of all AIDS cases. Half the adolescent women with AIDS in New York City were IV drug users or their sex partners.

With IV drug use concentrated in the city's poorest neighborhoods, the AIDS epidemic is hitting minorities the hardest. Thirty-one percent of the city's AIDS cases are among blacks; 23% are among Hispanics. Eighty-six percent of male IV drug users with AIDS and 90% of mothers of children with AIDS are black or Hispanic (Fig 4).

AIDS PROJECTIONS

The best current estimates project that by the end of 1991, over 43,000 people will have developed full-blown AIDS in New York City; 32,000 will have died (Fig 5). More AIDS cases will have been diagnosed here in 1991 alone than have shown up from 1981 through 1986 (Fig 6).

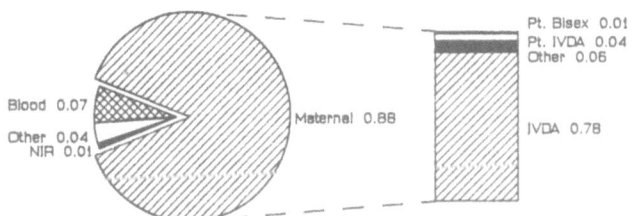

FIGURE 3. New York City pediatric AIDS cases by risk groups, March 1987.

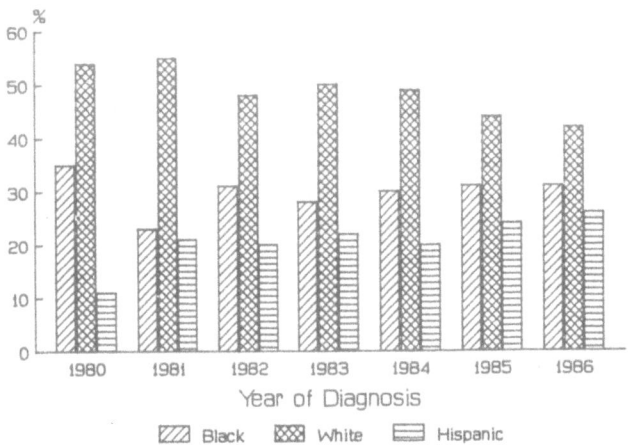

FIGURE 4. AIDS incidence in New York City by race/ethnicity.

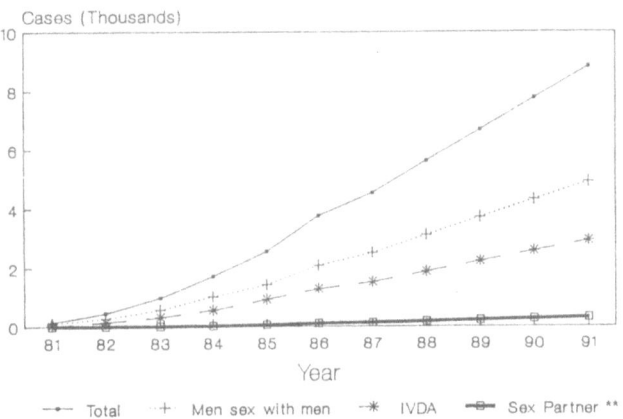

FIGURE 5. AIDS incidence in New York City, 1981–1991.

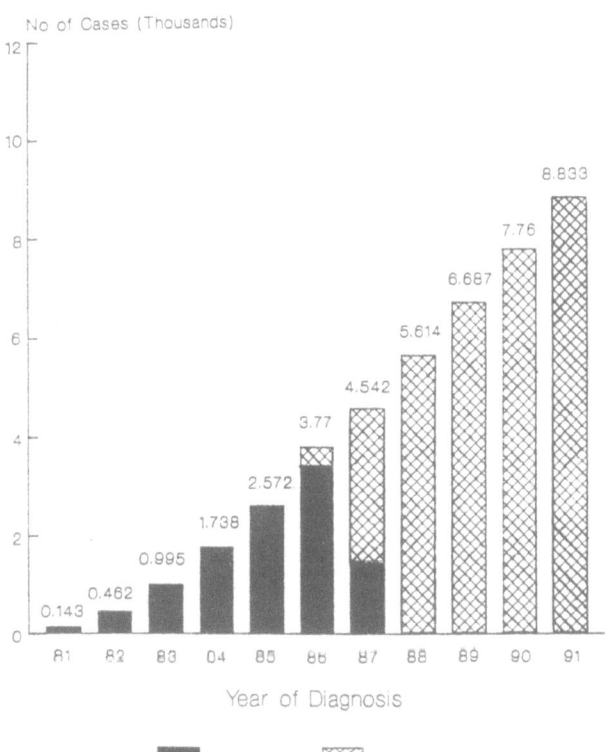

FIGURE 6. AIDS incidence in the total population (August 17, 1987).

Among men, close to 37,000 cumulative AIDS cases are projected for 1991, compared with 6,000 for women (Fig 7). By 1991, women will have accounted for 13% of the total cases, compared with 11% presently (Fig 8). Homosexual men will represent 24,000 cases, 56% of the total (Fig 9); 14,500 cumulative cases are projected among IV drug users, 34% of the total (Fig 10). Almost 2,800 cumulative cases are projected among young people aged 13 to 24 years (Fig 11).

These projections assume that the rates of the last six months will remain constant over the next four years. They reflect only cases already counted, using the current standard case definition. They do not include the newly reported figures that reflect the undercounting of mortality among addicts. These would greatly inflate the current number of persons ill with HIV infection and the deaths from HIV-related illness, as well as increase the projections for the future by as much as 150% for drug abusers.

These estimates challenge us to understand the patterns of infection, control the spread of the virus, protect people from AIDS-related discrimination, and provide medical care and social service support to those sick from the disease. Long term resource requirements for clinical care and social, mental health, housing, hospice, and respite services are major concerns. If a vaccine or effective treatment were developed, resource demands would still intensify as the number of people with AIDS continues to rise.

HOSPITAL SERVICES

Hospital services in particular will be strained by the increase in AIDS incidence. On any day, more than 1,200 people with AIDS or AIDS-related illnesses occupy city hospital beds, including 420 in municipal hospitals. The

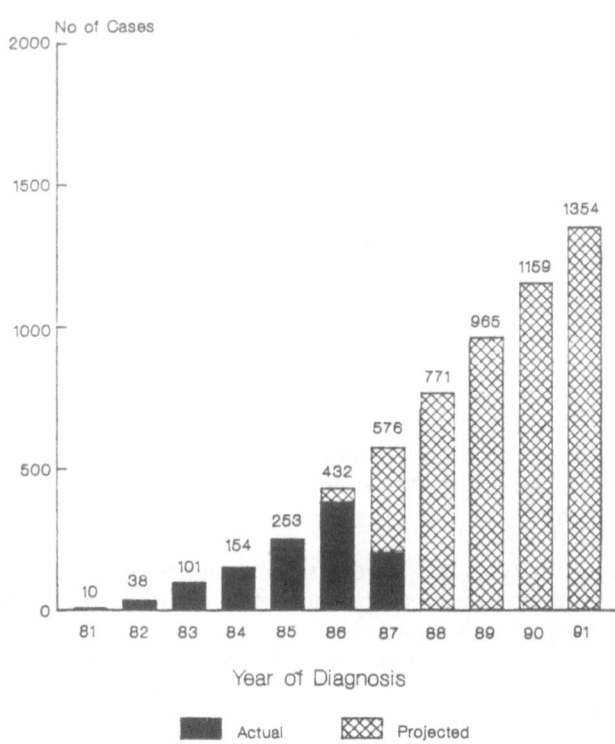

FIGURE 8.   AIDS incidence in the female population (August 17, 1987).

annual cost of treating AIDS patients here is projected to reach $1 billion a year by 1991.

The HIV-related patient census in the Health and Hospitals Corporation (HHC) is expected to rise at least 20%

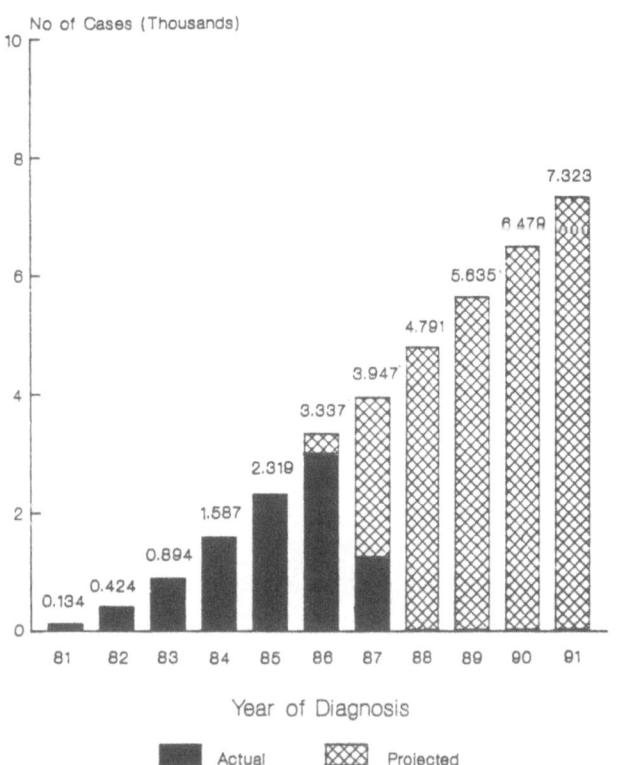

FIGURE 7.   AIDS incidence in the male population (August 17, 1987).

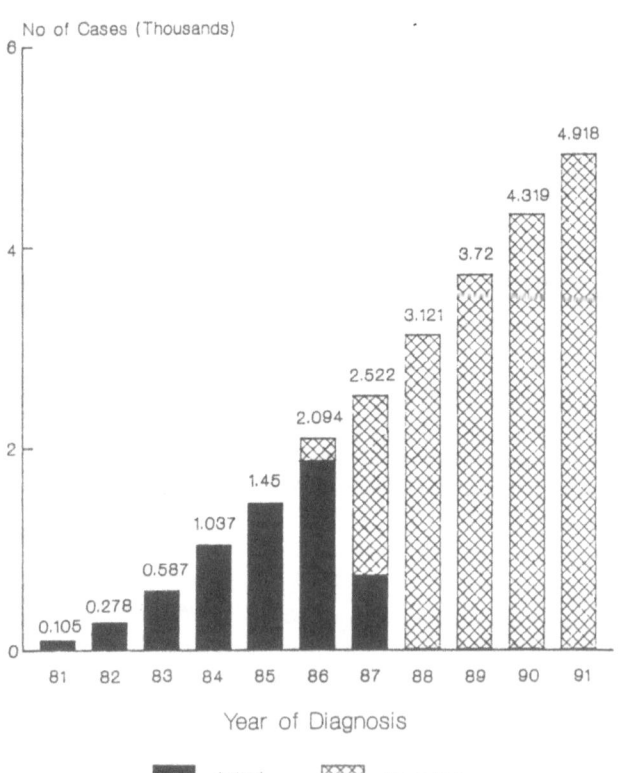

FIGURE 9.   AIDS incidence in the male homosexual, non-intravenous drug abuser population (August 17, 1987).

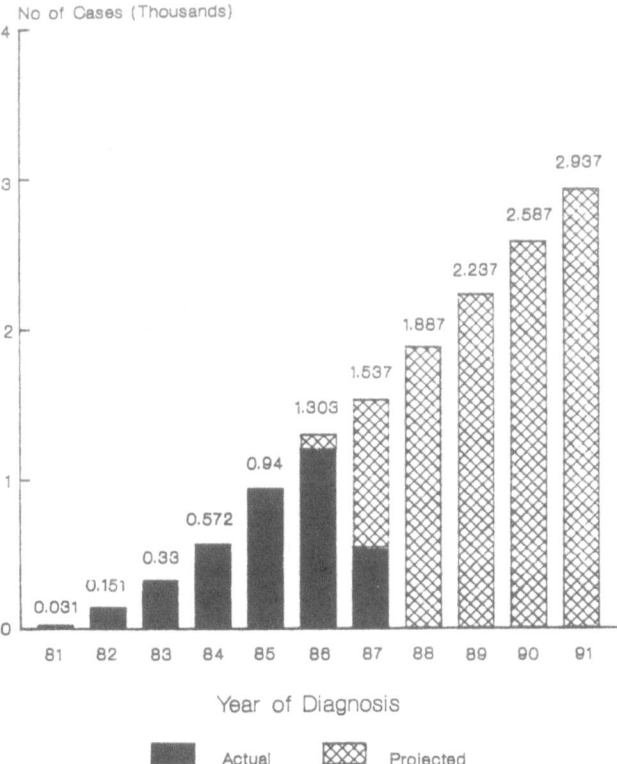

FIGURE 10. AIDS incidence in the intravenous drug abuser population (August 17, 1987).

annually, including a large share of substance abusers with poorer health status. Already, 75% of AIDS patients at HHC hospitals contracted the virus from IV drug use,

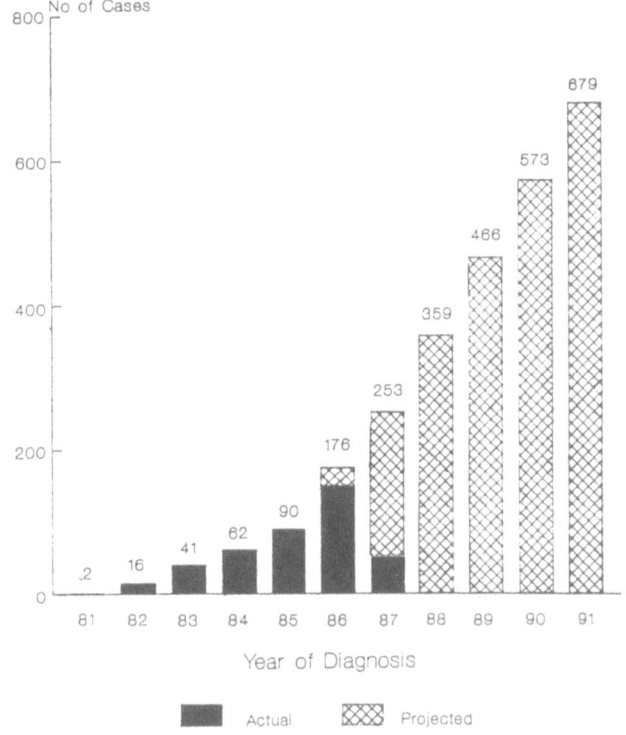

FIGURE 11. AIDS incidence among persons aged 13–24 years (August 17, 1987).

including direct drug use, sexual contact with a drug user, or being born to an intravenous drug abuser or sex partner. With inadequate federal and state reimbursement, the burden of funding for unreimbursed care for AIDS patients will continue to fall on the city, and especially its public hospitals.

For the increasing numbers of patients with AIDS, HHC provides AIDS-related clinical assessment, complete inpatient and outpatient medical care, and extended care services. The Human Resources Administration provides emergency shelter and assists in housing matters and AIDS-related problems with family and children's services. The Department of Mental Health is developing outpatient clinics and day-treatment services for persons with AIDS, and for families and friends affected by AIDS. The AIDS Discrimination Unit of the City Human Rights Commission is handling an increasing number of complaints of AIDS-related discrimination.

PUBLIC HEALTH EDUCATION

A pattern of discrimination against people known to be or even suspected of being infected with HIV has emerged in employment, education, housing, and health care and financial services. To eliminate this, AIDS education efforts must be increased, and legislation supported that protects against discrimination and unauthorized or inappropriate disclosures of confidential health records.

New York City has mounted an all-out effort to stop the spread of HIV infection. This effort includes several elements.

First, the New York City Department of Health is increasing public health education risk reduction efforts. In fiscal 1988, projected spending for the department's AIDS prevention activities will be $8.4 million. This includes $7.1 million for a range of public health education programs that direct education to the general public and target special programs to people engaged in high-risk sex and drug behavior.

Recently, the department launched the second in a series of frank multimedia advertising campaigns, this one directed at intravenous drug users. The first series promoted the use of condoms among heterosexuals to prevent the spread of AIDS. A third campaign will soon promote abstinence among adolescents, and a fourth will reinforce the prevention message to homosexual men.

The department is increasing its outreach program to people practicing high-risk behaviors. Public health educators take the message of prevention into neighborhoods where IV drug use is high to reach drug users and their sex partners. This complements the state's activities in directly providing AIDS education to intravenous drug users in treatment programs, shooting galleries, and on the streets. The outreach program is expanding from nine to 15 communities and works with many citywide and local groups to reach those at risk through drug abuse.

Half of the roughly 100,000 people who move through the city correctional system each year are current or former IV drug users, and 50–60% of these are estimated to be HIV-positive. A Health and Correction Departments program educates city jail inmates about AIDS and distributes condoms to those at highest risk of infection to slow transmission in and out of jail. Prison Health Services offers inmates risk-reduction counseling and voluntary, confidential HIV testing.

To reach people before they take part in unsafe sex, public health educators distribute educational literature and condoms at sex clubs, massage parlors, and other places where patrons seek multiple sex encounters or unsafe sex.

RISK-REDUCTION COUNSELING

A critical element of prevention efforts is an aggressive, extensive program to increase voluntary, confidential risk-reduction counseling and HIV antibody testing. The New York City Department of Health's intensive voluntary, confidential counseling and HIV antibody testing helps to increase people's awareness of their risk and encourages them to change their behavior to reduce the chance of becoming infected or infecting others.

Testing is available at free, anonymous test sites, including the department's three Anonymous Counseling and Testing Sites (to expand to five in fiscal 1988), through any licensed physician, and at the department's sexually transmitted disease clinics. In fiscal 1987, the department's Bureau of Laboratories performed a total of 108,635 tests, approximately 13 times as many as in fiscal 1986. In fiscal 1988, the department will be able to test more than 450 specimens a day because of increased funding; currently, an average of 300 samples are tested daily.

The department's contact notification program actively helps HIV-infected people to notify their contacts. This service will soon be offered to the AIDS/ARC patients of private physicians.

The department's counseling and testing policy recommends that physicians routinely discuss AIDS infection and risk-avoiding behavior with their patients, and offer counseling and testing to patients at risk. Thus far, this has not occurred to the extent mandated by the epidemic; fewer than 3,000 of the 25,000 city physicians have sent blood specimens of at least one of their patients to the department's laboratory for testing. Physicians must assume a greater role in helping to contain the spread of HIV infection.

REFUSAL TO TREAT AIDS PATIENTS

A small number of physicians and other health care workers have refused to treat patients known or thought to be infected with the AIDS virus. This threatens the assumptions on which our health care system is based and cannot be tolerated. Comprehensive education programs must destigmatize AIDS among health workers. The department has been working with health providers to ensure that they understand the CDC precautions.

CONCLUSIONS

The latest statistics on AIDS and drug abuse-related deaths must signal a renewed effort to break the AIDS-IV drug connection. The problems of narcotic addiction make it difficult to apply traditional public health measures to control the spread of infection in this population.

Critical to the prevention effort must be linking AIDS public health education programs to drug treatment programs. Currently, there are only 225 inpatient drug detoxification beds in the city, and only 30,000 methadone maintenance slots. Waiting periods for admission range from weeks to months. There are currently only 3,800 beds for those needing long-term residential treatment after detoxification.

I have advocated expanded drug treatment programs to prevent AIDS since the beginning of my tenure as Commissioner of Health. Although we have seen modest increases from the state government, and the promise of innovative federal programs, the effort to prevent the spread of AIDS through drug treatment programs is currently insufficient.

According to the New York State Department of Substance Abuse Services, 8% of seronegative persons who are IV drug abusers seroconvert each year. We need to approach drug treatment interventions in HIV prevention with a greater urgency. We continue to advocate a needle exchange program with the New York State Commissioner of Health; while we must explore this option, the most important step would be the rapid and large-scale expansion of capacity in substance abuse treatment facilities.

The New York City Department of Health is also expanding its efforts to investigate the nature of HIV and its transmission, as well as to assess how well risk-reduction messages change behavior. It is attempting to eliminate the false dichotomy between civil liberties and public health. Opposition to mandatory antibody testing is based on sound public health principles. With no effective treatment available, mandatory testing would inefficiently use resources and would drive people away from the public health system.

Finally, the department is increasing coordinated planning and funding at the federal, state, and local levels. An interagency task force coordinates the city's AIDS programs and services. Spending for treatment, testing, counseling, education, and other programs in fiscal 1988 will be over $385 million, of which $98 million is city funds. This is up from $250 million, $75 million of which was city tax levy, in fiscal 1987. In 1989, we project continuing increases in city funding for AIDS programs, as well as a rise in AIDS funding for the city from federal sources.

Even this will not be enough to keep up with the epidemic. We have been fortunate in this city to have the vigorous support of the mayor for our policy and program initiatives. Analogous leadership has not come at the federal level. A significant federal commitment is long overdue. We need nothing less than a bold and comprehensive national prevention strategy. It must inhibit the spread of the virus among heterosexuals, and reduce the toll among homosexual men and intravenous drug abusers and their sex partners and children.

Implementing a national prevention strategy is already within our reach. The strategy should include three major elements:

- A massive national public health education program consisting of an "outer shell" of information to the general public and an "inner shell" of targeted education for people practicing high-risk behavior.

- Rapid expansion of voluntary, confidential counseling and HIV antibody testing into every public and private clinical facility, including physicians' offices, hospital outpatient departments, sexually transmitted disease clinics, family planning and abortion clinics, and anonymous test sites.

- Major efforts to curtail AIDS transmission via the intravenous drug user. Efforts must range from interdiction at the international level, to law enforcement at all levels, to more education programs, increased and liberalized methadone maintenance, and rapid and massive detoxification programs, plus availability of clean needle exchange.

A national prevention strategy demands a "moon-shot" approach to federal resource commitment, guided by aggressive, articulate, and visible leadership from the highest levels of the federal administration. With the exception of Surgeon General Koop, that leadership has so far been lacking.

Without a vigorous, comprehensive national prevention program within the next 18 to 24 months, we will fall behind in the epidemic among heterosexuals, as we have with homosexual men and intravenous drug users. Seizing the opportunity now would save large numbers of lives and substantially reduce the enormous burdens and costs of the epidemic into the mid-1990s.

REFERENCES

1. New York City AIDS surveillance data, New York City Department of Health, 1987. Unless otherwise noted, all New York City surveillance data are generated by the Department of Health.
2. Stoneburner RL, Des Jarlais DC, Guigli P, et al: Increasing mortality among intravenous drug users in New York City and its relationship to the AIDS epidemic: Evidence for a larger spectrum of HIV-related disease. Presented at the Annual Meeting of the American Public Health Association, New Orleans, La, October 18, 1987.

Chapter 22
The impact of AIDS on the health care system in New Jersey

STEVEN R. YOUNG, MSPH

The goal of the New Jersey State Department of Health (NJSDH) with regard to an acquired immunodeficiency syndrome (AIDS) health care delivery system is to "develop an integrated network of AIDS health services that will provide for acute care and cost-effective, post-hospitalization, community-based care for AIDS/ARC patients, families and significant others." This is a lofty goal which will require much more effort before it is reached.

The issues surrounding this goal can be viewed from three broad perspectives: the cost of that care to New Jersey's system of health care and service delivery; the direct impact on persons and institutions who have a role and legal responsibility in providing treatment and care; and the broad spectrum of health and social service needs of persons with AIDS (PWAs).

In addition, the financial burden of AIDS has caused widespread concern. Despite this, data on expenditures for services are surprisingly scarce. In New Jersey, several programs are presently studying this issue. The Robert Wood Johnson Foundation–AIDS Health Services Program for Newark and Jersey City will be studying cost-effectiveness and appropriateness of community-based services, as will New Jersey's "Home and Community-based Services Model Waiver for Persons with AIDS or ARC," administered by the Department of Human Services. Several institution-based studies are taking place in an effort to document costs of AIDS acute care and to develop an AIDS-specific diagnosis related group (DRG) rate for reimbursement. Service programs, such as a residential AIDS drug treatment program and a pediatric AIDS residential/respite/foster care facility, both funded by the NJSDH, will be subject to cost-effectiveness studies. Most recently, the Health Research and Education Trust, an affiliate of the New Jersey Hospital Association, approached the NJSDH to assist in the formulation of a study proposal focused on utilization and cost of services for PWAs.

The purpose of this chapter is to describe the interrelationship between financing care, the delivery of needed services, and education for providers and the public alike, not only for prevention, but to sensitize people to the important issues so that they will be more supportive of the services that need to be operationalized. The one benefit of our experience with an ever-increasing caseload is that more and more persons are being personally touched by the disease and have become committed to the effort.

OVERVIEW OF AIDS IN NEW JERSEY AND ITS IMPACT ON THE PROVISION OF CARE

In New Jersey, a majority of human immunodeficiency virus (HIV) infection is intravenous (IV) drug related. Nearly 41% of the state's 2,500 reported AIDS cases have occurred among male intravenous drug users, and nearly 10% have been among female IV drug users. Another 7%

Mr Young is Coordinator of AIDS Health Services, New Jersey State Department of Health, Trenton, NJ.

of New Jersey's AIDS cases have resulted from heterosexual transmission, and nearly 3% more have involved children with an infected parent. Drug use is implicated in a majority of these cases as well, bringing the total percentage of drug-related AIDS cases in the state to over 60% (Fig 1). New Jersey's proportion of AIDS cases in each of these drug-related categories (male IV drug user, female IV drug user, heterosexual transmission, child with parent at risk) is roughly double that found in the United States as a whole. In New Jersey's largest city, Newark, more than 70% of the AIDS cases are among IV drug users, exclusive of sexual partners or children.

The delivery of services to people with AIDS or AIDS-related complex (ARC) in New Jersey is complicated by three factors. The first is discrimination against people with AIDS that results from ignorance and fear on the part of the public and providers alike. Among its consequences are eviction from housing, loss of employment, refusal of ambulance services, and denial of medical services.

Poverty is a second factor that stands between many people with AIDS and the services they need. In New Jersey, poverty is especially severe in inner-city minority populations. The infant mortality rate in Newark, for example, which can be taken as an indicator of the general state of nutrition and health, is about 18/1,000, or nearly twice the New Jersey average.[1] These figures suggest that this population in general lacks a wide range of services, including timely and appropriate health care; shelter and food; social and community support, both emotional and material; and help in conducting daily activities. If these basic human needs (the last generally applying only to the young, the old, and the infirm) frequently go unmet in Newark's non-HIV-infected population, they are certain to pose even more serious problems for those who are infected. The latter category includes a disproportionate number of blacks. Overall, Newark's population is 56% black, 19% Hispanic, and 23% white, but its reported AIDS cases are 80% black, 12% Hispanic, and 7% white.[2]

A third factor that complicates service delivery to New Jersey's people with AIDS is that many of them are IV drug users. A number of problems arise when AIDS is associated with drug use. It is difficult to gain access to IV drug users, partly because their activity is illegal. Once they have entered the treatment system, there is a need to treat their addictions as well as their HIV-related illnesses. IV drug users frequently live on the streets, and this complicates their placement from acute care hospitals following episodes of severe illness. More than other people with AIDS (many of whom experience dementia), IV drug users suffer from impaired judgment as a result of their drug use. The deficits of community support, good nutrition, and good health that are typical in the inner city are amplified for IV drug users. Indeed, IV drug users typically present themselves at acute care facilities relatively late in the course of their HIV infections, resulting in medical complications more severe and lifespans shorter than those of other people with AIDS. And like most of the unemployed, IV drug users typically lack private insurance or personal resources to cover the costs of their health care.

Similar problems are experienced by children born with AIDS or ARC. Many have unstable home situations: Their parents may be IV drug users, deceased, poor at parenting, or unable to cope with AIDS. As with IV drug users, this results in longer-than-necessary hospital stays following episodes of acute illness. Because children with AIDS have poorly developed immune systems, they experience different and more frequent illnesses than adults with AIDS/ARC.

Due to the IV drug use-AIDS connection in New Jersey, extreme pressures exist to provide and finance care. Additional specific factors include the presentation of different medical problems among IV drug users, including a higher incidence of *Pneumocystis carinii* pneumonia, which requires more intense hospital care; and the inability to appropriately discharge IV drug users due to lack of homes and community services to support them. This increases length of stay, which is reported to be anywhere from 12 days to 26 days in New Jersey hospitals with a range of three days to over one year, and acute care costs, since much of that care is inappropriate. Outpatient services need to be carefully structured to provide effective service for those that do not have a community placement. Another factor is the growing number of pediatric AIDS cases, which also require more care than adult cases.

In the absence of a cure or vaccine for AIDS, every effort must be made to prevent the spread of HIV infection. In New Jersey, this is best accomplished through the prevention and control of drug abuse. In the current fiscal year, funding for drug treatment in New Jersey has increased 33% to support increased treatment slots and enhanced reimbursement for those slots. Of course, more money for more drug abuse treatment is a simplistic approach that does not take into consideration how to increase slots, how to get more people into treatment via outreach, and the development of new treatment approaches. The Treatment and Community Support Unit, Division of Narcotic and Drug Abuse Control, has been among the innovators in AIDS prevention among IV drug users. NJSDH initiatives conceptualized and developed by this group include:

- the use of ex-addict street educators to take AIDS prevention messages to current addicts;
- the use of AIDS coordinators to give risk reduction messages to IV drug users in treatment, serve as a community education resource, provide training for other drug treatment center staff, and provide advocacy for patients;

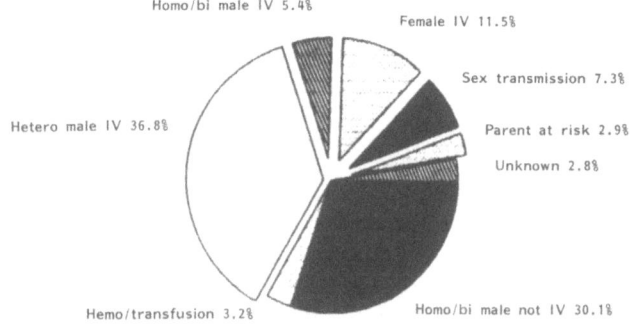

FIGURE 1.   New Jersey AIDS cases by risk factor, as of December 1, 1987.

- a coupon program to entitle addicts not recently in treatment to a free initial drug detoxification and an AIDS prevention class; and
- mobile outreach vans to go to areas frequented by IV drug users and give basic health examinations, prevention information, and referrals.

In light of the AIDS epidemic, new strategies for treatment that are more attractive to addicts need to be developed. In fact, drug treatment centers may need to become primary care centers with a full complement of AIDS professionals.

FINANCIAL IMPACT ON HOSPITALS AND HEALTH CARE PROVIDERS

The clinical course of AIDS is characterized by a progressive decline in immune system competence and repeated episodes of severe opportunistic infections which lead to hospitalization for diagnosis and therapy. The episodic nature of the disease necessitates a full spectrum of health and social support services. A large share of the rapidly escalating costs for such services in New Jersey will fall on Medicaid and uncompensated care. Approximately 50% of patients in northern New Jersey hospitals are enrolled in the State Medicaid Program. Through New Jersey's hospital rate setting and uncompensated care system, paying hospital patients and insurers (private and public) have had to bear financial responsibility for the state's uninsured PWAs.

New Jersey's system operates on the basis of prospective hospital payments that are determined by a patient's admitting diagnosis. The reimbursement rates that correspond to DRGs are the same for all payers, though they vary from one hospital to another. (No DRGs have yet been established specifically for people with AIDS.) The reimbursement system has one other outstanding feature: No patient is turned away from a New Jersey hospital because of an incapacity to pay for his or her care. To cover the costs of care for those who cannot afford it, New Jersey has instituted a system whereby all payers to hospitals (patients, insurance companies, state, etc) pay a surcharge on each calculated rate to cover the costs of uncompensated care. The uncompensated care system operates only for acute care facilities; it does not cover the costs of nursing facilities or home care, for example.

The cost of AIDS, direct and indirect, has been relatively low to date when compared with the economic costs of all other illnesses. However, the cost of AIDS treatment per case is at the top of the list of major diseases, along with other expensive illnesses such as renal disease and the terminal stages of certain cancers. Estimated lifetime treatment costs have ranged from $29,000 to $147,000. This wide variation is due, in part, to differences in length of hospital stays in different geographic areas of the country. One of the factors holding down treatment costs in New Jersey is that IV drug user patients present late to the health care system and die quickly. This is not a comforting measure of cost control. On the other hand, there is less likelihood that IV drug users with AIDS will be discharged home between acute episodes. In addition, the cost of care for pediatric AIDS cases, of which there are a significant number, is estimated by the Centers for Disease Control (CDC) to be 140% of the cost of care for adults.[3]

The real financial significance of AIDS is that the costs have not been anticipated, since those afflicted are primarily young persons with historically low rates of sickness and death. By adding a layer of unexpected cost, AIDS has confounded risk assessment and prediction for all payers and disrupted established patterns for distributing the cost burdens among them. The AIDS scene is rapidly changing in regard to the demographics of patient groups, medical interventions, treatment models, and development of state policies, making cost estimates "calculated guesses." What is certain, however, is that given the health and social service needs of PWAs, the barriers to service, and the financial implications of what is occurring, high priority must be placed upon developing a continuum of services outside of hospitals for PWAs.

INTERRELATIONSHIPS BETWEEN THE FINANCING OF CARE AND THE DELIVERY OF SERVICES

Acute care for AIDS patients has fallen disproportionately on public and church institutions in inner-city areas of northern New Jersey. This phenomenon has been referred to as the "ghettoization of PWAs." Green[4] has indicated that by 1991, 2% of all medical/surgical beds will be occupied by AIDS patients. In New Jersey, the rate at one institution is currently at 50%. Five hospitals have cared for more than 100 AIDS patients, six hospitals have cared for 50–100 patients, 15 hospitals have cared for 25–50 patients, and most other hospitals have cared for at least one patient. Much of this trend is due to the demographics of the disease; however, to some extent we are aware of the inappropriate referrals of PWAs. Patient referral may sometimes be due to the "inability to provide appropriate care." Inappropriate referrals which essentially deny access to care, and are the result of HIV routine testing without informed consent or suspicion of positivity, are clearly unethical and intolerable.

High caseloads—ones that are rapidly increasing—cause concern about the operational aspects of hospitals. Similar concerns exist in other community-based health care agencies. There are staffing concerns; institutions have recognized the difficulty in recruiting teams of professionals necessary to work with PWAs. Ongoing training and support systems are necessary. The development of multidisciplinary care teams for PWAs is one of the greatest challenges facing the health care system.

Communities in New Jersey have accepted the fact that PWAs are treated in hospitals. But what about the future? As caseloads increase disproportionately in some hospitals, they may lose other patients who have freedom of choice and choose not to be treated in an "AIDS hospital."

The NJSDH has maintained that acute care should be shared throughout institutions as defined by their service area and patient profile. However, as public and church institutions become hospitals of last resort, their financial viability may be threatened. Even with Medicaid and uncompensated care reimbursement, there is potential for calamitous AIDS cost burdens. Clearly, the public role of financing is increasing but inadequate. As the total bill for AIDS increases, there is a need to divide the responsibility of paying among patients, families, private payers, and government health plans. So far, the New Jersey system of reimbursement is keeping hospitals afloat financially.

In addition, there is a broad spectrum of issues related to patient care, employee safety, and provider services that may affect a hospital's liability insurance. In fact, this has already been witnessed in other AIDS care settings such as drug treatment centers and transitional homes for children.

In the long run, however, a positive approach and outlook must be maintained on New Jersey's treatment capability for PWAs. The large number of empty hospital beds in New Jersey makes it unlikely that the AIDS epidemic will completely overload the state's hospital capacity, except possibly in high impact communities such as Newark, Jersey City, and Paterson. In these cities, AIDS care has contributed to an increasing occupancy rate. Building new hospitals for AIDS may be a necessity in the future. Clearly, hospitals will not default due to the previously described reimbursement mechanism and the fact that state and local leaders realize the political fallout from such occurrences.

Increased availability of alternative levels of care is essential. In the short term this will increase costs due to startup expenses, but in the long term will be a more cost-effective approach. In fact, hospitals may choose to provide alternative levels of care themselves. Conversion of unused acute care beds, identification of "swing" beds, or use of decertified beds may be viable options. Politically and clinically, linking a continuum of care with acute care makes sense.

Hospitals in New Jersey have filed formal requests for higher reimbursement for their AIDS caseloads and a $600 increase for AIDS-related DRG admissions has been adopted. Hospitals will be strained but will not go out of business due to AIDS. What is ultimately needed is a network of providers to share responsibility for a continuum of health services that are adequately funded via existing reimbursement systems to relieve some of the burden felt on the acute care side.

NEW JERSEY PLANS

Since most of the burden of financing medical care for persons with AIDS who lack sufficient coverage now falls on the state, we will continue to develop innovative strategies in providing appropriate care. Methods used include the following:

- seed money for start-up demonstration programs;
- providing financial support for AIDS staff through contracts;
- provision of training and consultation to local agencies' staff in order that they may assume AIDS-related functions;
- creation of enhanced reimbursement rates.

The major barriers in developing a continuum of care fall into two broad categories:

- lack of political/community support;
- lack of adequate financing mechanisms.

The broad range of services needed indicates the complexity of caring for persons afflicted with this disease. In some instances, completely new types of resources must be created and questions arise as to how they can be licensed and reimbursed for operational costs. A description of New Jersey's programmatic efforts is presented in *AIDS in New Jersey: A Report from the Department of Health.*[5] The report illustrates the wide range of services and their potential funding source. Services include case management, outpatient ambulatory care, medical day care, dental care, home health care, skilled nursing, personal care assistance, therapy, hospice, pediatric residential/respite/foster care, residential AIDS drug treatment, adult residential housing, long term care, volunteer buddy support, early intervention (children), transportation, counseling/mental health, legal counsel, pastoral care, and drug abuse home treatment. Many services are not reimbursed, and some are reimbursed at an inadequate level. Reimbursement sources include federal, state, third party Medicaid, and private foundation monies.

In New Jersey, an uncompensated care pool has been used to share the financial risk among acute care hospitals and third party payers. Our State Medicaid Program instituted a "Home and Community-based Services Model Waiver for Persons with AIDS or ARC," which provides for reimbursement of cost-effective services that meet some of the needs of our patient population: case management, skilled nursing at home, personal care assistance, medical day care, drug abuse treatments at home, and foster care for children. The program, along with a system of in-hospital case management, is attempting to reduce the need for hospitalization, thus reducing costs and enhancing the quality of life for AIDS patients. It is currently too early to provide a demonstration of success. On the negative side, there are many instances where there are no options for case management and referral of clients—institutionalized hospice, long term care, housing, or subacute unit.

There are many programmatic areas where further attention is needed. The NJSDH proposes in the near future to:

- coordinate a planned effort to educate, train, and desensitize primary care physicians, nurses, aides, social workers;
- study the costs of care, the medical procedures that contribute to those costs, and the methods of payment used by people with AIDS;
- implement a statewide mass media/public education campaign not only for purposes of prevention, but to elicit support for the necessary complement of health services;
- conduct feasibility studies to determine providers/sites of alternative levels of care. Such a study has taken place for the City of Newark, in conjunction with both the city and the New Jersey Health Care Facilities Financing Authority, and conducted by a private, independent consulting firm;
- conduct a periodic census of hospitals to determine the demand for AIDS-related care and identify inappropriate referral patterns.

SUMMARY

The New Jersey State Department of Health will continue to facilitate the creation of health care sites outside of hospitals for people with AIDS. This will relieve some of the burden carried by acute care inner-city institutions and provide more appropriate and humane care. In addition, we are urging hospitals to work with us in performing prospective studies to determine reliable cost estimates.

Important questions remain unanswered. How will cost burdens be shared among individuals, private hospitals, HMOs, local/state/federal governments, and insurance companies and their investors? In Chicago, the AIDS Medical Resource Center is doing some innovative work in cost determinations based on patients' needs and negotiating for a prepaid lifetime reimbursement with third party payers. Services are provided via a network of providers who are contractually linked and who share the financial risk should their costs exceed the negotiated fee. Will access to care be equitable? Will we have appropriately trained health care workers for many settings? Will the shortage of nurses affect our ability to provide care? Will insurance companies require HIV testing for new policyholders, thereby resulting in an increase in patients without coverage, or will such testing be prohibited, with insurance companies raising their charges for all so as to cover risk? Some people will then not be able to afford a health insurance policy.

These issues deserve consideration from a variety of health professionals, especially in regard to their role and responsibility in addressing them.

REFERENCES

1. *Vital and Health Statistics—1986*. Trenton, New Jersey State Department of Health, 1987.
2. *Monthly AIDS Surveillance Report*. Trenton, New Jersey State Department of Health, 1987.
3. Hardy AM, Rauch K, Echenberg D, et al: The economic impact of the first 1,000 cases of acquired immunodeficiency syndrome in the United States. *JAMA* 1986; 255:209–211.
4. Green J, Singer M, Wintfeld N, et al: Projecting the impact of AIDS on Hospitals. *Health Affairs* Fall 1987, pp 19–31.
5. *AIDS in New Jersey: A Report from the Department of Health*. Trenton, New Jersey State Department of Health, 1987.

Chapter 23

Barriers to the modification of sexual behavior among heterosexuals at risk for acquired immunodeficiency syndrome

KAROLYNN SIEGEL, PHD, WILLIAM C. GIBSON, MA

Acquired immunodeficiency syndrome (AIDS) may no longer be viewed as a disease that only poses a significant threat to homosexual men and intravenous drug users. About 7% of cases diagnosed in 1986 were from among three groups in which the majority of cases are thought to result from heterosexual transmission: heterosexual contacts; persons born outside of the US; and persons with no identified risk factor. The proportion of cases accounted for by these groups is projected to increase to 10% in 1991.[1] If one considers only the cases acquired through heterosexual contact, it is projected that the proportion of all cases in this category will increase from 2% in 1986 to 5% in 1991.[1]

It is difficult to arrive at a reliable estimate of the prevalence of human immunodeficiency virus (HIV) infection within the heterosexual community. One strategy for deriving such an estimate from available data yields a rate of HIV infection of 45 per 100,000 (or 0.045%) among the US adult population with no known risk factor.[2] In a sample of 185 self-described heterosexuals attending a sexually transmitted disease clinic, two, or slightly less than 1%, were positive for HIV.[3] Among 134 members of a Minnesota-based social/sexual club, none of the 75 male members and two of the 59 female members tested positive for HIV antibodies.[4] This constitutes a seroprevalence rate of 3% among the female club members. When 92 prostitutes in Seattle, Washington, were tested, 5% were found to be HIV antibody positive; similarly, when 25 prostitutes in Miami, Florida, were tested, 40% of this group were seropositive.[5] In one study,[6] testing of seven female sex partners of men with AIDS or AIDS-related complex (ARC) yielded HIV antibody in 71%. Another study of 42 women who had had sex with men suffering from AIDS or ARC found a 47% seropositivity rate.[7] Finally, of 21 female sex partners of men with hemophilia who were either HIV positive, had lymphadenopathy, or had AIDS, 10% tested seropositive themselves.[8]

Whatever the true prevalence of infection, it is reasonable to assume that the rate is higher in cities with large, established risk group populations (since it is in these cities that the greatest opportunity for transmission to heterosexuals exists). The rate of infection would also presumably be higher among individuals who have a pattern of sexual behavior that includes unprotected intercourse with multiple partners; and higher among those subgroups that traditionally have been regarded as risk groups for other sexually transmitted diseases (STDs) such as syphilis, gonorrhea, hepatitis, and herpes. A higher infection rate would

From the Department of Social Work, Memorial Sloan-Kettering Cancer Center, New York, NY.

also be expected among blacks and Hispanics, who are greatly over-represented among AIDS cases in the United States, especially in the categories of heterosexual contacts, women with AIDS, and perinatal transmission.

It is now generally accepted that bidirectional heterosexual transmission can occur, although female-to-male transmission is less well documented and may be less efficient.[5,9-16] It is also recognized that many, if not most, infected heterosexuals are probably unaware of their status and therefore are unlikely to be taking precautions to protect their sexual partners.

The AIDS epidemic has progressed to such a point that all sexually active individuals not in a long-standing monogamous relationship—regardless of sexual orientation—must be considered potentially at risk for the disease. However, there is evidence that many heterosexuals likely to be at increased risk for AIDS are not altering their sexual behavior. A recent study[17] of a random probability sample of high-risk adults in San Francisco (defined as having had two or more partners in the past year or awareness of sexual relations with a homosexual or bisexual male, an intravenous drug user, or a prostitute) found evidence of widespread persistence in recognized risky behaviors. Of those respondents who had ever engaged in vaginal intercourse without a condom, 59% said that they currently did so about as often as in the past, while 22% did so even more often. Of those who had ever had sex with a homosexual or bisexual man, 28% said they currently did so as often as in the past, while 11% said they did so more often. When asked to rate on a scale from 1 to 10 how much impact the AIDS epidemic had had on their sexual behavior or lifestyle (1 = no impact at all, 10 = a great deal of impact), 68% of the respondents chose a score of 5 or less; a full 33% selected 1.

These data suggest that many heterosexuals at increased risk for HIV infection do not yet recognize their susceptibility or are not motivated to adopt behavioral modifications, circumstances that create the potential for significant spread of the virus in the general population. In response to this realization, we have begun to see a shift in public health educational efforts toward a greater emphasis on targeting sexually active heterosexuals. As these preventive activities begin to accelerate, it is useful to ask what barriers might impede the adoption of safer-sex recommendations among at-risk heterosexuals. This chapter focuses on an analysis of those barriers. Recommendations for surmounting or alleviating existing obstacles to change and for more effectively achieving adoption of safer-sex recommendations are also offered.

BARRIERS TO BEHAVIOR MODIFICATION

Perceptions of Low Vulnerability. Most models of preventive health behavior regard a feeling of personal susceptibility to an illness as a necessary condition for an individual to adopt a preventive health action.[18] That is to say, most heterosexuals will not be motivated to modify practices that could place them at risk for infection with the AIDS virus if they do not perceive themselves to be vulnerable to the disease. It has already been documented that a general tendency exists for people to believe that they themselves will not be victims of negative life events—including serious illness.[19-21] People tend to distort reality in a positive direction in order to avoid the anxiety that would result from a more realistic assessment of their vulnerability. Thus, apart from other factors (discussed below) that may contribute to a faulty appraisal on the part of many heterosexuals of their risk for infection, public health educational efforts must also confront a common defensive mechanism that fosters an unfounded optimism regarding personal invulnerability to health (and other) threats.

Unfortunately, several features of the way we have communicated about AIDS both in the media and in public health messages may have inadvertently contributed to a perception on the part of many heterosexuals that they have little cause for personal concern. For example, the widespread emphasis on anal intercourse as a principal mode of sexual transmission may lead many heterosexuals who refrain from this practice to evaluate their risk of infection as being low. Similarly, the emphasis early in the epidemic on a large number of partners as a risk factor may have led many who have had only a small number of partners to feel unthreatened by the disease. In reality, of course, while the probability of infection increases with the number of partners, the possibility of becoming infected exists with even a single partner if unprotected sex occurs.[22] The focus on "risk groups" as opposed to "risk behaviors" is still a feature of communications that contributed to a false sense of security among many who engage in practices that are associated with transmission of the AIDS virus.

Further, people also evaluate their risk of experiencing a negative life event by employing stereotypes, or what Tversky and Kahneman[23] have called the "representativeness" heuristic. That is, people tend to have a preconception in their minds of the typical sort of person who experiences a particular kind of negative event—such as acquiring a venereal infection. They appraise their own vulnerability based on their evaluation of how much or little they resemble their mental representation. Because the victims they imagine tend to be stereotypes, they generally judge themselves as very different and therefore at low risk.

Misperception of the Efficacy of Adaptive Behaviors. While AIDS is a relatively new disease, sexually transmitted diseases have been around for centuries. In 1917, the Venereal Disease Control Division of the Public Health Service was founded to stem the spread of STDs. It has become apparent in the intervening years that while a variety of prophylactic methods (social, mechanical, chemical, and systemic) have been identified, significant barriers to their utilization exist.

In the case of AIDS, the only prophylactic measures believed to be potentially effective at this time, if one continues to engage in risky sexual practices, are reducing one's number of partners, being more selective in the choice of partners, and using condoms.

The reduction of partners, in the absence of condom use, is only effective if the rate of infection in the population from which one selects his or her partners is still quite low. If, on the other hand, the prevalence of infection is high, little protection is conferred by this strategy. For example, in cities with large homosexual male communities, where it is estimated that the rate of infection may be as high as 68%,[24] reducing one's number of partners from, say, 20 to two, still presents a 90% risk of exposure.

Being more selective in the choice of one's partners implies that one has a means of evaluating the probability that a potential partner is infected. However, this necessitates an extensive knowledge of the potential partner's sexual and medical history: Is he or she a member of an established risk group; has he or she been the partner of a member of an established risk group; has he or she had multiple partners during the past several years; has he or she had a blood transfusion during the past several years? Few individuals are likely to possess such knowledge of prospective partners, or to feel comfortable obtaining this information.

Some heterosexuals believe that if they can feel confident that their partner is not a bisexual male or an intravenous drug user, they run little danger of infection. Others believe that if in addition to avoiding these risk group members they also select only partners who are white, middle class, and who hold professional or white collar jobs, they are unlikely to risk exposure to the AIDS virus.

The inadequacies of these strategies for avoiding infection are obvious. First, it is not possible to reliably determine who currently, or within the past ten years, may have engaged in homosexual behavior or intravenous drug use. Many homosexual men have been able to "pass" their entire adult life because they do not fit the stereotypical image of a gay man. Similarly, as our awareness of the pervasiveness of drug use in our society has grown, it has become evident that there are many "respectable" people who have used drugs for years without friends or coworkers learning of their behavior.

Similarly, social class variables are not reliable screening criteria for partner selection. Drug abuse and bisexuality occurs among all social classes, races, and ethnic groups. Recipients of contaminated blood, who are unaware that they may be infecting others, are also represented in every social strata as well as all races.

Barriers to the Adoption of Condoms. Condoms offer a more useful method of controlling the spread of HIV infection. Their efficacy in preventing many of the traditional STDs is already well documented.[25,26] Preliminary data, while inconclusive, also seem to support their efficacy in preventing the transmission of the AIDS virus.[27] It remains to be seen whether heterosexuals will be more motivated to use condoms to prevent AIDS than they have been to use them to prevent other venereal diseases. For despite condoms' efficacy and safety as a technique of STD control, estimates of condom use among STD clinic patients range only from 3% to 20%, and among the general male population, condom use usually does not exceed 25%.[25]

The barriers to the use of condoms have been well documented. These include the following: the belief that condoms compromise the pleasure of intercourse;[28-30] the tendency to view the condom primarily as a contraceptive device rather than as a means of prophylaxis against STD; [31-32] the belief that condom use is unnatural; [28-29] the tendency to underestimate the personal risk of infection present in a situation; [25,33,34] the failure to anticipate and/or prepare in advance for sexual activity;[25,33-35] the belief that one's partner would be offended if a condom were

introduced; [32,33,36,37] the belief that safe, effective treatment is available and, therefore, prevention is not important;[31,33] the use of alcohol or drugs before or during sex, which leads to a failure to use condoms or improper usage; [33-35] the stigmatization of condom use through their popular associations with promiscuity, prostitution, and extramarital sex;[37-40] the belief that condoms are ineffective or unreliable;[25,41] the embarrassment or discomfort of purchasing condoms;[42-44] the belief that using condoms makes sex seem premeditated and not spontaneous.[40]

Confusion Regarding the Magnitude of the Threat to Heterosexuals. While there has been intermittent discussion in the mass media about the potential danger of the growing spread of AIDS beyond the established risk groups into the wider heterosexual community, there have also been periodic reassurances that the proportion of AIDS cases accounted for by non-risk-group members has remained relatively stable over time. Such seemingly conflicting messages have resulted in a sense of confusion among many regarding the actual magnitude of the risk of infection to most heterosexuals.

Similarly, while bidirectional transmission of the virus is accepted as possible, the relatively small number of cases of female-to-male transmission that have been documented has contributed to the perception that heterosexual males may incur a low risk of infection from unprotected intercourse. Because it is still often left to males to introduce the use of condoms, a man's low sense of vulnerability may serve as a barrier to his doing so.

The Interpersonal Nature of Sexual Activity. Because of the interpersonal nature of sexual intercourse, decisions to engage in or refrain from risky sex must be "negotiated." To effectively practice safer sex the partners must agree on limits and the use of condoms whenever the opportunity for the exchange of body fluids exists. Whereas with most other health-related behaviors it is only necessary to persuade a single individual to change his behavior to bring about the desired outcome, in the case of "unhealthy" sexual behavior, two individuals must be convinced of the necessity of modifying their actions. When one partner is not motivated to practice safe sex, he or she may not cooperate with the other partner in having a safe encounter. Or the unmotivated partner may undercut the resolve of the other partner to avoid unsafe sex by persuading him or her that no risk exists in unprotected intercourse or by failing to cooperate in the proper use of condoms.

The Stigma of AIDS. Sexually transmitted diseases have always been stigmatized in our society. Venereal infections are widely regarded as the outcome of sexual excess and low moral character. Historically, these diseases have been associated with dirt and uncleanliness.[45] So strongly are sin and moral depravity tied together with STDs in the popular mind that, as has been pointed out, victims of these diseases feel compelled to deny their condition or assert their innocence (eg, "I got it from a toilet seat.")[46]

AIDS, of course, has been no exception. In fact, its association with two of the most stigmatized groups in society—homosexuals and drug abusers—has only served to accentuate the stigma attached to the disease. As a result, the need to dissociate oneself from AIDS or even from the implication that one could possibly be infected may be very great. If introducing a condom might be construed to mean that one acknowledges that one may be at risk, individuals may be unwilling to do so. Further, if doing so is felt to impugn the character of one's partner, one also may resist the use of condoms.

The stigma associated with AIDS may also make individuals unwilling to seek out information—including prevention-related information—about the disease. The wish to deny that the problem has any personal relevance is so strong among many that it may serve as a barrier to their obtaining needed education about the disease.

HEALTH EDUCATION IMPLICATIONS

As can be seen from the foregoing discussion, several barriers exist to heterosexuals' adoption of safer sex practices. Taken singly and in combination, these barriers appear to be formidable, indeed, and overcoming them will not be an easy task. Nevertheless, we present several recommendations for removing or reducing the obstacles to behavior change.

Careful attention must be given to the varying meanings and implications individuals will assign to certain language that may be used in educational materials. For example, communications should focus on risk behaviors (eg, engaging in intercourse without a condom) rather than risk groups (eg, homosexual or bisexual men and intravenous drug users). Talking about risk groups permits most of the public to defend against a sense of personal vulnerability, which may be necessary for the adoption of behavioral modifications; because these individuals do not belong to or identify with the groups, they will not identify with the threat. For the same reason, health educators must work to break down traditional stereotypes about the kinds of people who get sexually transmitted diseases. Such myths may lead many at-risk individuals to underestimate their own susceptibility.

The use of the terms "multiple partners" and "sexually active" are other examples of language that may seem clear and straightforward to health educators but has different meanings to different individuals. It is important to clarify for the public that "multiple partners" refers to two or more partners in a specified time frame—eg, within the last year. It must also be understood that "multiple partners" refers not only to situations in which the individual has two or more partners concurrently, but also to a pattern of serial monogamy, in which the individual has only one partner at a time, but each for a relatively brief period of time (eg, less than a year).

Finally, the term "sexually active" will be interpreted in varying ways. Because early in the epidemic AIDS was identified with homosexual men practicing "fast lane" sex, characterized by a large number of partners, AIDS has become associated in the popular mind with sexual promiscuity. As a result, many people will equate the expression "sexually active" with "promiscuous" or having multiple partners. Thus, when they hear that sexually active heterosexuals are at risk and must adopt certain prophylactic actions, they may assume that the messages do not apply to them. If by sexually active we mean, for example, anyone with two or more partners during the past year, we should state that. It is also important to recognize that patterns of sexual behavior and sexual norms may vary somewhat across racial and ethnic groups. Individuals will appraise how risky or active their behavior is by comparing it to the prevailing norms of their social group. If they regard themselves as only typical or even less active than typical, they are likely to judge themselves as sexually conservative and at little risk for AIDS or other STDs regardless of a pattern of multiple partners.

The efficacy of condoms as a prophylactic for STD must be emphasized, and their accessibility, especially to those who are most likely to have unprotected sex, should be increased. Availability of condoms has been shown to influence their use. For example, one study found that distributing condoms to a group presumably at risk for STD (inner-city adolescent males) resulted in an overall increase in condom use from 19% to 68%, with use in the last sexual encounter increasing from 20% to 91%.[47] Health educators also need to promote a change in image for condoms. As was noted above, condoms are often associated in the minds of many with promiscuous or "illicit" sexual activity. Further doubts exist concerning their reliability. Individuals must be shown that proper and consistent use of condoms provides not only contraception, but also an effective and generally reliable prophylaxis for STD. Additionally, through statements by health educators and in the media, condom use must be shown to be acceptable and appropriate among heterosexuals in stable relationships. Finally, since in some cities women now purchase approximately 40% of the condoms sold,[48] this information should be directed at women as well as men.

As was noted above, individuals tend to assume that they can evaluate the riskiness of a potential sexual encounter and will consequently take or not take appropriate preventive action based on these evaluations. The language employed in some health recommendations may promote this tendency. For example, a communication may tell individuals to use condoms if they know or suspect that a potential sexual partner is a risk-group member or has had sexual contact with a risk-group member. This encourages individuals to rely on their judgment or intuition to evaluate the potential risk a prospective partner is likely to represent. Such judgments will usually be based on distorted traditional stereotypes of the "types" of people who are likely to be risk-group members or to contract an STD.

Rather, individuals must be shown that *anyone* can be infected, that they cannot rely on their judgments, and they should thus take appropriate prophylactic steps such as condom use on every sexual encounter. They should also be made aware that they cannot take a sex history and thus rule out risky partners. This is a flawed and unreliable method for assessing risk. Even assuming a potential sexual partner is able (and willing) to recall and relate everything he or she has done sexually in the past seven to ten years, it is extremely unlikely he or she will know about the behaviors and riskiness of his or her past partners.

As has been done in the male homosexual community, heterosexuals should be educated in the process of negotiating limits with potential sexual partners. They must be given the skills to communicate effectively with their partners about their unwillingness to engage in certain risky sexual practices. The greater assertiveness of women in interpersonal matters that has emerged in recent years should be encouraged in sexual negotiations. Both men and women should feel they have both the right to insist on protection as well as the responsibility for providing appropriate prophylactics. Both should be instructed in the proper use of condoms. Above all, this must be done, not in an atmosphere of suspicion, but in one of mutual respect, concern, and caring.

One must, however, be sensitive to the special cultural barriers that may exist. For example, within the Hispanic subculture, sex roles in sexual matters are more rigidly prescribed. For a woman to appear too knowledgeable about sexual matters can call her character into question. Special strategies must be developed for these communities. Grass-roots involvement of community leaders will be essential to the success of educational efforts.

Finally, individuals must be shown and convinced that AIDS and other STDs are no respecters of age, income, race, or social class. Not only poor, non-white, "out-group" members, but also wealthy, white, and socially well-positioned individuals have contracted and died of these diseases. To this end, AIDS must be destigmatized and its depiction as a disease limited to gay men and drug abusers shown to be false. Perhaps as AIDS continues to move beyond these stigmatized groups, the disease itself may lose some of its stigma. This may largely be a function of time. However, to the extent that health educators are responsible for enlightening the public, they can perhaps focus on showing that AIDS is not just a disease of homosexual men and drug abusers. AIDS sufferers deserve neither moral condemnation nor mere pity, but support and concern. AIDS is not due to a weakness in character, but is a blood-borne disease that happens to be transmitted by sexual contact.

It addition to this health education approach, another source of health communications can be opened. This would involve the use of "opinion leaders," well known and respected individuals whom the public trust and to whom they will listen. Because these individuals are respected, the public is interested in their views on controversial matters and will often seek to emulate their values and attitudes. We should explore the use of opinion leaders to raise public awareness of the problems AIDS poses, to encourage a collective sense of purpose in combating the epidemic and in reshaping sexual norms.

CONCLUSION

Although a reliable estimate of the prevalence of HIV infection among the general heterosexual population (excluding risk group members and their partners) is not available at this time, it is likely that it is still quite low. This circumstance should not promote a sense of complacency, but rather should be regarded as representing an opportunity to significantly limit the spread of the epidemic.

As described in this chapter, multiple barriers exist to persuading at-risk heterosexuals to modify sexual behaviors implicated in the spread of infection. While knowledge about risky and safe practices is a prerequisite to the adoption of safer sex practices, it is not usually a sufficient condition. As we have shown, many of the barriers to behavior change that exist are perceptual and attitudinal.

This means that health education in the case of AIDS must mean more than merely transmitting information, it must also alter perceptions and modify attitudes. We have offered recommendations for accomplishing these objectives.

It appears that the AIDS epidemic will be with us for some years to come. Unfortunately, at this time little empirical data exist for guiding our health education efforts aimed at the general population. Research on the factors that influence heterosexuals' tendency to modify their sexual behavior in response to the threat of AIDS must be assigned a high priority by the government. We need fundamental data on people's high-risk sexual practices, beliefs, and perceptions regarding AIDS to mount an effective national public health campaign.

REFERENCES

1. Morgan WM, Curran JW: Acquired immunodeficiency syndrome: Current and future trends. *Public Health Rep* 1986; 101:459–465.
2. Sivak SL, Wormser GP: How common is HTLV-III infection in the United States? [letter]. *N Engl J Med* 1985; 313:1352.
3. Whittington WL, Kraus SJ, Lee F, et al: The prevalence of HTLV-III/LAV antibodies in heterosexuals [letter]. *JAMA* 1986; 255:1702–1703.
4. Centers for Disease Control: Positive HTLV-III/LAV antibody results for sexually active female members of social/sexual clubs—Minnesota. *MMWR* 1986; 35:697–699.
5. Centers for Disease Control: Heterosexual transmission of human T-lymphotropic virus type III/lymphadenopathy-associated virus. *MMWR* 1985; 34:561–563.
6. Redfield RR, Markham PD, Salahuddin SZ, et al: Frequent transmission of HTLV-III among spouses of patients with AIDS-related complex and AIDS. *JAMA* 1985; 253:1571–1573.
7. Harris CA, et al: Human T-lymphotropic virus type III/lymphadenopathy associated virus infections and acquired immunodeficiency syndrome in heterosexual partners of AIDS patients. Presented at the 25th Interscience Conference on Antimicrobial Agents and Chemotherapy, 1985.
8. Kreiss JK. Kitchen LW, Prince HE, et al: Antibody to human T-lymphotropic virus type III in wives of hemophiliacs. Evidence for heterosexual transmission. *Ann Intern Med* 1985; 102:623–626.
9. Jones P, Hamilton PJ, Bird G, et al: AIDS and haemophilia: Morbidity and mortality in a well defined population. *Brit Med J* 1985; 291:695–699.
10. Redfield RR, Markham PD, Salahuddin SZ, et al: Heterosexually acquired HTLV-III/LAV disease (AIDS-related complex and AIDS). Epidemiologic evidence for female-to-male transmission. *JAMA* 1985; 254:2094–2096.
11. Calabrese LH, Gopalakrishna KV: Transmission of HTLV-III infection from man to woman to man [letter]. *N Engl J Med* 1986; 314:987.
12. Padian N, Pickering J: Female-to-male transmission of AIDS: A reexamination of the African sex ratio of cases [letter]. *JAMA* 1986; 255:590.
13. Pearce RB: Heterosexual transmission of AIDS [letter]. *JAMA* 1986; 256:590–591.
14. Schultz S, Milberg JA, Kristal AR, et al: Female-to-male transmission of HTLV-III [letter]. *JAMA* 1986; 255:1703–1704.
15. Wyckoff RF: Female-to-male transmission of HTLV-III [letter]. *JAMA* 1986; 255:1704–1705.
16. Redfield RR, Wright DC, Markham PD, et al: Female-to-male transmission of HTLV-III [reply]. *JAMA* 1986; 255: 1705–1706.
17. Research and Decisions Corporation: Designing an effective AIDS risk reduction program for San Francisco: Results from the first probability sample of multiple/high-risk partner heterosexual adults. San Francisco, 1986.
18. Cummings KM, Becker MH, Maile MC: Bringing the models together: An empirical approach to combining variables used to explain health actions. *J Behav Med* 1980; 3:123–145.
19. Weinstein ND: Unrealistic optimism about future life events. *J Personality Social Psych* 1980; 39:806–820.
20. Weinstein ND: Unrealistic optimism about susceptibility to health problems. *J Behav Med* 1982; 5:441–460.
21. Perloff LS: Social comparison and illusions of invulnerability to negative life events, in Snyder CR, Ford C (eds): *Clinical Social Psychological Perspectives on Negative Life Events*. New York, Plenum (in press).
22. Francis DP, Chin J: The prevention of acquired immunodeficiency syndrome in the United States: An objective strategy for medicine, public health, business, and the community. *JAMA* 1987; 257:1357–1366.
23. Tversky A, Kahneman D: Judgment under uncertainty: Heuristics and biases. *Science* 1974; 185:1124–1131.
24. Curran JW, Morgan WM, Hardy AM, et al: The epidemiology of AIDS: Current status and future prospects. *Science* 1985; 229:1352–1357.
25. Hart G: Role of preventive methods in the control of venereal disease. *Clin Obstet Gynecol* 1975; 18:243–253.
26. Stone KM, Grimes DA, Magder LS: Personal protection against sexually transmitted diseases. *Am J Obstet Gynecol* 1986; 155:180–188.
27. Conant M, Hardy D, Sernatinger J, et al: Condoms prevent transmission of AIDS-associated retrovirus [letter]. *JAMA* 1986; 255:1706.

28.   Darrow WW: Attitudes toward condom use and the acceptance of venereal disease prophylactics, in Redford MH, Duncan GW, Prager DJ (eds): *The Condom: Increasing Utilization in the United States*. San Francisco, San Francisco Press, Inc, 1974, pp 173–185.

29.   Felman YM, Santora FJ: The use of condoms by VD clinic patients. A survey. *Cutis* 1981; 27:330–336.

30.   Condoms. *Consumer Reports* 1979; 44:583–589.

31.   Cutler JC: Prophylaxis in the venereal diseases. *Med Clin North Am* 1972; 56:1211–1216.

32.   Arnold CB: The sexual behavior of inner city adolescent condom users. *J Sex Res* 1972; 8:298–309.

33.   Curjel HE: An analysis of the human reasons underlying the failure to use a condom in 723 cases of venereal disease. *J Roy Nav Med Serv* 1964; 50:203–209.

34.   Wittkower ED, Cowan J: Some psychological aspects of promiscuity. Summary of investigation. *Psychosom Med* 1944; 6:287–294.

35.   Hart G: Factors influencing venereal infection in a war environment. *Br J Vener Dis* 1974; 50:68–72.

36.   Fiumara NJ: Ineffectiveness of condoms in preventing venereal disease. *Med Aspects Hum Sex* 1972; 6:146–150.

37.   Yacenda JA: Knowledge and attitudes of college students about venereal disease and its prevention. *Health Serv Rep* 1974; 89:170–176.

38.   Free MJ, Alexander NJ: Male contraception without prescription. A reevaluation of the condom and coitus interruptus. *Public Health Rep* 1976; 91:437–445.

39.   Sherris JD, Lewison D, Fox G: Update on condoms—products, protection, promotion. *Pop Rep* 1982; (Sept.–Oct.):121–156.

40.   Armonker RG: What do teens know about the facts of life? *J School Health* 1980; 50:527–530.

41.   Rainwater L: *And the Poor Get Children*. Chicago, Quadrangle, 1960.

42.   Yarber WL: Teenage girls and venereal disease prophylaxis. *Br J Vener Dis* 1977; 53:135–139.

43.   Yarber WL, Williams CE: Venereal disease prevention and a selected group of college students. *J Am Vener Dis Assoc* 1975; 2:17–24.

44.   Finkel ML, Finkel DJ: Sexual and contraceptive knowledge, attitudes and behavior of male adolescents. *Family Plan Perspect* 1975; 7:256–260.

45.   Brandt AM: *No Magic Bullet: A Social History of Venereal Diseases in the United States Since 1880*. New York, Oxford University Press, 1985.

46.   Darrow WW, Pauli ML: Health behavior and sexually transmitted disease, in Holmes KK, et al (eds): *Sexually Transmitted Diseases*. New York, McGraw Hill, 1984.

47.   Arnold CB, Cogswell BE: A condom distribution program for adolescents. The findings of a feasibility study. *Am J Public Health* 1971; 61:739–750.

48.   Menzies HD: Back to a basic contraceptive. *NY Times*, January 5, 1986, p C15.

Part III
Current Issues and Opinions

Chapter 24
AIDS: The eleventh year

In his novel *The Plague,* Albert Camus observed that "Epidemics like wars always seem to take people by surprise."[1] A number of the chapters in this volume address the latest "surprise" of acquired immunodeficiency syndrome (AIDS)—the significance of heterosexual transmission in the United States. While our finest biomedical scientists struggle to understand and gain some control over this "new" virus, the known risk groups are benign decimated by disease and the number of new cases, many involving heterosexual transmission, seems to grow inexorably, and ultimately will certainly affect all of society.

In June 1986, the US Public Health Service held a meeting on AIDS in Berkeley Springs, West Virginia.[2] Among the predictions coming from that meeting were that, by 1991, only four years from now, the cumulative number of cases of AIDS will exceed a quarter of a million. It was also predicted that in 1991, the tenth year of the epidemic, we in the US will have to care for 150,000 people who are sick with AIDS, approximately ten times the number in care today—a number already straining health care resources in many cities.

Finally, it was predicted that by 1991, in the absence of a dramatic breakthrough in treatment, at least 54,000 more people will have died of AIDS, approximately the same number of Americans who died in the 15 years of the Vietnam War. This will bring the cumulative number of AIDS deaths in the US to 179,000 in the decade since AIDS was first reported in 1981.

By some cruel irony of history, the year 1992, the 11th of AIDS in the US, will also be the 500th anniversary of Columbus' first voyage across the Atlantic. This historical event, important both to our civilization and to the modern world, is also one of profound biological significance. The year 1492 is full of meaning because it marks the end of the almost total isolation of a huge portion of humanity, a natural quarantine imposed by two great oceans for over 20,000 years. The historian Alfred Crosby calls this event and its aftermath *The Columbian Exchange,*[3] the moment in which two long-separated worlds were reunited, with enormous consequences for both. Aside from all the gold and the silver, the slaves and the soldiers, potatoes and tobacco, tomatoes and maize (all the things which we were schooled to associate with the discovery of the New World), there was also a great biological mingling and the reestablishment of a global system of health and disease which has shaped our world ever since.

The Europeans brought smallpox, typhus, and cholera to the New World, and these killed more native Americans than all the Conquistadores' muskets and cannons. And, in exchange, on the very first ship of Columbus' expedition returning to Barcelona in 1493 traveled the syphilis treponema, a deadly stowaway. Whether it was in one of the crew members or in one of the Indians returned as captives to Europe does not really matter. Syphilis, unknown in Europe at that time, would, within a dozen years, spread to the rest of the Old World and take a fearful toll.

Five hundred years ago, when it first struck Europeans, syphilis was, for them, a new disease, as AIDS is for us today. It appears to have been far more virulent and far more dangerous than the syphilis we see now. The first risk groups for syphilis were soldiers and sailors, and warfare provided the means for its rapid spread via sexual transmission to the entire population of 16th century Europe and beyond.

Crosby says of the spread of syphilis in Europe:

Charles the 8th of France crossed the Alps into Italy with an army of about 50,000 soldiers (of French, Italian, Swiss, German and other origins) bound for the capture of Naples. The army trailed its column of the usual camp followers and engaged in the usual practices of rape and sack. But, Ferdinand and Isabella, anxious to prevent the establishment of French power in Italy, sent Spanish troops. So Charles packed his bags and marched back to France and the whole process of battle, rape and sack was repeated in reverse. Syphilis, hitherto spreading slowly and quietly across Europe, flared into epidemic in Italy during this invasion. Charles arrived back at Lyon in November of 1495 and disbanded his army. Its members, with billions of treponemas in their blood streams, scattered back to their homes in a dozen lands or off to new wars. With the dispersal of this army, the lightning spread of syphilis across Europe and the rest of the world became inevitable.[3]

Syphilis appeared in Germany by the summer of 1495; in Switzerland and France later that same year; in Holland, England, Greece, and Hungry in 1496. It reached Russia by 1499, and by 1505 it had reached China, 11 years after its first appearance in Spain.[3] As we consider the 11th year of AIDS, are there parallels to draw?

At the second International Conference on AIDS held in Paris in June 1986, one could see the conjunction of the work of many investigators studying the heterosexual transmission of AIDS and the latest data on the prevalence of infection in cities around the world. The most startling data concerned the high levels of infection among intravenous drug users in Europe: Barcelona, 70%; Edinburgh, 42%; Bologna, 52%; Milan, 30%; Toulouse, 58%; Paris, 65%; Vienna, 35%; Belgrade, 48%—levels which must grow given the lack of drug treatment and the continued illegality of providing sterile needles for drug users in all of these cities. These are rates of infection which have ominous implications, not only for the addicts themselves but, given the usual heterosexual character of the group, for all of their many sexual partners. Indeed, intravenous drug abusers are potentially a bridge to the heterosexual population at large.

The major studies on heterosexual transmission discussed in Paris—especially the work from the University of Miami,[4] Montefiore Medical Center in the Bronx, NY,[5] and Walter Reed Army Hospital in Washington, DC,[6] had all been presented at other scientific meetings and some had already appeared in print. Further, if one chose to apply the findings, reports of the experience with AIDS in Haiti and Africa also seemed to shed light on heterosexual transmission. However, the time lag associated with publication seemed poorly attuned to the pace of a rapidly growing epidemic and threatened to create a serious gap in understanding both within the scientific community and between that community and the general public. For these reasons some exchange of information and viewpoints more in "real time" seemed appropriate. Clearly there is a need for dialogue between those conducting the primary research and surveillance, those whose responsibility it is to care for the patients, and those involved in shaping public policy aimed at prevention.

Several different surveys have indicated low levels of public confidence in our communications about AIDS. People feel that they are not being told "the whole story." This lends some urgency to the need to both establish the truth about sexual transmission of AIDS and to fully communicate it to the public in the clearest possible terms and as soon as possible. One cannot leave a vacuum to be filled by anxieties and fears and those who pander to them. While we may be dimly aware of the dangers associated with rousing public fears about AIDS, few of us have had the experience of a epidemic of this sort, and we do not fully understand the hazards of doing the reverse—which is to remain silent while the process slips beyond our control. Indeed, in many areas this may already have happened.

Modern epidemiology can help if one uses it as the imaging and teaching tool that it can be. In discussing John Snow's work on cholera, Wade Hampton Frost of Johns Hopkins wrote in 1936 that epidemiology is "something more than the total of its established facts and includes chains of inference which *extend beyond* the bounds of direct observation."[7] We have before us today a good deal of direct observation about AIDS and, more importantly, new forms of knowledge about this disease, based on new technologies, which extend our vision very far indeed. These allow us, in essence, to see into the future of this epidemic. The chapters included in this volume amass much useful evidence on the question of the heterosexual transmission of AIDS and reveal something of the means and the potential magnitude of that route of infection. The studies presented cross international boundaries and differences of race and social class. They do, I believe, deal a blow to the concept of "risk groups," as opposed to "risk behavior," for the acquisition of this disease. For a time these groups served as a guide to help focus our preliminary research. However, in retrospect, they also appear to have been as much a psychological maneuver as a public health strategy, a maneuver which lulled many into believing they were not at risk and thereby ultimately failed to protect us.

The purpose of some of the chapters in this volume is to examine the notion that AIDS is a disease which has human sexuality at its fulcrum, not a disease of homosexuals or drug addicts, Haitians or Africans, although these groups have suffered significantly from its spread. These chapters provide a basis for evaluating this judgment and a basis for considering some of its implications for our future.

ERNEST DRUCKER, PhD
Associate Professor
Department of Epidemiology and
Social Medicine
Montefiore Medical Center/
Albert Einstein College of Medicine
Bronx, NY 10467

1. Camus A: *The Plague*. New York, Alfred A. Knopf Inc, 1947.
2. US Public Health Service: Coolfont Conference on AIDS. Washington, DC, June 1986.
3. Crosby A W Jr: *The Columbian Exchange: Biological and Cultural Consequences of 1492*. Westport, Conn, Greenwood Press, 1975, pp 149–151.
4. Fischl MA, Dickinson GM, Scott GB, et al: Evaluation of heterosexual partners, children, and household contacts of adults with AIDS. *JAMA* 1987; 257:640–644.
5. Harris C, Small CB, Klein RS, et al: Immunodeficiency in female sexual partners of men with the acquired immunodeficiency syndrome. *N Engl J Med* 1983; 308:1181–1184.
6. Redfield RR, Markham PD, Salahuddin SZ, et al: Frequent transmission of HTLV-III among spouses of patients with AIDS-related complex and AIDS. *JAMA* 1985; 253:1571–1573.
7. Frost WH (ed): Introduction, in *Cholera*. Baltimore, Md, Johns Hopkins University Press, 1936, p ix.

Chapter 25

AIDS in New York City: Moving ahead on effective public health approaches

The relentless tragedy of acquired immunodeficiency syndrome (AIDS) is nowhere more starkly felt than in New York City. As of the end of February 1987, 9,188 people in New York City had been diagnosed with AIDS; 58% have died. AIDS is the leading cause of death in New York City for men 25 to 44 years of age, and for women aged 25 to 29.[1]

Half a million people in New York City are estimated to be infected with human immunodeficiency virus (HIV) today. Homosexual and bisexual men make up the largest percentage of cases, though the proportion of AIDS cases among this group has fallen from 73% in 1981 to 55% in 1986, while the proportion of cases among intravenous (IV) drug abusers has risen from 22% in 1981 to 36% in 1986. From 50% to 60% of the city's estimated 200,000 heroin users are thought to be HIV-infected.[1]

IV drug abusers have been, and will likely continue to be, the major source of the spread of HIV infection to women and children in New York City. Of the 932 women diagnosed with AIDS in New York City since 1981, 80% have been IV drug abusers or the sex partners of IV drug abusers. One hundred seventy-eight cases of AIDS have occurred in New York City in children, the vast majority of these having been infected perinatally by their mothers. Ninety-two percent of mothers who infected their children were IV drug abusers or the sex partners of IV drug abusers.

AIDS is also having an increasing impact on New York City's minority communities. More than half of all AIDS victims in New York City are black or Hispanic. Eighty-six percent of male IV drug users with AIDS are black or Hispanic; 91% of mothers of children who have AIDS are black or Hispanic.[1]

By the end of 1991, more than 40,000 people will have developed AIDS in New York City alone; 30,000 will have died. These projections are based on a five-year horizon; no one knows the ten- or 20-year clinical outlook for those now infected. Nor do we know what long-term burdens will be posed by HIV-associated illnesses, such as tuberculosis (TB) or lymphoma. The impact of HIV immunodeficiency on the trends of other important diseases is under study and as yet is incompletely understood.

Against this background, and as the epidemic spreads in New York City, a number of public health policy issues are emerging as critical.

First, intensive public education efforts need to be implemented, without creating irrational anxiety and hysteria. Presently, the only feasible way to alter the course of the AIDS epidemic is by educating the public, training health and social service professionals, and offering counseling for personal risk reduction and antibody testing. Health professionals, educators, and the media must discuss AIDS issues appropriately, facing the facts about AIDS squarely, with honesty about our areas of uncertainty, and in explicit, understandable language.

Second, vigorous public health actions need to be increased while resisting ineffective measures of social control. Pressures are mounting for measures such as universal or mandatory AIDS antibody screening programs, as well as for isolation and quarantine of AIDS victims. At a conference sponsored by the Centers for Disease Control (CDC) held in Atlanta in February 1987, virtually all public health officials from the areas of highest AIDS prevalence agreed that forcing people to learn their serostatus, when no treatment is available, and when confidentiality may not be assured, would be unwise and counterproductive.

Third, increases in available resources for research and education must support the broad range of clinical, public health, and social service needs. The federal government has been very reluctant to recognize the true dimensions of and propose an adequately funded federal response to AIDS. It must do much more to support the unprecedented demands for AIDS treatment, human services, public health initiatives, and human rights resources, without sacrificing the research and education efforts that are so necessary.

To translate these policy issues into measures for controlling the spread of AIDS, in the current absence of effective treatment, we must rapidly increase confidential, voluntary counseling and testing. The New York City Health Department is moving aggressively to make voluntary, confidential HIV antibody counseling and testing much more widely accessible. The Department has published a counseling and testing policy containing guidelines for health professionals involved in the prevention and treatment of HIV infection as well as education of those at risk.[2] The policy states that anyone should be able to know his or her antibody status, provided the test results will be kept confidential, testing is voluntary, and pre- and post-test counseling is available. We strongly recommend that physicians actively consider whether their patients may be at risk of AIDS infection, discuss risk-avoiding behavior as part of routine medical care of all patients, and offer counseling and, if appropriate, antibody testing to patients at risk.

To support the confidential, voluntary aspects of counseling and testing, we have adopted a course of action known as contact notification. With this approach, the Health Department is urging, and directly and actively assisting when asked, people who are seropositive to notify their contacts.

We must increase access to substance abuse treatment programs for IV drug addicts. This is one of the most critical options for halting the spread of AIDS among addicts and to women and children. Currently, New York City has long waiting lists for methadone maintenance programs; drug-free rehabilitation programs are full to capacity. The federal government must consider drug rehabilitation programs as one of our important priorities, and provide more federal dollars through states and communities so that more addicts may find treatment for their addiction.

The Department of Health, in conjunction with the Divison of Substance Abuse Services of New York State, has developed a proposal to explore an additional strategy for reducing the spread of HIV among drug users: a research project to determine the effect of the availability of clean needles to a small, carefully selected and monitored group of IV drug addicts awaiting entry into drug treatment programs. If approved by the State Health Commissioner, the research study will serve as the basis for evaluating the efficacy of this approach in halting the further spread of the AIDS virus, while avoiding promotion of IV substance abuse.

Efforts to expand our knowledge base must be increased. Research needs to be expanded to investigate the nature of HIV and its transmission. Health Department researchers are collecting data for two studies, a survey of hospital patients suspected of having AIDS to identify associated risk factors, and a study of risk factors for transmission of AIDS in heterosexual couples in which one partner contracted AIDS from a blood transfusion. In another project, Department researchers and five participating hospitals are studying HIV transmission from infected mother to child. A series of blind and anonymous serosurveys is planned, to shed greater light on current infection patterns, especially among women of childbearing age.

Massive public health education risk-reduction efforts must be increased. For the present, the most effective way to reduce the spread of HIV infection is a multifaceted prevention and risk-reduction strategy directing education at the general public, plus targeting information and outreach for people engaged in high-risk behavior. Such a strategy is currently being undertaken by the Health Department's program of AIDS education and counseling. The Health Department has launched a $1 million campaign to promote latex condom use in all appropriate circumstances. The campaign includes a plan to distribute a million condoms next year along with educational material. The Department has also been working with two advertising agencies to develop multimedia public health advertising campaigns that will begin in the spring of this year.

The false dichotomy between civil liberties and public health must be eliminated. Stands on issues such as contact tracing and mandatory antibody testing have at times been portrayed as sacrificing public health in the name of civil liberties. Yet the approaches taken in New York City are based on sound public health principles; virtually all public health professionals agree that public health would be hindered by control measures such as mandatory testing. HIV-infected people—already facing devastating discrimination in housing, employment, and insurance—would not cooperate with our counseling, education, and testing if they feared that society was considering measures that could lead to quarantine, isolation, and additional forms of discrimination.

Funding at the federal, state, and local levels must be increased. Last year, the National Academy of Sciences called for a $2 billion AIDS research and education effort. The Academy recommended that $1 billion a year be newly appropriated for extensive basic and applied biomedical investigations of the disease.[3] Another $1 billion would go for a massive continuing education campaign to increase public awareness of the ways of protecting against infection. The money would also be applied to other necessary public health measures, such as screening the blood supply, voluntary confidential testing, and increased efforts in treatment and prevention of IV drug use. The Academy's call must herald an increase in the national commitment against the massive problem of AIDS.

The epidemic, and our understanding of it, is growing and changing constantly. Responsible policy must be continually reexamined against these changing conditions, and modified if necessary.

Education, health promotion, and risk reduction—these will remain the critical weapons in the fight against AIDS for at least the next several years. Those of us in a position to influence policy must do all we can to advance these weapons against this mounting health problem in New York City, across the United States, and around the world.

STEPHEN C. JOSEPH, MD, MPH
Commissioner of Health
City of New York
New York, NY 10013

1. Analysis of New York City AIDS surveillance data, New York City Department of Health, 1987.
2. New York City Department of Health HIV counseling and testing policy, March 1987.
3. Institute of Medicine, National Academy of Sciences: *Confronting AIDS: Directions for Public Health, Health Care and Research*. Washington, DC, National Academy Press, 1986, pp 33–34.

Chapter 26
The prevention of AIDS

The chapters in this volume dealing with acquired immunodeficiency syndrome (AIDS) constitute an urgent call to action. The problem is: What action? In this rapidly changing field, controversy surrounds detailed proposals, but the principles on which action should be based are, or at least ought to be, unchanging.

First of all, there must be a massive effort in public education. Other countries do it well. Sweden, which I will use as an example several times, offers intense education on sexual health and other health issues in the public schools, beginning at the earliest possible age.[1] That public education process continues, using every conceivable medium of information, throughout the lifetime of every citizen. We in the United States permit massive advertising for cigarettes and other forms of self-destruction and encourage television programs and films that implicitly encourage sex without responsibility, but do not use the same channels to reach our people about the perils that surround us and how they can be avoided.

There must be a massive expansion of relevant prevention and treatment services. Industrialized countries like Sweden, with approximately the same GNP per capita as the US, provide significantly more public services through higher rates of taxation, the proceeds of which are applied to human rather than military purposes.[2] Condoms, to take a highly relevant if relatively inexpensive example, are supplied extremely cheaply at multiple easily-accessible sites, including public vending machines.[3] Counseling and other preventive services are far more accessible than in the United States. Treatment services, including immediate availability for every drug user or other at-risk person who wants to use them, are viewed as an urgent public responsibility. We, as a rich country, can do no less.

There must be a far greater role in the formulation of public policy for those most affected and those most at risk. As an example, Sweden, after an extensive public education campaign, conducted a national referendum on the future of nuclear power; an extraordinarily large part of the electorate, compared to our levels of voting, took part.[4] More locally, most Swedish health service policies are set at the county level and almost all health service funding is collected and controlled at the local level.[2] We must begin, in our own heterogeneous nation—sharply divided between those who have wealth and power and those who do not—to find ways to involve people much more directly in the development and implementation of policies that directly affect their lives. For example, the needle-exchange program in Amsterdam is a coordinated project developed jointly by public health authorities and

the organized "Association of Drug Addicts."[5] Greater involvement of those directly afflicted will not only lead to more effective policies but the resulting reduction in feelings of alienation and powerlessness will have reverberations for improvement of health and well-being throughout our society.

Any society that wishes to use repressive measures, such as various forms of quarantine, against its people must justify those actions not only on utilitarian grounds but also in terms of fairness or justice. In short, the society must earn the right to use such measures. To use the example of Sweden yet again, the Associated Press reported in February 1986 that an intravenous drug user "who tested positive for the virus believed to cause AIDS was involuntarily detained in a Stockholm hospital after continuing to share needles with other drug users and to have sex without taking precautions to protect his partner."[6] Without taking a position on the complex question of the usefulness, not to speak of the desirability, of involuntary detention in our society, the more important point is that Sweden may have earned the right to limit civil liberties in certain ways for the protection of others. The extraordinary nature of its health and human services, its emphasis on services for minorities and for others in its population who are least well off, its other social concerns for its people, and the many other areas in which it is working for the public health, may give it that right. We in the United States are only beginning to earn the right to selectively limit civil liberties for the protection of others from AIDS. We still permit tobacco advertising and smoking in public places; we still do not require passive restraints in automobiles; we fail to protect the public health in any number of appropriate ways. For us to single out certain vulnerable groups or certain areas of human behavior for Draconian restriction is morally unacceptable.

To again cite a specific example, in October 1985 the New York State Public Health Council adopted an addition to the state health code that defined "high risk sexual activity" as anal intercourse and fellatio, labelled any commercial facilities in which such activity takes place "a public nuisance dangerous to the public health," and permitted their closing by health authorities.[7] I was the only member of the Council to vote against the regulation. My dissent was based on two grounds. First, many knowledgeable groups argued that it was precisely in those kinds of establishments that some of the best education on sexual health issues was taking place, and that the recent fall in surrogate measures of "high risk" sexual activity, such as the incidence of gonorrhea, demonstrated that. Second, and more important, intravenous drug use appeared to represent a greater risk factor for AIDS transmission than fellatio or anal intercourse, particularly in New York City, and it is increasingly clear that vaginal intercourse is an important mode of transmission. Yet here was a measure that was restrictive in only one area of risk, not surprisingly directed against people and acts that some powerful people find repugnant, but which did nothing to attempt to deal with more important risk factors. Similar issues are raised by involuntary blood testing for antibodies (which it has recently been suggested should be applied as broadly as for all those applying for marriage licenses and for all those admitted to hospitals), and of course by job, school, or insurance denial for those who are antibody-positive. Even if such actions could be shown—as they have not so far been—to be rational they present extremely difficult problems. The point is that if our society wants to limit civil liberties in certain areas for the protection of public health, it must do so equitably and justly. Picking out certain groups for special restriction—particularly if they are socially and politically weak and vulnerable—or subjecting large groups to testing which is of questionable predictive or therapeutic value, may be a greater danger to our society than is AIDS.

The nature of AIDS and the recent evidence on the routes of its communicability pose an enormous challenge to our society. The question is whether we will meet that challenge using methods that improve human rights and the quality of life for all—in short, whether we will use the crisis to move toward being a more democratic and just nation, or whether our response will further erode the already bruised and tearing fabric of our society.[8,9]

VICTOR W. SIDEL, MD
Distinguished University Professor
of Social Medicine
Montefiore Medical Center/
Albert Einstein College of Medicine
Bronx, NY 10467

1. Swedish sex education and its results. *Current Sweden* 1984; no. 315.
2. Sidel VW, Sidel R: Sweden—Planned pluralism, in *A Healthy State: An International Perspective on the Crisis in United States Medical Care*, rev ed. New York, Pantheon Books, 1983, pp 118–141.
3. *Instruction Concerning Interpersonal Relations.* Stockholm, National Swedish Board of Education, 1977, p 175.
4. *Energy and Energy Policy in Sweden.* Stockholm, The Swedish Institute, 1986.
5. Buning EC, Coutinho RA, Jan Brussel GHA, et al: Preventing AIDS in drug addicts in Amsterdam. *Lancet* 1986; 1:1435.
6. HTLV-III carrier detained in Sweden. *Am Medical News*, February 7, 1986.
7. Official Compilation of Codes, Rules and Regulations of the State of New York, Title 10 (Health), Chapter 1 (State Sanitary Code), Part 24 (AIDS), Subpart 24-2 (Prohibited Facilities).
8. Sidel R, Sidel VW: Toward the twenty-first century, in Sidel VW, Sidel R (eds): *Reforming Medicine: Lessons of the Last Quarter Century.* New York, Pantheon Books, 1984, pp 267–284.
9. Sidel VW: The fabric of public health. *Am J Pub Health* 1986; 76:373–378.

Chapter 27
Fear of AIDS

Americans in general are still influenced by the fear of acquired immunodeficiency syndrome (AIDS). This fear, often uninformed and unwarranted, has an impact on many of the issues discussed in some of the chapters in this volume. A number of these chapters focus on the issue of sexual transmission, a subject which is of great concern. The fear of other routes of transmission persists, including those that either do not exist or, if they do, are really inconsequential in terms of the total AIDS epidemic. To some extent we have been hampered in our efforts to deal with the disease by an obsessive fear of transmission by nonsexual, "casual" contact. What appear to be really important factors in terms of human immunodeficiency virus (HIV) transmission are sexuality and substance abuse. Yet there is a great deal of difficulty in publicly and intelligently dealing with these particular aspects of basic human existence in the context of the AIDS epidemic. We are all sexual beings, and many in our society are abusers of either legal or illegal drugs. These behaviors are deeply embedded in our psychology and our culture, making them difficult to approach in such a way that behavior can be changed.

A basic issue that relates to the fear of AIDS, and which has diverted attention from concentrating on sex and drugs, is the continuing irrational belief among some that a virus that causes such a terrible disease in young people must be very easily transmitted. In fact the accumulated information, supported by the facts, indicates that the disease is not easily transmitted. Studies of both household contacts of AIDS patients[1] and hospital workers caring for AIDS patients[2] make this clear. In terms of heterosexual transmission, it is noteworthy that the majority of long-standing sexual contacts of infected individuals remain uninfected, even after hundreds of sexual encounters.[3]

The fear of AIDS is also related to the fact that we tend to concentrate on isolated transmission events rather than on the probability of transmission. The overall literature on AIDS and some of the chapters in this volume provide information from population-based studies that permit a determination of rates of risk.[1–5] Rather than observing that an event can occur, one should reflect on how frequently it occurs and from this begin to approach the factors that are associated with its occurrence.

We remain uninformed about the current patterns of

HIV transmission. It we think in terms of infection and not disease, there is at least a five-year lag period in documenting and understanding transmission patterns. This is the result of the prolonged incubation period of the disease.[6] In order to understand what is currently occurring one must perform seroprevalence surveys in populations not known to engage in the traditional high-risk behaviors of intravenous drug abuse and homosexual sex. An illustration is the occurrence of female-to-male sexual transmission. Documentation of this form of transmission does not appear in AIDS case surveillance data but may be present in seroprevalence surveys. The virus first entered predominately male populations in US society—homosexual men, intravenous (IV) drug abusers, and those suffering from hemophilia. Therefore the pool of infected women able to transmit infection to men was quite small five years ago. Since the number of infected women is increasing, seroprevalence surveys among sexually active heterosexuals might disclose increasing rates of female-to-male transmission at present, whereas AIDS case surveys do not because they document the results of transmission events that occurred many years ago. However, because of the fear of AIDS and the resultant consequences of seropositivity, such as isolation and stigmatization, loss of jobs and health insurance, elimination of sexuality, and the burden of uncertainty about the future, it is difficult to perform seroprevalence surveys. There is little incentive for serologic testing for individuals. Seroprevalence surveys, contact tracing, and knowledge about who is infected and how transmission is occurring have all thereby been impeded. Further, to characterize current heterosexual transmission patterns, one must determine the rate of seropositivity among adolescents and sexually active young adults in geographic areas of extensive IV drug abuse, since IV drug abuse and heterosexual transmission are clearly linked. But this must be done with appropriate concern for confidentiality and the protection of individuals' rights.

The availability of chemotherapy in the future will substantially change the situation and make individual serologic testing valuable by enabling early treatment. If one looks at the history of sexually transmitted disease in this society in the last century, it is clear that it was only the availability of specific therapy with penicillin that made contact tracing for syphilis and gonorrhea a viable public health tool. To expect individuals to be tested, we must have something more to offer them than bad news, particularly if that news is accompanied by stigmatization and other social dilemmas. The possibility of offering a treatment in the future, with some degree of cautious optimism, might change this situation.

Finally, it is important to emphasize how essential it is to understand the behavior and the culture in which transmission occurs. The biologic model of disease or of virus infection inadequately explains transmission. In order to understand transmission, one must know what people do, how and where they do it, how frequently, and why. One must understand the culture in which these events take place in order to gain access to changing behavior. The papers by Hein[7] about adolescent sexuality and Des Jarlais[8] about prostitution make this clear. The same detailed understanding of patterns of IV drug use is essential to influence behavior.

To interrupt the transmission of HIV, information and education remain the most important tools.

GERALD FRIEDLAND, MD
Associate Professor
Department of Medicine
Department of Epidemiology and
Social Medicine
Montefiore Medical Center/
Albert Einstein College of Medicine
Bronx, NY 10467

1. Friedland GH, Saltzman BR, Rogers MF, et al: Lack of transmission of HTLV-III/LAV infection to household contacts of patients with AIDS or AIDS-related complex with oral candidiasis. N Engl J Med 1986; 314:344–349.

2. McCray E: The cooperative needlestick surveillance group, occupational risk of acquired immunodeficiency syndrome among health care workers. N Engl J Med 1986; 314:1127–1132.

3. Saltzman BR, Harris CA, Klein RS, et al: HTLV-III/LAV infection and immunodeficiency in heterosexual partners of AIDS patients. Presented at the International Conference on AIDS, Paris, France, June 1986.

4. Burke DS, Brundage JF, Bernier W, et al: Demography of HIV infections among civilian applicants for military service in four counties in New York City. NY State J Med 1987; 87:262–264.

5. Quinn TC: AIDS in Africa: Evidence for heterosexual transmission of the human immunodeficiency virus. NY State J Med 1987; 87:286–289.

6. Lui KJ, Lawrence DN, Morgan WM, et al: A model-based approach for estimating the mean incubation period of transfusion-associated acquired immunodeficiency syndrome. Proc Nat Acad Sci 1986; 83:3051–3055.

7. Hein K: AIDS in adolescents: A rationale for concern. NY State J Med 1987; 87:290–295.

8. Des Jarlais DC, Wish E, Friedman SR, et al: Intravenous drug use and the heterosexual transmission of the human immunodeficiency virus: Current trends in New York City. NY State J Med 1987; 87:283–286.

Chapter 28

Human immunodeficiency virus
antibody testing:
Time for clinicians
to use it

In 1985 the enzyme-linked immunosorbent assay (ELISA) to detect antibody to the human immunodeficiency virus (HIV) was licensed by the Food and Drug Administration. Used in conjunction with appropriate confirmatory tests such as the Western blot, it was now possible to identify individuals who had been infected with this virus. The use of these tests was immediately and universally adopted by blood banks in this country. However, their use in the clinical setting was limited by a number of unanswered questions raised by clinicians, advocacy groups, and public health officials. These issues are nearing resolution, and it is now time to place HIV testing in wider clinical use.

There were four critical issues that impeded the wider use of HIV antibody testing. First, effective pre- and post-test counseling programs had yet to be developed and implemented. The accuracy of HIV testing in various populations needed to be defined. The meaning (clinical implications) of a confirmed positive test needed to be completely understood. Finally, no clear therapeutic options were available to clinicians caring for the seropositive patient who had not yet developed clinical acquired immunodeficiency syndrome (AIDS). Our clearer understanding of these issues is now a compelling reason for using HIV testing on a more active basis.

The need for effective counseling in conjunction with HIV testing has now been recognized.[1] Effective counseling programs, including both pre- and post-test counseling, have now been developed and implemented around the country. These programs have been instituted in diverse settings including hospitals, family planning clinics, methadone maintenance clinics, anonymous testing sites, and sexually transmitted disease clinics.[2]

The greatest impediment to the development of counseling programs is the lack of financial resources and an inadequate pool of trained counselors. This was demonstrated most clearly in Illinois when the introduction of required premarital HIV testing overwhelmed the few established public programs.[3] The Illinois experience is also instructive in reinforcing the concept of concentrating testing and counseling resources on high-risk groups. Diffusing scant resources to large populations delays their use for those populations that need it most.

The accuracy of HIV testing in various populations has been clarified in the past two years. Controversy around the issue of false-positives has really surrounded the use of the ELISA, an initial screening exam.[4] Under standard testing protocols all positive ELISAs are repeated, then confirmed by a Western blot (a far more specific if more costly test) prior to the patient's being notified that he or she is antibody positive. A positive confirmatory test is considered evidence of HIV infection. The sensitivity of the currently licensed ELISA tests is 99% or greater.[5] Given this performance, the probability of a false-negative test result is remote, except during that period prior to the development of antibodies. The specificity of a repeatedly reactive ELISA is approximately 99%.[5] The use of a supplemental test such as the Western blot markedly increases this specificity. Under ideal conditions, the probability that a testing sequence will result in a false positive in a population with a low rate of infection ranges from less than one in 100,000 to five in 100,000.[5] While some concern has been expressed about the rate of false positives in such low risk populations, it is important to recognize that in higher risk populations (where the seroprevalence of HIV rises above 5%), a positive test sequence should be considered exactly that, positive for HIV antibody.

The clinical implications of a confirmed positive antibody test have been clarified during the last 24 months by several studies. A confirmed positive test means that an individual is infected, potentially infectious, and has a high probability of developing symptomatic illness within seven years of infection. In adults, the best data have been generated from the San Francisco City Clinic cohort study, comprising a group of homosexual and bisexual men who were enrolled in a hepatitis B virus study in the late 1970s. Of 155 men with long term HIV infection (approximately 88 months), 36% have progressed to AIDS, while more than 40% had other signs or symptoms of infection; only 20% have remained completely asymptomatic.[6] These epidemiologic observations have been supported by other studies which have noted a clear and progressive decline in T-helper cells in 90% of individuals after at least three years of HIV infection.[7] Hence it appears that HIV infection is associated with an inexorable decline in cell-mediated immunity.

One of the initial arguments against HIV testing was the lack of therapeutic options for the seropositive patient. Clinical developments have now progressed to the point that practitioners can intervene to avoid some of the complications of HIV-induced immunosuppression. The clinical use of T4 (helper) lymphocyte enumeration plays an important role in this evaluation. As the number of T4-cells decreases, one's chance of developing one of the opportunistic infections increases. For example, it appears that when T cells decrease below a level of $200/\text{mm}^3$, one is at increased risk of developing *Pneumocystis carinii* pneumonia (PCP).[8] Several studies have demonstrated the effectiveness of various regimens in preventing PCP.[9,10] At least one additional study has demonstrated its use in asymptomatic seropositive individuals with T4 cell depletion.[11] The approach to patients who are tuberculin positive will also vary depending on the patient's HIV status. For example, the American Thoracic Society has recommended that isoniazid (INH) prophylactic therapy should be instituted in patients who are seropositive and have positive tuberculin skin tests.[12] Tuberculosis is a serious problem in many patients with HIV infection. Although most patients with severe HIV-induced immunosuppression are anergic, many are not. Application of tuberculin skin tests prior to the development of anergy can allow the clinician to determine whether to institute INH prophylaxis in hosts that may undergo further depression of cellular immunity. An additional clinical indication is based on recently completed studies in New York State which have shown a rate of HIV seropositivity in newborns of 1.5 to 2.5%.[13,14] In light of these data, the Centers for Disease Control (CDC) has suggested that women living in communities where there is known high prevalence of HIV infection be offered information and education about AIDS as well as testing. Finally, and most critically, even though all individuals should examine and alter their own personal behavior, an awareness of serostatus serves as an additional incentive to protect loved ones.

In New York State, the state with the highest incidence of AIDS, utilization of HIV testing is among the lowest of any state.[15] Clearly testing can be used to prevent further spread, to anticipate clinical problems in specific patients, as well as to help women make informed decisions about pregnancy. All testing should continue to be provided in a manner that ensures confidentiality. As physicians we need to understand the full implications of HIV testing so that we can adequately counsel our patients. Finally, we must reject all calls for mandatory (or routine) testing of populations. In an era of limited resources HIV testing should be done for clinical indications, not to pursue ideological goals. Nonetheless, it is now clear that all clinicians must become comfortable in nonjudgmentally inquiring about both a patient's drug and sexual history in order to determine whether they might benefit from HIV testing. The application of broader, selective testing will contribute greatly to patient survival as well as to preventing the spread of HIV disease.

JACK A. DeHOVITZ, MD, MPH
Assistant Professor
Departments of Preventive Medicine and
Community Health and Medicine

SHELDON H. LANDESMAN, MD
Associate Professor
Department of Medicine
State University of New York
Health Science Center at Brooklyn
Brooklyn, NY 11203

1. Centers for Disease Control: Public Health Service guidelines for counseling and antibody testing to prevent HIV infection and AIDS. *MMWR* 1987; 36:509–515.

2. DeHovitz JA, Witt MD, Altimont TJ (eds): *The AIDS Manual: A Guide for Health Care Administrators*. Baltimore, National Health Publishing, 1988.

3. Wilkerson I: Prenuptial AIDS screening: A strain in Illinois. *NY Times*, January 26, 1988, p 1.

4. Meyer KB, Pauker SG: Screening for HIV: Can we afford the false positive rate? *NEJM* 1987; 317:238–241.

5. Centers for Disease Control: Update: Serologic testing for antibody to human immunodeficiency virus. *MMWR* 1988; 36:833–845.

6. Curran JW, Jaffe HW, Hardy AM, et al: Epidemiology of HIV infection and AIDS in the United States. *Science* 1988; 239:610–616.

7. Melbye M, Biggar RJ, Ebbesen P, et al: Long-term seropositivity for human T-lymphotropic virus type III in homosexual men without the acquired immunodeficiency syndrome: Development of immunologic and clinical abnormalities. *Ann Intern Med* 1986; 104:496–500.

8. Lane HC, Masur H, Gelmann EP, et al: Correlation between immunologic function and clinical subpopulations of patients with the acquired immune deficiency syndrome. *Am J Med* 1985; 78:417–422.

9. Gottlieb MS, Knight S, Mitsuyasu R: Prophylaxis of *Pneumocystis carinii* infection in AIDS with pyrimethamine-sulfadoxine. *Lancet* 1984; 2:398–399.

10. Metroka CE, Lange M, Braun N: Successful chemoprophylaxis of *Pneumocystis carinii* pneumonia with dapsone in patients with AIDS and ARC. Proceedings of the Third International Conference on AIDS. Abstract #THP. 231. Washington, DC, 1987.

11. Veira J: Fansidar prophylaxis of *Pneumocystis carinii* pneumonia. Proceedings of the Third International Conference on AIDS. Abstract # TP.221. Washington, DC, 1987.

12. American Thoracic Society/Centers for Disease Control: Mycobacterioses and the acquired immunodeficiency syndrome. *Am Rev Respir Dis* 1987; 136:492–496.

13. Lambert B: One in 61 babies in New York City has AIDS antibodies, study says. *NY Times*, January 12, 1988, p 1.

14. Landesman S, Minkoff H, Holman S, et al: Serosurvey of human immunodeficiency virus infection in parturients. *JAMA* 1987; 285:2701–2703.

15. Centers for Disease Control: HTLV-III/LAV antibody testing at alternate sites. *MMWR* 1986; 35:284–287.

Chapter 29

The new horizon: Programmatic responses to the HIV epidemic

Although the current epidemic of human immunodeficiency virus (HIV) infection has been recognized for at least seven years, in many respects we are just beginning to appreciate the sobering consequences of its impact. There is hardly an analyst familiar with the demographics of HIV infection who has not predicted substantial outlays for the medical care of the many infected individuals who will become symptomatic within the next decade. Researchers persist in their attempts to develop effective medical treatments, but even the most optimistic of them believe that there is no cure or vaccine on the immediate horizon. It is clear that many of our citizens will suffer prolonged, expensive, and untimely deaths as a result of the immune damage wrought by this viral infection.

Dr Steven Joseph, New York City's Commissioner of Health, has been quoted as saying, "the way mankind responds to crisis is first disbelief, then denial, then the third stage is mobilization, and we're at the horizon of that now.[1] Perhaps the surest proof of that statement is the influence that epidemic HIV infection is having on organizations within our society. The media, business corporations, public and private educational institutions, correctional facilities, religious institutions, and health care organizations of all types, regardless of their source of funding, scope of services, or geographic location, are mobilizing to confront the issue of acquired immunodeficiency syndrome (AIDS). While such activity is preferable to the tepid organizational response that characterized the early years of the epidemic, this activity, in and of itself, will not insure a comprehensive or coordinated response to the problem of HIV infection. Because of the federal government's lack of a comprehensive plan of action in response to the AIDS epidemic in its early years, much of the burden for strategic planning and programmatic development fell to state and local governments, health care facilities located in high incidence areas, and a host of community organizations which sprang up to meet the needs of infected clients. Although the manner in which these entities confronted the epidemic—often with little support, sympathy, or funding—is laudable, it was not a substitute for a comprehensive, coordinated national plan of action against the virus. The federal coordination of a programmatic response to HIV infection is no less important than the coordination of a similar response with regard to biomedical research and vaccine development. This response should include initiatives to prevent the further transmission of the virus, to expand health care and related services in areas of the country with substantial numbers of cases, to modify existing systems of health care financing to meet the needs of individuals who have lost all of their assets to this infection, and to create mechanisms which would subsume a share of the financial burden for the out-of-hospital care of AIDS patients, which has, in many instances, been placed upon the nonprofit sector.[2]

As noted by Novick et al,[3] the proportion of incident AIDS cases reported in "high incidence" areas will continue to decrease as more cases are reported in "low incidence" areas. Centralizing our attack on AIDS will facilitate information and resource sharing such that providers in areas currently designated as "low incidence" can develop adequate programmatic structures in advance of the epidemic. They will not have to relive all of the frustration endured by "high incidence" communities in the first years of the epidemic in order to profit from their experience. Not only will centralization of strategy help to insure a similar level of quality across disparate communities, it will also minimize the local, often untoward, political response which AIDS-related programs sometimes generate, especially in the area of prevention services. Of all the programmatic challenges we face as a result of the AIDS epidemic, the creation of effective, targeted prevention programs is among the most difficult.

At least in theory, there appears to be broad-based support for the concept of preventing the further transmission of HIV. There are, however, important variables that influence the manner in which we approach the subject of HIV prevention, and which subsequently have an impact on the way in which we mount programs to actualize these objectives. Because substantial resources will be consumed in the process of providing care for those already infected, it is conceivable that funding for prevention initiatives will have to compete with funding for treatment. Culturally, we have a strong bias toward biomedical solutions to health problems, and this may also serve to minimize the resources that are designated for serious prevention efforts. It is readily apparent that it is far easier to reach a consensus on the appropriateness of developing an effective antiretroviral chemotherapeutic agent than it is to obtain endorsement of the aggressive promotion of an explicit message about sexual prophylaxis, or an evaluation of programs that would enable intravenous drug abusers to participate in sterile needle exchanges.[4] In the absence of an effective treatment or vaccine against HIV, programs for the prevention of infection must not limit themselves to the "seek and treat" mentality which has become the bulwark of disease control within the public health establishment for the past two decades. If our objective is to interrupt viral transmission, we must be willing to design programs that have a reasonable chance of achieving that goal.

There are other barriers to prevention as well. AIDS is a burden which is not equally distributed across society. The burgeoning analysis of this epidemic indicates that it is actually a series of "subepidemics" which are related but unequal.[5] Specific groups are overrepresented within the "dole," groups whose behaviors may not conform to societal notions of propriety or whose day-to-day living circumstances may be completely alien to the average citizen. In order to effectively prevent transmission of virus within these subpopulations, we must develop messages and modalities that are acceptable to them, which they can understand, and which they can ultimately come to accept as normative. Risk-reduction campaigns that have been effective among homosexual men are not ipso facto acceptable to sexually active inner-city youths, nor to the female sexual partners of intravenous drug abusers. To promote HIV prevention within these populations we must develop strategies that specifically "reflect the special characteristics, needs, and preferences of these target groups."[6] When AIDS prevention messages are homogenized to a level that makes them acceptable to a general audience, or are arbitrarily transferred from one "risk group" to the next, they may lose their appeal to the target audience for which they were designed.

An ongoing misunderstanding appears to be in the differentiation of public education campaigns from targeted prevention programs. Although the general public requires information about AIDS, and how the virus is transmitted, individuals who are at particular risk of infection will require more substantial, more intensive efforts to promote the modification of those behaviors that place them at risk for HIV infection. While the frequent airing of public service announcements about AIDS and media attention to the subject of HIV infection are integral components of the basic education we must undertake, they should not be mistaken for risk reduction interventions. The latter, while they incorporate an informational component, also address germane psychological, behavioral, and situational characteristics of the target population in an effort to promote behavioral change. Legislators, educators, and the panoply of individuals who are positioned to influence the development of prevention programs must be made to understand that risk reduction programs are based on social science theory and sound public health practice—not on whether or not they will be palatable to the public at large. This is not to negate or minimize the controversy that often attends such proposals, only to underscore the fact that we cannot afford to "politicize" the process of program development, especially in the area of prevention services.[7]

At this phase of the epidemic, AIDS has become a ubiquitous acronym, and for many of us, it is difficult to remember a time when it was not part of our consciousness or our vocabulary. Clearly there are those who still view it as the disease of "outsiders," as something they know of only indirectly. But as more people succumb to their infections, as more households and families become touched by the reality of sickness and death, this perception will become the luxury of the fortunate few. Certainly, AIDS is not the end of mankind, and those individuals or groups who have chosen to describe it as the 20th century bubonic plague have fortunately been proven wrong. Nonetheless, the epidemic is bound to have a lasting impact on our society. Not only will it influence the scope and direction of current biomedical research and medical therapeutics—it will also affect our cultural mores, our attitudes about death and dying, and many of our basic assumptions about the primacy of technology as a solution to problems. Although epidemics are first and foremost medical phenomena, they are also extraordinary catalysts for societal change. At this juncture, as expenditures are being designated for programs to meet the needs of the infected and the at-risk, it is essential that we plan our strategy carefully, with special attention to the circumstances and needs of the clients whom we wish to serve, and that we capitalize on the lessons we have learned in the past seven years.

RONALD O. VALDISERRI, MD
Director
Falk Clinic Laboratories

Associate Professor of Pathology
University of Pittsburgh
School of Medicine

Assistant Professor of Infectious Diseases
University of Pittsburgh
Graduate School of Public Health
Pittsburgh, PA 15213

1. Lambert B: U.S. confronting AIDS with sense of realism. *NY Times*, February 17, 1988, pp A1, B10.
2. Arno PS: The non-profit sector's response to the AIDS epidemic: Community based services in San Francisco. *Am J Public Health* 1986; 76:1325–1330.
3. Novick LF, Truman BI, Lehman JS: The epidemiology of HIV in New York State. *NY State J Med* 1988; 88:242–246.
4. Fineberg HV: Education to prevent AIDS: Prospects and obstacles. *Science* 1988; 239:592–596.
5. Curran JW, Jaffe HW, Hardy AM, et al: Epidemiology of HIV infection and AIDS in the United States. *Science* 1988; 239:610–616.
6. APHA Technical Report: Criteria for the development of health promotion and education programs. *Am J Public Health* 1987; 77:89–92.
7. Osborne JE: AIDS: Politics and science. *N Engl J Med* 1988; 318:444–447.

Chapter 30

Acquired immunodeficiency syndrome as a paradigm for medicolegal education

In the fall semester of 1987, I attempted to introduce pre-clinical second-year medical students at the State University of New York Health Science Center at Brooklyn to the range of medicolegal issues that would confront them as they entered the clinical phase of their training. For many medical students, and for many in medical practice, "medicolegal issues" previously meant the issue of medical malpractice, in particular the risk that one might be sued. All students in the entire class (220 students) were introduced to this topic with two one-hour lectures which are part of a required course in health services taught by the Department of Preventive Medicine and Community Health.

By means of a lottery, students are assigned to seminar groups that meet for two hours once a week for eight weeks. A total of 14 seminar topics are offered, and most students are given their first choice.[1]

The seminar under discussion, "Legal Issues in Medicine," was specifically designed to introduce a small group of students to some other legal issues in medicine. A total of 13 students participated in the seminar.

The initial seminar session was devoted to legal issues raised by acquired immunodeficiency syndrome (AIDS), including concerns regarding antibody testing programs, confidentiality, and discrimination. The second seminar session addressed issues of biomedical research, including how studies might be designed to be both ethical and scientifically useful. The remaining six seminar sessions dealt with a variety of other topics, including the regulation of unsafe manufactured products, issues in forensic psychiatry, access to health care, legal protection of children's welfare, and patients' refusal of treatment.

Several of the seminar discussions revolved around hypothetical fact situations, similar to the "case method" often used in legal education. This method was chosen to allow the students to get a feel for the task of applying abstract rules to particular cases, to help them anticipate how difficult this might prove in the future in dealing with actual rather than hypothetical patients.

The written assignment for the seminar drew on the material presented in the first two seminar sessions. It called on the student to consider how to design a research proposal to study an AIDS vaccine. At the same time, initial reports of the first US trial of an AIDS vaccine were appearing in the press, and it was hoped that this would lend a further sense of immediacy and reality to the assignment.

One of the strongest impressions I carried away from the seminar was of the desire of many of the students for rules and certainty. Attempts to discuss what they thought would happen in a given hypothetical situation sometimes led to requests for more information about the relevant medical facts, and/or what the law said should be done. I think that here, as in other aspects of clinical medicine, one of the most difficult things for students to deal with is the need to decide and act in the face of uncertainty.

It was not my goal to try to produce legal experts, merely to alert the students to the fact that they might in the future sometimes benefit from seeking legal advice. Quotations from New York statutes and court cases were sometimes helpful in illustrating one state's attempts to grapple with some of these issues, and also in demonstrating how broadly stated rules can have considerable ambiguity when the attempt is made to apply them to particular cases.

In the end, much of our discussion of the law focused not so much on what the law is, but on what the students thought it should be. One useful exercise in this regard was to move from discussion of a hypothetical fact situation and how the students thought it should be handled, to discussion of how to formulate a general rule that would produce a just result in the given hypothetical case as well as in other future cases. My hope was that this would give the students a better appreciation of how difficult a task this can be.

In the process of making therapeutic decisions for patient care, the medical students in their clinical years will be exposed to the difficulty of choosing a course of action in the midst of uncertainty. One of the main points I hoped to convey was that some of these same problems arise as the law interacts with medicine.

There are several sources of uncertainty. In some cases, the law is reasonably clear, and the problem is primarily the physician's lack of information. As such, the solution is the clearcut one of seeking legal advice. In other cases, the law is phrased in terms of a general rule (eg, exercise "reasonable care"), while the application of that rule to the facts of a given case is ambiguous.

There are also more fundamental sources of uncertainty in the law, which arise primarily because legislators have chosen not to address issues that have long been recognized in medicine. These may range from defining the circumstances under which a patient may refuse life-sustaining treatment to the mechanics for making health care decisions on behalf of incompetent patients.[2] In many jurisdictions the trend has been away from unbridled discretion by the attending physician toward greater legal involvement in these matters, but this trend has not always been accompanied by clear guidance on what legal rules are to be applied.

Just as many courts and state legislatures have begun to deal with some of the thorniest medical-legal issues of the 1960s and 1970s, the AIDS epidemic has erupted. AIDS has intensified the concern over some of these issues, as AIDS patients consider how vigorously they wish to be treated, as well as who will make medical decisions for them if their mental status should be impaired by AIDS dementia, lymphoma of the brain, or opportunistic CNS infection. AIDS has also sparked a revival of interest in some issues that had nearly been forgotten in this country, particularly how one should balance the individual patient's rights against a societal interest in infection control measures.[3]

In summary, there are useful purposes that can be served by instruction in legal issues in medicine. First, it can afford an appreciation that there is more to the topic than malpractice law. Second, it is another way of introducing preclinical students to the difficulty of making decisions in the face of incomplete information. Third, by focusing not just on the question of what the law is but on what it should be, discussions such as these introduce medical students to society's role in addressing questions of medical ethics. Finally, it is my hope that this background will prove useful to medical students, as they prepare to begin clinical training and to confront the legal and ethical issues raised by AIDS.

NEIL J. NUSBAUM, MD, JD
Assistant Clinical Professor
Department of Preventive Medicine
and Community Health
State University of New York
Health Science Center at Brooklyn

Department of Medicine
The Brookdale Hospital Medical Center
Linden Blvd at Brookdale Plaza
Brooklyn, NY 11212

1. Imperato PJ, Feldman J, Nayeri K: Second year medical student opinion about public health and a second year course in preventive medicine and community health. *J Community Health* 1986; 11:244–258.
2. New York State Task Force on Life and the Law: *Life-Sustaining Treatment: Making Decisions and Appointing a Health Care Agent.* Albany, July 1987.
3. Rosenberg CE: *The Cholera Years: The United States in 1832, 1849 and 1866.* Chicago, University of Chicago Press, 1962.

Chapter 31
AIDS and the origin of species

Any sudden catastrophe forces us initially to view its effects in the short term—the immediate threat to ourselves and to loved ones, and the damage to society. But a few moments' reflection on the more profound implications of a calamity may allow us to profit from the lessons that it teaches.

The current epidemic of acquired immunodeficiency syndrome (AIDS) does not as yet compare in its effects with the European epidemics of bubonic and pneumonic plague in the 14th and 17th centuries, or the pandemic of influenza in 1918, or the continuing endemic of malaria in many countries. But the insidious, unrelenting, lethal characteristics of AIDS have laid an icy hand upon society. Accusations of moral misbehavior against the victims of the current AIDS epidemic tend only to divert attention from the useful lessons we can learn from consideration of other aspects of the problem.

In all likelihood the abrupt appearance of this illness would have been no surprise to Charles Darwin. A rereading of his *Origin of Species*[1] suggests that not only would he have anticipated such an event for a number of speculative reasons which I will mention, but he probably would have suggested that a parallel condition must have occurred in the extremely remote past, long before records of such events could have been kept.

Darwin concluded that each successive generation of a species produces variants of the original organism, usually over the very long term and with small increments of change, but sometimes with abruptly evident effects. Those variants which are better adapted to their environment than their forebears or their contemporaries tend to survive; those less well adapted tend to vanish. He believed that without variation within its many species, life itself would not have survived the widely differing and frequently changing conditions on this planet. In Darwin's view, even those variants that best fit a particular environment would disappear if the environment itself were to change significantly. Further, even those variants that are well suited to a particular environment are often subject to very narrow limits of behavior, which the organism ignores at its peril.

In explaining the biological interactions between living organisms, Darwin offers a complex scenario which appears to fit many aspects of AIDS.

The sexual form of reproduction appears to allow the offspring within a species to have access to a diverse gene pool and to a wide opportunity for variation. The act of sexual intercourse involves the transmission of cells and secretions from one sexual partner to the other; hence it must involve some modification of the recipient's immune system in order to avoid antibody production that would prevent effective insemination.

It is possible that currently existing sexual species are those variants which happened to evolve a controlled or reduced immune reaction in the lower genital tracts of the females, whereby the inseminating cells (spermatozoa) are not attacked by antibody production, despite repeated inseminations. At the same time that spermatozoa are left relatively intact, microorganisms invading the female genital tract generally are dealt with effectively by usual host-defenses. The immunologic mechanisms no doubt evolved side-by-side with the common genital-to-genital patterns of direct sexual contact between male and female partners.

During embryonic development, the cloaca differentiates to form the urogenital sinus and the rectum-anus. Postnatally, both vagina and rectum-anus must adjust to colonization by different groupings of microorganisms. The columnar epithelium of the lower colon and rectum adjusts immunologically to the presence of some 400 or more different bacterial species, and to other microorganisms.[2] By contrast, the vaginal squamous epithelium, the cervix, and no doubt the endometrium adjust to different groupings of organisms.[3-5] As long as sexual intercourse occurs in the usual fashion, the receptive site can deal appropriately with the entry of many foreign proteins, spermatozoa, and microorganisms.

When sexual contact does not follow the usual pattern, a variety of effects may result. In the case of oral-genital sexual contact, the immunologic defenses of the squamous epithelium of the upper respiratory and alimentary tracts might be effective in preventing invasion by unanticipated microorganisms, since from the moment of birth these points of entry have adjusted to a wide spectrum of microorganisms and foreign proteins. In addition, the swallowing process quickly invokes the destructive effects of gastric acidity and proteolytic enzymes.

By contrast, when genital-anal penetration occurs, spermatozoa together with an unaccustomed set of microorganisms now come in contact with columnar intestinal mucosa that may not yet have evolved adequate immunologic barriers against them.[6] The result may be easier invasion of microorganisms into the mucosal cells and thence into the internal milieu of the recipient sexual partner. In most cases, the latter's systemic immunologic defenses then generate adequate responses.

Let us vary this scenario by adding the factor of numerous and promiscuous genital-anal intrusions, during either homosexual or heterosexual contacts.[7] In other settings one can take into account the factor of excessive frequency and promiscuity of sexual contacts, as with prostitutes; or the more obvious transmission of contaminated materials by the intravenous route. Darwin in all likelihood would have suggested that sooner or later, in one or more locations on this Earth, these situations would give a special environmental advantage to one or more variants within species of microorganisms. The inevitable results would be ready invasion of the host by the variant or variants, unchecked proliferation within the host, and a variety of destructive consequences, including widespread geographic dissemination. The AIDS virus appears to be such a variant, able to penetrate colonic cells and ultimately to spread to many different types of cells in the human body. It invades the vulnerable T-cell, often though not always destroying its capacity to defend the host, and leaves the host a prey for the invasion of still other microorganisms.

When this coincidence of circumstances involving unusual host exposure to an especially capable invader occurs, death of the host is inevitable, unless effective therapeutic interventions can be developed. This pattern of destructive invasion, in the course of which the invader kills the susceptible host and as a consequence destroys

itself, is common to many epidemics; it suggests that the course of the AIDS "epidemic" may be self-limited over time, though at what ultimate cost in human lives and personal distress cannot be imagined.

Darwin might have suggested a corollary hypothesis. From the early beginning of the process of evolution, the more complex evolving life-forms must have been attacked by a broad spectrum of microorganisms. Those variants of these complex life-forms that developed the ability to cope effectively with such microorganisms were the ones that survived. One mechanism of coping which these variants developed could have been the immune system as we know it. Darwin very likely would have suggested that the apparently unusual organisms that we identify as secondary invaders in AIDS today—*Pneumocystis carinii*, *Mycobacterium avium-intracellulare*, *Candida*, cytomegalovirus, cryptosporidium, cryptococcus, toxoplasma, and others—are the same or similar organisms which millions of years ago were destructive to our early biological ancestors, until the latter developed variants with effective immunologic means of coping with them. Now that the HIV virus can destroy that same segment of the immune system which originally dealt with these organisms, we are again witness to the invasions and destructiveness of these same ancient predators.

We have much to learn about the process that leads to the production of variants within a species. Such a process brings with it many advantages for survival but also limitations on behavior. Of necessity, we must treat with respect those biological patterns which Nature has found most effective and most efficient for our survival in the present environment of this planet. This is not a moralistic precept; Darwin himself was attacked as a destroyer of human moral systems, even though it is likely that many moral codes originated, in part at least, in a wise accommodation to the requirements of Nature.

At some risk, we may by scientific effort alter Nature's patterns. Until we do, those of us who do not adapt appropriately to current patterns face the threat of extinction, to be replaced by life-forms whose biological conduct conforms to requirements worked out slowly and painfully by Nature over the last half-billion years.

JOHN T. FLYNN, MD
Consulting Editor

Associate Chief
Department of Medicine
The New York Infirmary-Beekman
Downtown Hospital
170 William St
New York, NY 10038

1. Darwin C: *The Origin of Species*. New York, Macmillan Publishing Co, 1962.
2. Moore WEC, Haldeman LV: Discussion of current bacteriologic investigations of relationships between intestinal flora, diet, and colon cancer. *Cancer Res* 1975; 35:3418.
3. Bartlett JG, Onderdonk AB, Drude E, et al: Quantitative bacteriology of the vaginal flora. *J Infect Dis* 1977; 136:271–277.
4. Ohm MJ, Galask RP: Bacterial flora of the cervix from 100 prehysterectomy patients. *Am J Obstet Gynecol* 1975; 122:683–687.
5. Gorbach SL, Menda KB, Thadepalli H, et al: Anaerobic microflora of the cervix in healthy women. *Am J Obstet Gynecol* 1973; 117:1053–1055.
6. National Institutes of Health: AIDS virus infection in colorectal cells. *JAMA* 1987; 257:1702.
7. Padian N, Marquis L, Francis DP, et al: Male-to-female transmission of human immunodeficiency virus. *JAMA* 1987; 258:788–790.

Part IV
Case Studies

Chapter 32

Coagulase-negative staphylococcal sepsis in drug-dependent newborns who may be HIV-positive

FRANCISCO MEDINA MEJIA, MD, STEPHEN R. KANDALL, MD

Neonatal sepsis due to coagulase-negative staphlylococci has been reported with increasing frequency in very low birth weight infants or infants subjected to invasive procedures or treatment.[1-3] We report two cases of coagulase-negative staphylococcal sepsis in passively addicted, but otherwise healthy, term infants who were not subjected to invasive procedures. One mother-infant pair was found to be serologically positive for human immunodeficiency virus (HIV); HIV status in the other pair is not known. Vertical perinatal transmission of acquired immunodeficiency syndrome (AIDS) from drug-dependent mothers to their infants[4-6] and newly described immunologic alterations in these infants[4] may render these neonates susceptible to infections with ubiquitous and indolent organisms.

CASE REPORTS

Case 1. A 2.72-kg female infant was born after a term gestation complicated by the mother's intravenous heroin abuse during the first six months of pregnancy. At 24 hours of age, the infant exhibited temperature instability, irritability, and tremors. A diagnostic workup for sepsis was performed, and therapy with ampicillin and gentamycin was started. The infant was also treated with camphorated tincture of opium (paregoric) for suspected opiate withdrawal.

Antibiotic therapy was discontinued on the third day of life, after negative blood, urine, and spinal fluid cultures were reported; the following day, a coagulase-negative staphylococcus susceptible to novobiocin was reported growing from the original blood culture. The isolated organism was

sensitive to ampicillin, penicillin, oxacillin, erythromycin, cephalothin, gentamycin, and chloramphenicol. On day six, a second blood culture was drawn which, four days later, grew a coagulase-negative staphylococcus with the same sensitivities as those of the first organism. On day ten, a third blood culture was drawn, and intravenous vancomycin, 45 mg/kg/day, was started; this blood culture also grew a coagulase-negative staphylococcus with the same antibiotic sensitivities. Vancomycin treatment was continued for ten days; blood cultures drawn during the treatment and following cessation of treatment were both negative. Drug withdrawal was managed with gradual reduction of the dosage of paregoric. The infant was discharged on the 28th day of life. No serious infections or hospital visits were noted at a nine-month follow-up evaluation.

Case 2. A 2.73-kg male infant was born after a 38-week gestation to a 32-year-old woman on maintenance methadone therapy who had abused injected cocaine during the pregnancy. On the second day of life, the infant had an elevated temperature, hypertonia, hyperreflexia, and tremulousness. Treatment with camphorated tincture of opium (paregoric) was started; on day 13, phenobarbital was added to control withdrawal. A diagnostic workup for sepsis was also performed at that time, and treatment with oxacillin and gentamycin was started. On day 16, the blood culture grew a coagulase-negative staphylococcus sensitive to vancomycin, tetracycline, and nitrofurantoin, and resistant to ampicillin, penicillin, oxacillin, erythromycin, clindamycin, cephalothin, and trimethoprim-sulfamethoxazole. A culture of cerebrospinal fluid (CSF) showed no growth. Blood cultures were repeated on day 16 and grew a coagulase-negative staphylococcus with the same antibiotic sensitivities. Blood and CSF cultures repeated on day 19 showed no growth.

Vancomycin therapy, 45 mg/kg/day, was started on day 19 and was continued for seven days. Blood cultures drawn during treatment and following cessation of therapy were negative. On day 33, HIV antibody studies were performed on both the mother

and the infant; both were positive as determined by Abbott EIA (enzyme immunoassay method). Neonatal withdrawal was managed with gradual reductions in paregoric and phenobarbital dosages, and the infant was discharged from the hospital on the 48th day of life. No serious infections or hospital visits were noted at a nine-month follow-up evaluation.

DISCUSSION

Despite a wide spectrum of morbidity,[7] an increased incidence of neonatal sepsis has not been reported in drug-dependent newborns. Recently, however, abnormal lymphocyte proliferation in response to mitogens and abnormal T4/T8 ratios have been documented in these infants.[4,8] These immunologic alterations may relate to subsequent development of AIDS, since most pediatric HIV infections and AIDS cases are acquired perinatally from infected mothers who used intravenous drugs during the pregnancy.[6] This same immunopathy could render such neonates susceptible to infections caused by bacteria of normally low virulence, such as coagulase-negative staphylococci.

Since sepsis can mimic neonatal drug withdrawal, the former should be considered when symptoms of withdrawal are not readily managed with appropriate medications. Despite low virulence, coagulase-negative staphylococcal infections can occasionally cause neonatal death.[2,9] The combination of maternal intravenous drug abuse, neonatal withdrawal, and isolation of coagulase-negative staphylococcus from neonatal cultures, even in a term infant, should prompt immediate institution of vancomycin therapy.

Acknowledgments. The authors thank Stacy B. Danheiser for her secretarial services.

From the Department of Pediatrics, Beth Israel Medical Center, Mount Sinai School of Medicine, New York.

REFERENCES

1. Munson DP, Thompson TR, Johnson DE, et al: Coagulase-negative staphylococcal septicemia: Experience in a newborn intensive care unit. *J Pediatr* 1982; 101:602–605.

2. Baumgart S, Hall SE, Campos JM, et al: Sepsis with coagulase-negative staphylococci in critically ill newborns. *Am J Dis Child* 1983; 137:461–463.

3. Stabile A, Assunta Pesaresi M, Currò V: Coagulase-negative staphylococcal septicemia in newborn babies [letter]. *Am J Dis Child* 1985; 139:541–542.

4. Rubinstein A, Sicklick M, Gupta A, et al: Acquired immunodeficiency with reversed T4/T8 ratios in infants born to promiscuous and drug-addicted mothers. *JAMA* 1983; 249:2350–2356.

5. Cowan MJ, Hellman D, Chudwin D, et al: Maternal transmission of acquired immune deficiency syndrome. *Pediatrics* 1984; 73:382–386.

6. Recommendations for assisting in the prevention of perinatal transmission of human T-lymphotropic virus type III/lymphadenopathy-associated virus and acquired immunodeficiency syndrome. *MMWR* 1984; 73:382–386.

7. Kandall SR, Albin S, Gartner LM, et al: The narcotic-dependent mother. Fetal and neonatal consequences. *Early Hum Dev* 1977; 1:159–169.

8. Culver KW, Ammann AJ, Partridge JC, et al: Lymphocyte abnormalities in infants born to IV drug abusers. *Pediatr Res* 1986; 20:389A.

9. Kumar ML, Jenson HB, Dahms BB: Fatal staphylococcal epidermidis infections in very low-birth-weight infants with cytomegalovirus infection. *Pediatrics* 1985; 75:110–112.

Chapter 33

An unusual presentation of lymphoma in a homosexual man

SANFORD DUBNER, MD, KEITH S. HELLER, MD

Reported cases of lymphoma in homosexual men have increased since the acquired immunodeficiency syndrome (AIDS) epidemic was first detected in the early 1980s. Lymphoma in the general population presents more commonly in the head and neck area than in any other anatomical region. Most patients are seen with disease arising in lymph nodes, but many exhibit disease originating in extranodal areas. Parotid lymphomas may arise either in the parotid parenchyma or in the lymph nodes within the parotid gland.[1] We discuss a case of lymphoma presenting as a parotid mass in a homosexual man with AIDS.

CASE REPORT

AIDS was diagnosed in a 40-year-old homosexual man when he presented with pneumocystis pneumonia six months prior to his current admission for a right-sided preauricular mass which had increased in size over the previous three months. The patient denied weakness, weight loss, night sweats, or any history of intravenous drug abuse. His history was significant for a splenectomy 20 years earlier for traumatic injury. On admission, the preauricular mass measured 5 cm × 7 cm, and there was no evidence of facial nerve paralysis. Laboratory studies revealed a white blood cell count of 6,700/mm³, with 56% lymphocytes, 33% segmented neutrophils, 10% monocytes, and 1% eosinophils.

The patient underwent surgical exploration of the parotid region. The mass was found to be within the substance of the parotid gland. Because of the suspicion of lymphoma, an incisional biopsy of the mass was performed. On gross examination the mass was firm and pale gray. Histologic examination indicated that the mass was a malignant lymphoma, diffuse type, with large cleaved lymphocytic cells. A postoperative workup included a computed tomographic scan of the abdomen and pelvis, which showed small inguinal lymph nodes but was otherwise unremarkable. The bone marrow was normal. Tissue and serum specimens studied at the National Cancer Institute revealed the patient to be antibody positive for the human immunodeficiency virus (HIV). The viral genome was not found in B cell tumor cells.

The patient received four courses of cytoxan, adriamycin, vincristine, and prednisone in one-month intervals. Radiation therapy was not administered. A follow-up examination after five months revealed complete remission, with total shrinkage and disappearance of the parotid mass.

DISCUSSION

The incidence of non-Hodgkin's lymphoma in patients with AIDS or AIDS-related complex (ARC) has been increasing since the AIDS epidemic began in 1980.[2] These patients frequently present with extranodal sites of tumor, particularly in the central nervous system, bone marrow, or abdomen. The frequency of extranodal tumor sites is greater than in patients without AIDS and more closely approximates the occurrence rates seen in patients with congenital or iatrogenic immunodeficiency.[3] In the non-AIDS population, approximately 5% of extranodal lymphomas are located in salivary glands, and as many as 90% of salivary gland lymphomas are parotid in origin.[4] A recent review noted that the frequency with which lymphoma occurred as an isolated parotid mass was between 0.6% and 2.4% of parotidectomy specimens.[1] Patients undergoing immunosuppressive therapy for transplantation surgery are likewise at increased risk for developing lymphomas; their risk is approximately 40 times that of the general population.

A four-year survival rate of 33% in the generalized population with non-Hodgkin's lymphoma has been reported.[5] To date, the majority of men with both AIDS and non-Hodgkin's lymphoma have died.[2] Non-Hodgkin's lymphoma and AIDS occurring concurrently in a given patient confers a poor prognosis, not only because of the sequelae of progressive lymphoma, but also because of an increased incidence of opportunistic infection.

Because of the increased risk of lymphoma, the management of AIDS patients should differ from the management of other patients with parotid tumors. In the non-AIDS patient, the presence of a parotid mass is an indication for parotidectomy, generally without a preliminary biopsy. In a patient with AIDS, incisional biopsy rather than parotidectomy may be the preferred initial procedure, particularly if a needle aspiration suggests a nonepithelial tumor. If frozen section reveals an epithelial tumor, parotidectomy may be performed. Otherwise, the procedure is terminated.

From the Head and Neck Service, Department of Surgery, Booth Memorial Medical Center affiliate of New York University Medical Center, Flushing, NY.

The surgeon who is aware of the possibility of lymphoma in the differential diagnosis of parotid gland enlargement in the patient with acquired immunodeficiency syndrome or immunosuppression may spare his patient an unnecessary parotidectomy and all of its concomitant risks.

REFERENCES

1. Nichols RD, Rebuck JW, Sullivan JC: Lymphoma and the parotid gland. *Laryngoscope* 1982; 92:365–369.
2. Ziegler JL, Beckstead JA, Volberding PA, et al: Non-Hodgkin's lymphoma in 90 homosexual men. Relation to generalized lymphadenopathy and the acquired immunodeficiency syndrome. *N Engl J Med* 1984; 311:565–570.
3. Frizzera G, Rosai J, Dehner LP, et al: Lym-phoreticular disorders in primary immunodeficiencies: New findings based on an up-to-date histologic classification of 35 cases. *Cancer* 1980; 46:692–699.
4. Hyman GA, Wolff M: Malignant lymphomas of the salivary glands. Review of the literature and report of 33 new cases, including four cases associated with the lymphoepithelial lesion. *Am J Clin Pathol* 1976; 65:421–438.
5. Freedman SI: Malignant lymphomas of the major salivary glands. *Arch Otolaryngol* 1971; 93:123–127.

Chapter 34
Oral candidiasis and AIDS

JEFFREY S. GELWAN, MD; BURTON M. GOLD, MD; HENRY J. SHIH, MD;
CRESCENS PELLECCHIA, MD

Candidal infections of the gastrointestinal tract are common in patients with acquired immunodeficiency syndrome (AIDS). Oral candidiasis, though not diagnostic of the syndrome, has been shown to carry a poor prognosis in patients in the prodromal stage, called AIDS-related complex (ARC).[1-3] In a prospective study of high-risk patients with unexplained oral candidiasis, Klein et al[1] found that 59% of these patients acquired a major opportunistic infection or secondary cancer at a median interval of three months. The authors concluded that in high-risk patients, oral candidiasis may represent an intermediate stage in the spectrum of disease that progresses from ARC to AIDS.

The association between oral and esophageal candidiasis in patients with AIDS and ARC has recently been investigated.[4-6] Since the presence of esophageal candidiasis fulfills the definition of AIDS as determined by the Centers for Disease Control (CDC), endoscopic evaluation of high-risk patients with oral candidiasis has been undertaken. Tavitian et al,[4] in a prospective study, evaluated 25 patients with oral candidiasis (eight with AIDS and 17 with ARC) to determine the presence of esophageal candidiasis. Esophageal candidiasis was found in all 25 patients, as determined by endoscopy and cytologic analysis, though six patients with moderate esophagitis were asymptomatic. The investigators concluded that in patients with AIDS or ARC, oral candidiasis indicates the presence of esophageal candidiasis. In a separate report, Tavitian et al[5] studied ten patients with AIDS and oral candidiasis and again found that all ten had evidence of esophageal candidiasis. Although our experience in general supports the relationship between oral and esophageal candidiasis, we have found three exceptions.

CASE REPORTS

Case 1. A 36-year-old man was referred to the gastroenterology service at Nassau County Medical Center for evaluation of odynophagia of two weeks' duration. He gave a history of intravenous drug abuse and exposure to a friend with AIDS. For the prior five months, he had noted generalized lymphadenopathy and whitish patches in the oral cavity unresponsive to oral mycostatin. Laboratory tests disclosed the following: culture of the buccal mucosa positive for *Candida albicans*; elevated globulin levels in the blood; the presence of antibodies to human immunodeficiency virus (HIV); and a normal esophagram. Esophagogastroduodenoscopy was performed to evaluate odynophagia and was entirely normal.

Case 2. A 26-year-old homosexual man underwent esophagogastroduodenoscopy for evaluation of pain on swallowing. His medical history was significant for gonococcal proctitis, *Campylobacter* enterocolitis, and exposure to AIDS. The patient has been followed in both infectious disease and gastroenterology clinics for oral thrush that was minimally responsive to oral nystatin and for chronic intermittent diarrhea. Recently, he was noted to have generalized lymphadenopathy and neutropenia. Both the esophagram and esophagogastroduodenoscopy were within normal limits. Ten months later, dysphagia developed, and endoscopy performed at that time confirmed the presence of candidal esophagitis.

Case 3. A 41-year-old man was admitted to Nassau County Medical Center for evaluation of progressive weakness, fever, night sweats, dysphagia, and weight loss. His medical history was significant for intravenous drug abuse, alcoholism, alcoholic liver disease, anemia, and sickle cell trait. One year prior to admission, the patient noted the onset of oral thrush, followed by the development of odynophagia and dysphagia to both solids and liquids. On admission, his physical examination was remarkable for a temperature of 102.3°F, oral thrush, generalized lymphadenopathy, and hepatomegaly. Laboratory data revealed the following: a throat culture positive for *Candida albicans*; anemia; neutropenia; hypergammaglobulinemia; elevated erythrocytic sedimentation rate; positive anergy panel; and a bone marrow biopsy demonstrating hyperplasia of erythrocyte, granulocyte, and megakaryocyte series, with a culture positive for *Mycobacterium avium intracellulare* complex.

An esophagram (Fig 1) done to evaluate odynophagia/dysphagia revealed a long mid-esophageal region showing irregular thickened folds suggestive of esophagitis. Subsequently, esophagogastroduodenoscopy was performed and revealed multiple areas of erythema and friability throughout the mid and distal esophagus. No exudate or discrete ulcerations were seen. Cytologic studies were interpreted as epithelia atypism, Pap class II-III, with probable viral inclusions suggestive of herpes. No fungal structures were seen. Pathologic examination (Fig 2)

From the Division of Gastroenterology (Drs Gelwan and Pellecchia) and the Departments of Radiology (Dr Gold) and Pathology (Dr Shih), Nassau County Medical Center, East Meadow, NY.

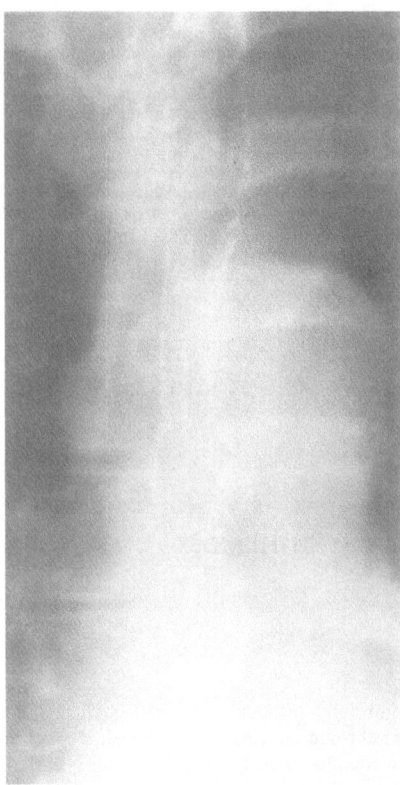

FIGURE 1. Fluoroscopic spot film of esophagram showing a long area of mid-esophagus with irregular thickened folds (Case 3).

demonstrated acute necrotizing inflammation with "ground-glass" and molded nuclei

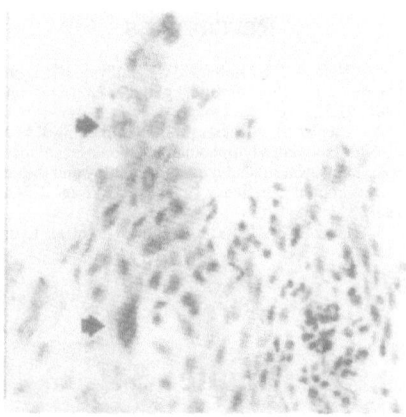

FIGURE 2. Esophageal biopsy demonstrating acute necrotizing inflammation with "ground-glass" and molded nuclei (upper arrow) forming a multinucleated giant cell (lower arrow) (hematoxylin-eosin stain, original magnification × 250) (Case 3).

forming a multinucleated giant cell suggestive of herpes.

DISCUSSION

Oral candidiasis can exist without esophageal candidiasis in patients with either AIDS or ARC, even in the presence of esophageal symptoms. In patients 1 and 3 presented in this report, odynophagia was present. Yet esophageal candidiasis was ruled out during esophagogastroduodenoscopy. Case 2

illustrates that oral candidiasis can exist in patients with AIDS or ARC for some time before esophageal candidiasis develops. These cases demonstrate the need for further investigation into the association between oral and esophageal candidiasis in patients with either AIDS or ARC. Meanwhile, early upper endoscopy should be considered in evaluating patients with either oral candidiasis and/or esophageal symptoms.

REFERENCES

1. Klein RS, Harris CA, Small CS, et al: Oral candidiasis in high-risk patients as the initial manifestation of the acquired immunodeficiency syndrome. *N Engl J Med* 1984; 311:354–358.
2. Romanowski B, Weber J: Oral candidiasis and the acquired immunodeficiency syndrome [letter]. *Ann Intern Med* 1984; 101:400–401.
3. Chandrasekar PH, Molinari JA: Oral candidiasis: Forerunner of acquired immunodeficiency syndrome (AIDS)? *Oral Surg Oral Med Oral Pathol* 1985; 60:532–534.
4. Tavitian A, Raufman J-P, Rosenthal LE, et al: Oral candidiasis indicates esophageal candidiasis in patients with AIDS and AIDS-related complex, in Abstracts submitted for 50th annual scientific meeting, American College of Gastroenterology. *Am J Gastroenterology* 1985; 80:867.
5. Tavitian A, Raufman J-P, Rosenthal LE: Oral candidiasis as a marker for esophageal candidiasis in the acquired immunodeficiency syndrome. *Ann Intern Med* 1986; 104:54–55.
6. Gelb A, Miller S: AIDS and gastroenterology. *Am J Gastroenterology* 1986; 81:619–622.
7. Kodsi BE, Wickremesinghe C, Kozinn PJ, et al: Candida esophagitis. A progressive study of 27 cases. *Gastroenterology* 1976; 71:715–719.
8. Epstein JB, Truelove EL, Izutzu KT: Oral candidiasis: Pathogenesis and host defense. *Rev Infect Dis* 1984; 6:96–106.

Chapter 35

Herpes simplex pericarditis in AIDS

ROBIN S. FREEDBERG, MD; AARON J. GINDEA, MD; DOUGLAS T. DIETERICH, MD;
JEFFREY B. GREENE, MD

Viral infection is the most common cause of pericarditis in healthy young adults and is frequently associated with clinical or occult myocarditis. Although numerous viruses can infect the heart in immunologically competent individuals,[1] herpes simplex virus has not been definitively identified as a cardiac pathogen.

From the Department of Medicine, New York University Medical Center, New York.

Pericardial effusions are common among hospitalized patients with acquired immunodeficiency syndrome (AIDS).[2] We describe a patient with AIDS in whom a pericardial effusion developed; herpes simplex virus was cultured from the effusion.

CASE REPORT

A 44-year-old homosexual man, with no known heart disease or risk factors for coronary artery disease and no history of oral or genital herpes, was admitted to New York University Medical Center with severe weight loss, and a one-week history of sharp

epigastric and substernal pain associated with several episodes of vomiting.

The physical examination was remarkable for cachexia, mild orthostasis, fever, and oral thrush. The hematocrit was 27%, the white blood cell count was 6,100/mm^3 with a relative lymphopenia, and the erythrocyte sedimentation rate was 100 mm/h. The electrocardiogram (including the QT interval) was within normal limits, although the QTc was mildly prolonged (450 msec). A chest film showed a normal cardiac silhouette and clear lungs. Lymphocyte subset studies revealed a marked depression of the helper population, with an OKT4/OKT8 ratio of 0.2, consistent with AIDS.

The patient received antacids and ketoconazole for oral candidiasis, and hydration was achieved with intravenous crystalloids and blood. Endoscopy of the upper gastrointestinal tract revealed esophageal ulcers. A biopsy showed multinucleated giant cells, some with intranuclear inclusions suggesting cytomegalovirus or herpes infection. Treatment with intravenous acyclovir (15 mg/kg/day) was begun, and the patient continued to receive this therapy throughout his hospital stay.

One month later, acute respiratory distress developed. A chest film showed diffuse interstitial infiltrates, which prompted empiric therapy with intravenous trimethoprim-sulfamethoxazole and erythromycin. Bronchoscopic biopsy was unrevealing, but because the patient failed to respond to the treatment regimen, trimethoprim-sulfamethoxazole was replaced with intravenous pentamidine for presumed refractory *Pneumocystis carinii* infection. Progressive pulmonary failure necessitated intubation and mechanical ventilation for one week.

Three days after extubation, the patient had an episode of ventricular tachycardia, which was terminated with a precordial thump. Electrolyte levels, including magnesium and calculated ionized calcium, were within normal limits. Arterial blood gas studies showed a P_{O_2} of 47 mm Hg and an A-a gradient of 63 mm Hg, and the patient agreed to reinsertion of the endotracheal tube. The electrocardiogram showed nonspecific T-wave flattening and a somewhat more prolonged QTc (480 msec).

Three days later, the patient had an episode of polymorphic ventricular tachycardia with loss of consciousness, which required electrical cardioversion. An electrocardiogram revealed a markedly prolonged QT interval (QTc 570 msec) and more dramatic changes in the precordial T-wave morphology (Fig 1). A chest film showed a globular cardiac silhouette with a small increase in the cardiothoracic ratio, and a bedside two-dimensional echocardiogram confirmed a small pericardial effusion with normal valves and wall motion (Fig 2). Serial cardiac enzyme determinations were normal. Doxepin was discontinued because of the possibility of tricyclic antidepressant-related repolarization abnormalities and ventricular irritability.

Initially, there were no recurrences of ventricular ectopy on a continuous infusion of bretylium. On the following day, however, the patient had multiple episodes of torsades de pointes (Fig 3) despite therapy with this agent and intravenous administration of magnesium sulfate. An isoproterenol infusion was begun, and further episodes of ventricular tachycardia were ultimately aborted by ventricular pacing at 120 beats/min.

The patient underwent open chest biopsy of the lung and pericardium under general anesthesia without complication. Two hundred cc of serous fluid was drained from the pericardial space. Pathologic examination of the lung showed chronic inflammation, and the pericardium showed fibrosis and congestion. Stains of both tissues for bacteria, mycobacteria, fungi, *P carinii* and *Legionella* were negative. Viral culture of the lung tissue grew cytomegalovirus, and viral culture of the pericardial fluid grew herpes simplex type I. The QTc remained prolonged, and attempts to discontinue overdrive pacing led to recurrent episodes of torsades de pointes. The patient experienced progressive pulmonary failure and, two months after admission, he died.

DISCUSSION

Many patients with AIDS suffer cardiac disorders. In an autopsy study of 41 patients who died of AIDS, ten were found to have cardiac involvement: four with Kaposi's sarcoma involving coronary arteries, myocardium and/or pericardium; three with culture-negative thrombotic endocarditis; two with nonspecific pericarditis; and one with cryptococcal myocarditis.[3] Noninvasive studies have demonstrated occult cardiac abnormalities to be common, with the echocardiographic incidence of pericardial effusion in hospitalized patients with AIDS reported to be 30%.[2]

In this patient, herpes simplex was

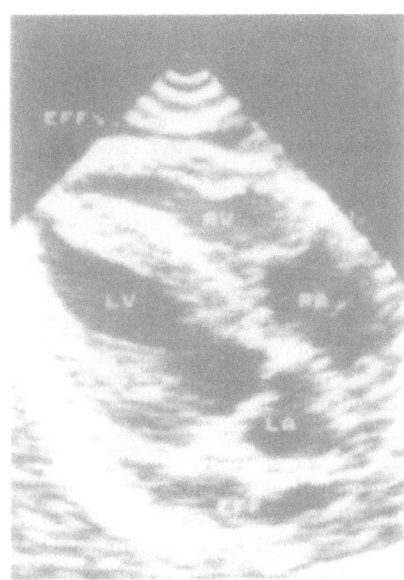

FIGURE 2. Bedside two-dimensional echocardiogram using subxiphoid approach shows small pericardial effusion (EFF) anteriorly and in the posterior atrioventricular sulcus (LA, left atrium; LV, left ventricle; RA, right atrium; RV, right ventricle).

recovered from the pericardial fluid, despite prolonged antiviral therapy with acyclovir. While a large number of prevalent viral pathogens are commonly implicated in pericarditis in otherwise healthy individuals, we are unaware of any cases of herpes pericarditis confirmed by culture findings. In one report of a healthy 22-year-old man whose pericarditis was associated with a concomitant rise in complement-fixing antibodies to both herpes zoster and herpes simplex, the authors presumed the latter to represent an anamnestic response to infection with the zoster virus.[4] Not surprisingly, in view of the fact that the viruses that commonly infect the pericardium are the same as those that typically cause myocarditis, herpes viruses have also rarely been invoked as etiologic agents in myocarditis. However, in one recent report of a patient with a cardiomyopathy that developed shortly after a varicella rash, herpes-like particles were found in a right ventricular biopsy specimen.[5]

Although arrhythmias are common in patients with pericarditis, those of ventricular origin are rare in the absence of underlying parenchymal heart disease.[6] The patient reported here, in whom no metabolic cause for repolarization abnormalities and torsades de pointes could be identified, may have had an associated myocarditis, which was solely manifested by these abnor-

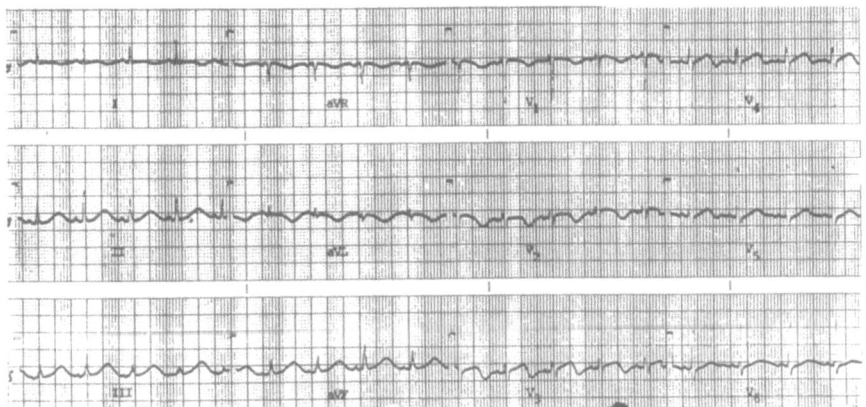

FIGURE 1. 12-lead electrocardiogram obtained after episode of symptomatic ventricular tachycardia demonstrated marked QT prolongation and repolarization abnormalities in the precordial leads.

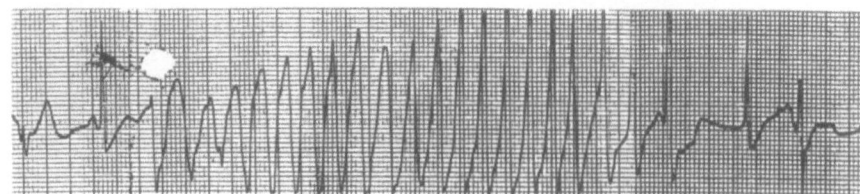

FIGURE 3. One of multiple episodes of torsades de pointes.

malities.[7,8] Although drug-related conduction abnormalities are the most frequent cause of torsades de pointes, the discontinuation of the only medication with a known association failed to correct the QT interval in this case. Given the limited experience with pentamidine, it is conceivable that this drug may have produced the detrimental QT prolongation. However, there is no report in the literature of any high-grade ventricular arrhythmia, such as torsades de pointes, associated with pentamidine.

Small pericardial effusions that lack hemodynamic significance are rarely cultured in critically ill patients. This case, however, suggests the possibility that immunocompromised patients with pericardial effusions may have a serositis caused by herpes simplex. We speculate that viruses causing self-limited illness in immunologically competent individuals may be the cause of some of the pericardial effusions found in patients with AIDS.

REFERENCES

1. Wenger NK: Infectious myocarditis. *Cardiovasc Clin* 1972; 4:167–185.
2. Reitano J, King M, Cohen H, et al: Cardiac function in patients with acquired immunodeficiency syndrome or AIDS prodrome [abstract]. *J Am Coll Cardiol* 1984; 3:525.
3. Cammarosano C, Lewis W: Cardiac lesions in the acquired immunodeficiency syndrome. *J Am Coll Cardiol* 1985; 5:703–706.
4. Winfield CR, Joseph SP: Herpes zoster pericarditis. *Br Heart J* 1980; 43:597–599.
5. Lowry PJ, Edwards CW, Nagle RE: Herpes-like virus particles in myocardium of patient progressing to congestive cardiomyopathy. *Br Heart J* 1982; 48:501–503.
6. Spodick DH: Arrhythmias during acute pericarditis: A prospective study of 100 consecutive cases. *JAMA* 1976; 235:39–41.
7. Gittleman IW, Thorner MC, Griffith GC: Q-T interval of electrocardiogram in acute myocarditis in adults with autopsy correlation. *Am Heart J* 1951; 41:78–90.
8. Karajalainen J, Viitasalo M, Kala R, et al: 24-hour electrocardiographic recordings in mid acute infectious myocarditis. *Ann Clin Res* 1984; 16:34–39.

Chapter 36
Fatal hemoptysis in a patient with AIDS-related complex and pulmonary aspergilloma

GERARD T. LOMBARDO, MD; NANARAO ANANDARAO, MD; CHING-SHEN LIN, MD; ANDRE ABBATE, MD; WILLIAM H. BECKER, MD

Hemoptysis is common in patients with pulmonary aspergilloma. Opinions vary as to its management. The underlying disease, the severity and frequency of hemoptysis, and the immune status of the patient have been proposed as factors to influence therapy. Unlike invasive aspergillosis, the behavior of cavitary disease in the immunocompromised host has not been fully described. This report describes a pulmonary aspergilloma in a patient with AIDS-related complex (ARC).

CASE REPORT

A 28-year-old man with a ten-year history of intravenous drug use was admitted to the Methodist Hospital several times during a 16-month period. The first admission was in March 1984 for right upper lobe pneumococcal pneumonia and was complicated by septicemia and a bronchopleural fistula. Closed tube thoracotomy resulted in complete reexpansion of the lung, although a thin-walled cavity remained in the right upper lobe.

Six months later, the patient presented with fever and cough. Sputum cultures showed no fungal or significant bacterial growth, and blood cultures were negative. The patient was anergic to skin testing with purified protein derivative and mumps antigen. His white blood cell count ranged from 4,000 to 5,000 cells/mm³, with a normal differential. The physical examination was normal, as were the blood chemistry studies and liver function tests. The patient's fever and cough improved with ampicillin therapy. A chest radiograph showed the cavity in the right upper lobe with apical capping and elevation of the right hilum. A computed tomographic (CT) scan showed that the cavity was empty and had a thick wall (Fig 1). The patient signed himself out of the hospital against medical advice.

Six weeks later he was readmitted because of hemoptysis of approximately 200 cc over a 24-hour period. He had lost ten pounds since the previous admission and was still using intravenous drugs. The patient was afebrile and appeared thin and unkempt. His respiratory rate was 14/min, and his blood pressure was 110/70 mm Hg. There were no skin lesions or adenopathy.

Examination of his ears, nose, and throat did not reveal a source of bleeding, but ex-

From the Departments of Pulmonary Medicine (Drs Lombardo, Anandarao, and Abbate), Pathology (Dr Lin), and Medicine (Dr Becker), the Methodist Hospital, Brooklyn, NY.

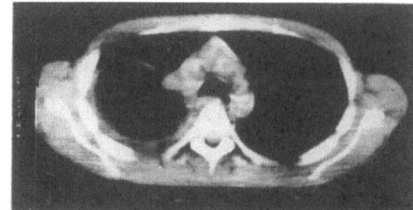

FIGURE 1. Computed tomographic (CT) scan showing an empty cavity in the right upper lobe.

tensive oral candidiasis was observed. Coarse bronchial breath sounds were heard in the right upper chest posteriorly. There were no cardiac murmurs. The abdomen and extremities were normal. The white blood cell count and differential had remained unchanged. There was a polyclonal hypergammaglobulinemia, and serum titers for cytomegalovirus antibody were positive. Sputum cultures subsequently grew *Aspergillus fumigatus*, *Candida albicans*, and *Mycobacterium avium intracellulare*. Blood and bone marrow cultures showed no bacterial growth. A chest radiograph and CT scan of the chest showed an irregular homogenous mass within the cavity (Figs 2, 3) suggestive of aspergilloma. Pulmonary function tests showed mild airflow restriction.

Because of continuous hemoptysis, bronchoscopy and surgical resection were advised, but the patient refused and signed himself out of the hospital. One month later, he was admitted to another hospital because of blood-streaked sputum. He was described there as a chronically ill cachectic man with oral candidiasis and diffuse lymphadenopathy. He again refused surgery. He returned to the emergency room at Methodist Hospital two months later complaining of blood-streaked sputum, had massive hemoptysis, and died one hour later. There was no clinical or laboratory evidence of coagulopathy.

An autopsy confirmed a large cavity measuring 10 cm in diameter within the right upper lobe, with fibrous adhesions to the aperture of the thoracic cage. The cavity contained an irregular, soft white and brown fungal mass mixed with clotted and fluid blood. The lining was uneven and gray-white or dark blue in color, with many small bronchi directly opening into the cavity. A 0.2-cm wide branch of the pulmonary artery had eroded into the wall of the cavity. The trachea and main bronchi contained large amounts of blood, which had been extensively aspirated in both lungs. The stomach contained 300 mL of blood. A smear and histologic sections of the cavity content showed septate and branched hyphae with budding

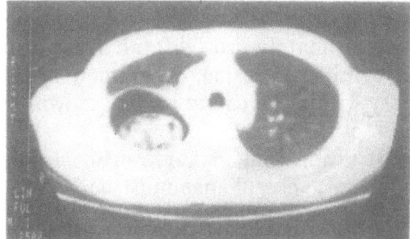

FIGURE 3. Repeat computed tomographic (CT) scan of the chest showing an intracavitary mass, six weeks after the first CT scan (Fig 1).

spores and conidiophores (fruit heads). The culture yielded *Aspergillus fumigatus*. The histologic sections of the cavity wall showed diffuse lymphocytic and plasma cell infiltration and a necrotizing artery with fibrin thrombus at the rupture site. There was no evidence of *Aspergillus* invasion into the blood vessels. The rest of the lung parenchyma showed severe, acute, and chronic bronchitis but no evidence of fungal, viral, bacterial, or protozoal infection. There was marked generalized lymphadenopathy.

DISCUSSION

Aspergillus fumigatus is a saprophytic fungus which can colonize pulmonary cavities and result in mycetoma. The pathogenesis and natural course of aspergilloma have not been well defined because of the broad spectrum of underlying diseases and conditions associated with the organism.

Features of aspergilloma include a solid, rounded mass on chest roentgenogram, positive sputum culture, and the presence of precipitating antibody against *Aspergillus* antigens. In immunocompetent patients, it is considered to be a slow-growing organism, although mycetomas measuring up to 3 cm have developed over several weeks.[1] Patients may be asymptomatic or have cough, dyspnea, malaise, or hemoptysis.

Hemoptysis is the most common symptom, occurring in 60–80% of cases.[1] The pathogenesis of hemoptysis may involve frictional forces within the cavity wall, hemolytic endotoxins, or proteolytic enzymes from granulocytes. The latter were implicated in the mechanism of cavitation and hemoptysis in a recent study of immunocompromised patients with acute leukemia and invasive aspergillosis.[2] As granulocyte numbers increase, there is a greater tendency for pulmonary cavitation and life-threatening hemoptysis; therefore, early operative intervention was suggested for this group. The influence of local factors and, in particular, granulocyte numbers in patients with AIDS-related complex or acquired immunodeficiency syndrome and aspergilloma has not been studied.

In cavitary aspergillomas, the incidence of fatal hemoptysis varies between 0% and 25%, depending on the population and the study design. This creates most of the controversy regarding management and especially indications for elective surgery. One study

TABLE I. Clinical Course of Reported Patients with Mycetoma and Fatal Hemoptysis

Author	Patient Number	Follow-up After Diagnosis of Mycetoma (yr)	Number With Fatal Hemoptysis (%)
Kaplan & Johns	12	7.1	1*(8)
Israel et al	24	2	4 (17)
Karas et al	20	—	4†(20)
Varkey & Rose	9	4.2	0
Faulkner et al	31	2.7	1 (3)
Butz et al	14	2.5‡	0
Reddy et al	10	3.9	0
Solit et al	19	6	5 (26)
Hammerman et al	33	1	5 (15)
Rafferty et al	18	4.5	3§(17)
Total	190		23 (12)
Mean		3.9	

* Patient had hepatic failure and a coagulopathy.
† All had complications of invasive aspergillosis; one had leukemia.
‡ Data given in only eight of 14.
§ Two patients had complications of invasive aspergillosis.

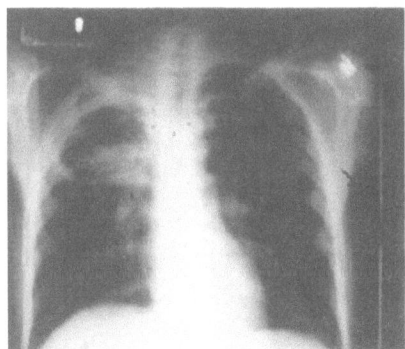

FIGURE 2. Posteroanterior roentgenogram of the chest showing an intracavitary mass.

suggested a nonoperative approach for patients with aspergilloma and sarcoidosis based on a low incidence of fatal hemoptysis,[3] while another study concluded that in the same population surgery was inescapable in 30% of cases.[4] For patients with chronic lung disease[5,6] and tuberculous cavities,[7,8] similar controversies exist. Table I summarizes the outcome of patients who were treated without surgery. The underlying diseases varied, and in some studies the immune status of the subject was not always clear. Additionally, the pathogenesis of hemoptysis remains obscure since details regarding ultimate size, rate of growth, and the local environment of the mycetoma were not discussed in the context of frequency or severity of hemoptysis. This makes the overall figure of 10% fatal hemoptysis difficult to interpret and to apply to indications for surgery.

In patients with AIDS and ARC, fungal disease is well recognized,[9] although to our knowledge mycetoma has not been described. A 6-cm mycetoma developed in the patient described here during a six-month period. Hemoptysis was variable over a five-month period and ultimately proved fatal. The cause of death was erosion of a pulmonary artery within the cavity wall as shown by autopsy.

It is apparent that treatment of pulmonary aspergillomas must be individualized based on the progression of disease and other host factors. Considering the degree of immune dysfunction and the severity of disease, rapid growth of a mycetoma and hemoptysis in a patient with AIDS-related complex may require surgery early in the course of treatment.

Acknowledgment.   The authors thank Ms Cathy Monahan for her secretarial assistance.

REFERENCES

1.   Bardana EJ: The clinical spectrum of aspergillosis—part 2: Classification and description of saprophytic, allergic, and invasive variants of human disease. *CRC Crit Rev Clin Lab Sci* 1981; 13:85–159.

2.   Albelda SM, Talbot GH, Gerson SL, et al: Pulmonary cavitation and massive hemoptysis in invasive pulmonary aspergillosis. *Am Rev Respir Dis* 1985; 131:115–120.

3.   Kaplan J, Johns JC: Mycetomas in pulmonary sarcoidosis: Non-surgical management. *Johns Hopkins Med J* 1979; 145:157–161.

4.   Israel HL, Lenchner GS, Atkinson GW: Sarcoidosis and aspergilloma: The role of surgery. *Chest* 1982; 82:430–432.

5.   Karas A, Hankins JR, Attar S, et al: Pulmonary aspergillosis: An analysis of 41 patients. *Ann Thorac Surg* 1976; 22:1–7.

6.   Varkey B, Rose HD: Pulmonary aspergilloma. A rational approach to treatment. *Am J Med* 1976; 61:626–631.

7.   Faulkner SL, Vernon R, Brown PP, et al: Hemoptysis and pulmonary aspergilloma: Operative versus nonoperative treatment. *Ann Thorac Surg* 1978; 25:389–392.

8.   Butz RO, Zvetina JR, Leininger BJ: Ten-year experience with mycetomas in patients with pulmonary tuberculosis. *Chest* 1985; 87:356–358.

9.   Armstrong D, Gold JWM, Dryjanski J, et al: Treatment of infections in patients with the acquired immunodeficiency syndrome. *Ann Intern Med* 1985; 103:738–743.

10.   Reddy PA, Christianson CS, Brasher CA, et al: Comparison of treated and untreated pulmonary aspergilloma. *Am Rev Respir Dis* 1970; 101:928–934.

11.   Solit RW, McKeown JJ Jr, Smullens S, et al: The surgical implications of intracavitary mycetomas (fungus balls). *J Thorac Cardiovasc Surg* 1971; 62:411–422.

12.   Hammerman KJ, Sarosi GA, Tosh FE: Amphotericin B in the treatment of saprophytic forms of pulmonary aspergillosis. *Am Rev Respir Dis* 1974; 109:57–62.

13.   Rafferty P, Biggs BA, Crompton GK, et al: What happens to patients with pulmonary aspergilloma? Analysis of 23 cases. *Thorax* 1983; 38:579–583.

Chapter 37

Lymphocytic interstitial pneumonitis in adult HIV infection

ROBERT Y. LIN, MD; PETER J. GRUBER, BA; RICHARD SAUNDERS, MD; ELLIOTT N. PERLA, MD

Pulmonary disease associated with acquired immunodeficiency syndrome (AIDS) is common and may be secondary to infectious and noninfectious processes.[1] One of the noninfectious processes is lymphocytic interstitial pneumonitis (LIP). LIP is an uncommon disorder that was first described by Carrington and Liebow[2] in 1966, and is characterized by a diffuse peribronchial and interstitial infiltration of the lung by lymphocytes and plasma cells.[3] LIP has been recognized as a common pulmonary complication in cases of pediatric AIDS and appears to be present in as many as 75% of these cases.[4] The present Centers for Disease Control (CDC) classification includes LIP as a diagnostic criterion for pediatric AIDS.[5]

The occurrence of LIP in adults with human immunodeficiency virus (HIV) infection has recently been noted.[6-10] In this report we describe two additional cases of LIP in adults with HIV infection. Also presented is an analysis from the literature of 14 cases of adults with LIP and HIV infection.

CASE REPORTS

Case 1. A 37-year-old man with a history of bisexuality and intravenous drug abuse was admitted to Metropolitan Hospital on March 11, 1987, with a two-month history of cough, shortness of breath, pleuritic chest pain, fever, and a 12-kg weight loss. His medical history was otherwise unremarkable.

On admission, the patient was afebrile. There was 1–2 cm diameter nontender lymphadenopathy in the cervical, axillary, and inguinal regions. Auscultation of the lungs revealed inspiratory rales and egophony in the right posterior and axillary

lung fields. Abdominal, skin, and joint examinations were within normal limits. The chest radiograph (Fig 1) showed right middle and lower lobe infiltrates with a prominent right hilum as well as a focus of previously noted left lung calcification. A panel of delayed type skin tests did not elicit any reaction.

A hemogram revealed a white blood cell count of 6,700/mm³; platelet count, 333,000/mm³; and hemoglobin, 10.9 g/dL. The differential white blood cell count showed 75% lymphocytes. Arterial blood gas levels were pH, 7.4; PCO_2, 35 mm Hg; and PO_2, 95 mm Hg. The IgG count was 4,000 mg/dL (normal, up to 1,700 mg/dL), the IgM was 68 mg/dL (normal, 30–360 mg/dL), and the IgA was 125 mg/dL (normal, 50–410 mg/dL). No monoclonal peak was detected on serum protein electrophoresis. A bone marrow aspirate was within normal limits. Antinuclear antibody, C3, C4, and rheumatoid factor levels were within normal limits. The Epstein-Barr viral capsid antigen (EB-VCA) IgG antibody titer was 1:320, while the cytomegalovirus IgG titer was 1:16. Peripheral blood studies showed a total helper T cell concentration of 1,240/mm³ with a T4/T8 ratio of 1:9 (both within normal reported limits). Pulmonary function tests showed a forced vital capacity (FVC) of 2.74 L (70% predicted), forced expiratory volume at one second (FEV_1) of 3.68 L (74% predicted), total lung capacity (TLC) of 4.58 L (74% predicted), and diffusion capacity for carbon monoxide (DLCO)

of 26.3% (98% predicted). HIV antibody was demonstrated by ELISA and Western blot techniques.

A transbronchoscopic biopsy of the right lower lobe showed infiltration of peribronchial areas and alveolar septae by mature small lymphocytes and scattered plasma cells with some areas of lymphocytic aggregates. Immunoperoxidase staining for light chains showed the presence of both kappa and lambda chains. This was interpreted as consistent with LIP. No *Pneumocystis carinii* or acid-fast organisms were found. A gallium scan showed bilateral lung uptake with more prominent uptake in the right lung (especially the right hilum). A computed tomogram of the chest showed right lung parenchymal consolidation with air bronchograms, as well as right hilar and mediastinal adenopathy (Fig 2). A mediastinoscopic biopsy of this lymph node showed a pattern of reactive hyperplasia with plasmacytosis and tangible macrophages within reactive follicular centers.

The patient was discharged from the hospital on prednisone, 60 mg/day. He was asymptomatic on 15 mg/day of prednisone at three months after discharge, and his chest film showed complete clearing of all infiltrates at that time. Steroid medication was completely tapered two weeks later, and the patient has remained asymptomatic six months after discharge. A repeat T lymphocyte analysis showed 412 T4 cells/mm³ and 900 T8 cells/mm³.

Case 2. A 31-year-old man with a history

From the Department of Medicine, Metropolitan Hospital, New York Medical College, New York, NY.

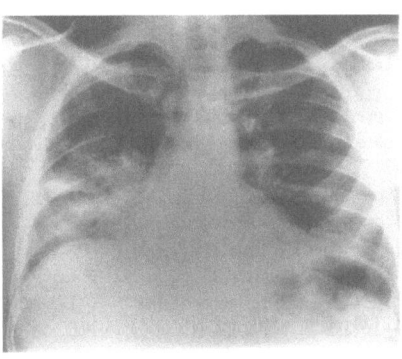

FIGURE 1. Posteroanterior chest film showing right middle and lower lobe infiltrates in case 1.

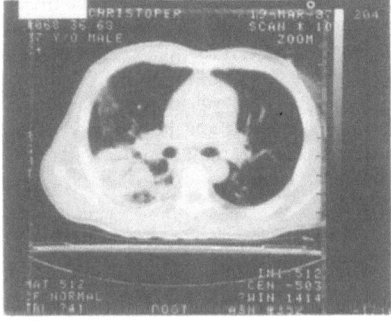

FIGURE 2. Computed tomograph of the chest demonstrating air bronchograms in the area of consolidation of the right lung in case 1.

of intravenous drug abuse (cocaine) was admitted to Metropolitan Hospital in March 1986 with complaints of fever, productive cough, hemoptysis, and a 14-pound weight loss over the past six months. His wife had recently died from AIDS.

On admission, he was febrile with a temperature of 38°C, he had cervical, supraclavicular, axillary, and inguinal adenopathy (1–2 cm), and he had rales in the posterior right lung fields. A chest radiograph revealed right middle and lower lobe alveolar infiltrates. The white blood cell count was 7,100/mm[3] with 24% neutrophils, 73% lymphocytes, and 3% eosinophils. The hematocrit was 35.8%. The serum asparate aminotransferase level was 90 U/L; albumin, 3.3 g/dL; and globulins, 7.0 g/dL. Arterial blood gas results on room air were pH, 7.43; PCO_2, 32 mm Hg; and PO_2, 87 mm Hg. Intermediate strength purified protein derivative was nonreactive, and sputum cultures for bacteria and mycobacteria were negative. HIV antibody testing was positive.

Right lower lobe transbronchial biopsy revealed diffuse infiltration of alveolar septae and peribronchial connective tissue with lymphocytic cells. No lymphoid follicles were identified. Light chain stains were polyclonal. No *Pneumocystis carinii* were identified in the biopsy or washings. Pulmonary function tests showed a FEV_1 of 3.37 L (82% predicted); FVC of 4.12 L (79% predicted), TLC of 5.71 L (90% predicted), and DLCO of 15.6% (60% predicted). A gallium scan revealed bilateral increased lung uptake.

The patient was treated with prednisone, 60 mg/day, with resolution of fever and cough and increase in body weight. The right lower lobe infiltrate resolved. He was admitted to the hospital in July 1986 for treatment of salmonella sepsis and in November 1986 for treatment of staphylococcal pneumonia.

On January 29, 1987, the patient was readmitted for headaches, changes in mental status, and fever. On admission, he was afebrile and found to have nuchal rigidity, cervical adenopathy, and a 2/6 systolic ejection murmur. The white blood cell count was 5,100 mm[3], and the platelet count was 240,000/mm[3]. The cerebrospinal fluid was positive for cryptococcal antigen at a titer of 1:1,024. The patient was treated with amphotericin and cefuroxime. On January 30, 1987, respiratory failure developed, and an endotracheal tube was inserted. The patient subsequently died on February 7, 1987. Post-mortem examination was not performed.

DISCUSSION

Sixteen cases associated with adult HIV infection,[6–10] including the two cases reported here, were reviewed. Three patients from one series[6] appear to have been reported previously in another report.[11] The characteristics of the reported adult LIP cases associated with HIV infection are shown in Table I.

LIP is thought to be part of a spectrum of benign lymphoid disorders of the lungs which diffusely involves alveolar septae.[12] Other lymphoproliferative disorders that can involve the lung (and have been described in association with AIDS) include non-Hodgkin lymphoma and angioblastic lymphadenopathy.[13,14] Benign lymphoid disorders of the lung such as LIP differ from lymphomatous involvement of the lung in that there is no evidence of light chain monoclonality, and the mononuclear infiltrates are always polymorphic in the former, whereas they may be monomorphic in lymphoma.[12,15] Both angioblastic lymphadenopathy and pulmonary lymphoma can have interstitial lymphocyte infiltration, and definitive differentiation between LIP and these two other disorders may on occasion require histologic evaluation of lymph nodes or more lung parenchymal tissue.

LIP is regarded as one of several chronic interstitial pulmonary patterns according to a schema of Liebow and Carrington.[3] In LIP, there is alveolar septal and peribronchial lymphocyte infiltration, as well as lymphoid aggregates that may contain micronodules often positioned around a central, thick-walled, periodic acid-Schiff-positive venule. Occasionally, germinal centers may be seen within the nodules, and epithelioid transformation of macrophages may be present within the germinal centers. Pulmonary fibrosis and noncaseating granulomas may be seen.[12] Similar histopathologic findings of lymphoid nodules, giant cells, and granuloma-like collections of mononuclear cells have been reported in a series of pediatric AIDS-associated LIP cases.[16] In the adult LIP cases reviewed

TABLE I. Patient Profiles of Adult HIV-Associated LIP

Patient No. (Ref. No.)	Chest Radiograph	H/S ratio (T4)	Age-yr (Race/ Nationality)	Infection	Lymphoid Involvement
1(6)	Diffuse reticulonodular	NS[†] (NS)	32 (African)	Five bacterial	RP,HA Sp,Hp
2(6)	Diffuse reticulonodular	0.23 (155)	53 (African)	Two bacterial	RP,PA
3(6)	Diffuse reticulonodular	0.27 (480)	28 (Haitian)		RP,PA
4(6)	Diffuse reticulonodular	0.28 (410)	40 (African)	One bacterial	RP,PA
5(6)	Diffuse reticulonodular	0.25 (310)	24 (Haitian)		RP,PA
6(6)	Diffuse reticulonodular	0.95 (450)	30 (Haitian)	Two bacterial	RP,HA PA
7(6)	Diffuse reticulonodular	0.60 (1,065)	32 (Haitian)		RP,PA
8(7)	Bilateral reticulonodular	0.2 (NS)	32 (Black)	*Mycobacterium avium/intracellulare*	PA,Hp Sp
9(7)	Bilateral reticulonodular	0.6 (NS)	56 (Black)	Presumed *mycobacterium tuberculosis*	Sp
10(7)	Bilateral reticulonodular	0.26 (NS)	46 (Black)	*Pneumocystis carinii*	
11(8)	Bilateral reticulonodular	0.7 (318)	43 (Not stated)	Esophageal candidiasis	Hp, Sp
12(present case)	Right middle and lower lobe infiltrates	NS	31 (Black)	Cryptococcus, Two bacterial	PA
13(present case)	Right middle and lower lobe infiltrates	1.9 (1,240)	37 (Black)	—	HA, PA
14(9)	Bilateral reticulonodular	0.45 (717)	30 (Black)	—	PA
15–16(10)	NS	NS	NS (Haitian)	NS	NS

* H/S ratio, T-helper to suppressor lymphocyte ratio; T4(CD4) lymphocytes per cubic millimeter; PA, peripheral adenopathy; HA, hilar adenopathy; Sp, splenomegaly; Hp, hepatomegaly; RP, retroperitoneal.
† NS, not stated.

herein, germinal centers, lymphoid nodule presence, and fibrosis in the pulmonary interstitium were reported, but there were no reports of giant cells, follicular or large cell hyperplastic changes, or granulomas. The evolution of adenopathic follicular hyperplasia into follicular involution/atrophy seen in HIV-associated peripheral lymph nodes[17] has not been reported in HIV-associated LIP. Recently, nonspecific pneumonitis has been described[1,18] as another noninfectious pulmonary manifestation of HIV infection which can be histologically distinguished from LIP because of a more mixed cellular infiltrative pattern with less well formed lymphoid aggregates, such as follicles and germinal centers. Two Haitian patients with miliary chest film patterns and diffuse lymphoid nodules on histologic analysis have been described in association with diminished CD4/8 (T4/8) peripheral blood lymphocyte ratios.[12] This may represent another pattern of pulmonary lymphoid involvement in HIV infection.

The clinical features of the patients reviewed in this report showed several interesting findings. The spirometric findings showed restrictive patterns in nine of ten cases studied (total lung capacity range, 44–90% predicted; DLCO range, 30–98% predicted) and obstructive patterns in one case.[6] On radiographic studies reported prior to the discovery of AIDS, LIP had been noted to have both interstitial and alveolar patterns.[12] The two patients described here showed lateralizing and discrete infiltrates, with documented air bronchograms in one. This confirms that both patterns (Table I) can occur in HIV-associated cases as well. In the 12 cases in which race was stated, all patients were black. None of the cases in the French series[6,9] was associated with intravenous drug abuse or homosexuality. Whether there is a genetic predisposition to LIP in adults is not clear. Four of the 16 patients had died at the time of the report (one each from failure to thrive, salmonella infection, cryptococcal infection, and *Pneumocystis carinii* pneumonia). Bacterial infections were sometimes recurrent and included salmonella, *Haemophilus influenzae*, staphylococcus, and streptococcus. Clinical AIDS[5] was described in three subjects at the time of diagnosing LIP; opportunistic infections consistent with AIDS were diagnosed after LIP in four patients, three of whom were treated with corticosteroids.

Treatment of LIP in the pre-AIDS era usually involved high-dose corticosteroid administration.[19] In the cases reviewed here, treatment and LIP response were not stated in all instances. Five patients were treated with corticosteroids, and their respiratory parameters and/or symptoms improved. In one series, patients' conditions were reported to be stable without steroid therapy. One case described by Grieco et al[8] had spontaneous improvement of respiratory symptoms and chest film appearance without steroid administration. In pediatric AIDS-associated LIP, both corticosteroids and gammaglobulin administration have been used with some success in improving respiratory parameters.[20] In the pre-LIP era, in LIP cases associated with hypogammaglobulinemia, there was reported improvement of LIP with gammaglobulin replacement therapy.[19]

The immunopathogenesis of LIP is not known, but pre-AIDS cases have often been associated with a variety of disorders with autoimmune components such as Sjögren syndrome, dysgammaglobulinemia, chronic active hepatitis, pernicious anemia, myasthenia gravis, and hypogammaglobulinemia. Polyclonal B cell stimulation and lymphoid tissue hyperplasia also seem to be common in LIP. In pre-AIDS literature on LIP, hypergammaglobulinemia was found in more than 90% of non-hypogammaglobulinemic patients in one series.[19] In our review, 92% (12/13) of patients with HIV-associated LIP had hypergammaglobulinemia. In this institution, hypergammaglobulinemia is seen in about 50–70% of the cases, while hypergammaglobulinemia in persistent generalized adenopathy secondary to HIV infection has been reported to occur in 31–88% of patients.[21] B cell tropic viruses are known to infect AIDS patients possibly secondary to an impaired T lymphocyte regulatory mechanism, and may be responsible in part for stimulating polyclonal immunoglobulin production[22] in these patients. Indeed, viral genomes such as Epstein-Barr virus DNA have been identified in some pediatric AIDS-associated LIP tissues.[23] Nine cases reviewed here were studied for EBV-VCA IgG, and five had titers of greater than 1:320.[6,23] Extrapulmonary lymphoid hyperplasia has been reported in pre-AIDS LIP cases.[19] This appears also to be present in HIV-associated adult LIP, with adenopathy/splenomegaly present in 13 of 14 cases reported. Whether LIP represents one of several sites of a generalized lympho-

proliferative response in HIV infection or whether there is a specific pulmonary immunogenic agent that provokes a localized response is a matter of speculation at this time.

Immunophenotypic studies of tissue sections in LIP have not shown any consistent patterns in pre-AIDS or HIV-associated cases. The latter have shown patterns ranging from mixed T and B cells,[24] to predominantly T cells with both T8 (CD8) and T4 (CD4) populations,[7] to predominantly T8 cells.[7,9] Pre-AIDS LIP cases have been reported with both T cell and B cell predominance.[8,9] Bronchoalveolar lavage findings in two HIV-associated cases[6,9] demonstrated decreased T4/T8 lavage lymphocyte ratios. Decreased ratios were identified in corresponding peripheral blood studies.

From this review of adult HIV-associated LIP, we submit an approach to managing patients in whom LIP is a diagnostic consideration—ie, those presenting with subacute or chronic respiratory symptoms and either lateralizing or bilateral infiltrates on chest radiographs. Since LIP is a diffuse interstitial process, transbronchial biopsy appears to be a reasonable first line method of obtaining adequate histopathologic and microbiologic specimens. Concurrent washings and specimens for mycobacterial cultures/stains, *Pneumocystis carinii* stains, and cytologic studies should be obtained. The biopsy specimens should be examined by periodic acid-Schiff staining as well as light chain immunoperoxidase stains to exclude malignant disorders. If uncertainty regarding malignancy still exists, a computed tomogram may detect mediastinoscopically accessible lymph nodes for further histopathologic examination, thus potentially obviating the need for open lung biopsy. Management considerations in these cases must take into account the observation that some patients will have spontaneous resolution and/or improvement of their pulmonary symptomatology. The administration of corticosteroids in an already immunocompromised patient should be individualized on the basis of concurrent disease, symptoms, and degree of respiratory impairment; and the length and dose of steroid therapy should be reviewed frequently and minimalized if possible. Although nonspirometric gauges of interstitial lung disease may be employed to follow these patients, such as quantitative bronchoalveolar lavage and gallium scanning,[25,26] concurrent infectious processes may complicate the interpretation of these tests. Clearly, it is of paramount importance to recognize and treat the infectious complications of AIDS in these patients. Also, the possibility of malignant transformation of de novo pulmonary lymphoma development should be considered.[12,15,27]

Because of the relatively few cases of adult HIV-associated LIP, many questions still exist regarding the prognosis, histopathology, and treatment of these patients. However, it seems clear that LIP constitutes part of the spectrum of pulmonary disorders that affect HIV-infected adults.

Acknowledgment. The authors thank Drs Simon, Alfelors, Connors, Ramaswammi, and Sadjadi.

REFERENCES

1. Stover DE, White DA, Romano PA, et al: Spectrum of pulmonary diseases associated with the acquired immune deficiency syndrome. *Am J Med* 1985; 78:429–437.

2. Carrington CB, Liebow AA: Lymphocytic interstitial pneumonia (abstract). *Am J Path* 1966; 48:36a.

3. Liebow AA, Carrington CB: The interstitial pneumonias, in Simon M, Potchen EJ, Le May M (eds): *Frontiers of Pulmonary Radiology: Pathophysiologic, Roentgenographic, and Radioisotopic Considerations.* New York, Grune & Stratton, 1969, pp 102–141.

4. Scott GB, Buck BE, Leterman JG, et al: Acquired immunodeficiency syndrome in infants. *N Engl J Med* 1984; 310:76–81.

5. Revision of the case definition of AIDS for national reporting—United States. *MMWR* 1985; 34:373–375.

6. Couderc LJ, Herve P, Solal-Celigny P, et al: Pneumonie lymphoide interstitielle et polyadenopathies chez des sujets infectés par le virus LAV/HTLV III. *Presse Med* 1986; 15:1127–1130.

7. Morris JC, Rosen MJ, Marchevsky A, et al: Lymphocytic interstitial pneumonia in patients at risk for the acquired immune deficiency syndrome. *Chest* 1987; 91:63–67.

8. Grieco MH, Chinoy-Acharya P: Lymphocytic interstitial pneumonia associated with the acquired immune deficiency syndrome. *Am Rev Respir Dis* 1986; 131:952–955.

9. Ziza JM, Brun Vezinet F, Venet A, et al: Pneumopathie lymphocytaire interstielle au cours d'un ARC. Preŝence du virus LAV dans le liquide de lavage broncho-alvéolaire. *Presse Med* 1986; 15: 1267–1269.

10. Saldana MJ, Mones J, Buck BE: Lymphoid interstitial pneumonia in Haitian residents of Florida. *Chest* 1983; 84:347.

11. Solal-Celigny P, Couderc LJ, Herman D, et al: Lymphoid interstitial pneumonitis in acquired immunodeficiency syndrome-related complex. *Am Rev Respir Dis* 1985; 131:956–960.

12. Kradin RL, Mark EJ: Benign lymphoid disorders of the lung, with a theory regarding their development. *Hum Path* 1983; 14:857–867.

13. Sifai B, Koziner B: Malignant neoplasm in AIDS, in De Vita VT Jr, Hellman S, Rosenberg SA (eds): *AIDS—Etiology, Diagnosis, Treatment, and Prevention.* New York, JB Lippincott Co, 1985, pp 213–222.

14. Sallahuddin SZ, Ablashi DV, Markham PD, et al: Isolation of a new virus, HBLV, in patients with lymphoproliferative disorders. *Science* 1986; 234: 596–601.

15. Turner RR, Colby TV, Doggett RS: Well differentiated lymphocytic lymphoma. A study of 47 patients with primary manifestation in the lung. *Cancer* 1984; 54:2088–2096.

16. Joshi VV, Oleske JM, Minnefor AB, et al: Pathology of suspected acquired immune deficiency syndrome in children: A study of eight cases. *Pediatr Pathol* 1984; 2:71–87.

17. Biberfeld P, Porwit-Ksiazek A, Böttinger B:

Immunohistopathology of lymph nodes in HTLV-III infected homosexuals with persistent adenopathy or AIDS. *Cancer Res* 1985; 45:4665S–4670S.

18. Suffredini AF, Ognibene FP, Lack EE, et al: Nonspecific interstitial pneumonitis: A common cause of pulmonary disease in the acquired immunodeficiency syndrome. *Ann Intern Med* 1987; 107: 7–13.

19. Strimlan CV, Rosenow EC 3d, Weiland LH, et al: Lymphocytic interstitial pneumonitis. Review of 13 cases. *Ann Intern Med* 1978; 86:616–621.

20. Silverman B, Charytan B, BenZion K, et al: Chronic interstitial pneumonitis in pediatric AIDS and AIDS related complex (prodrome). *Pediatr Res* 1984; 18:265.

21. Ziegler JL, Abram DI: The AIDS related complex, in DeVita VT Jr, Hellman S, Rosenberg SA (eds): *AIDS: Etiology, Diagnosis, Treatment, and Prevention.* New York, JB Lippincott, 1985, pp 223–234.

22. Bowen DL, Lane HC, Fauci AS: Immunologic features of AIDS, in DeVita VT Jr, Hellman S, Rosenberg SA (eds): *AIDS: Etiology, Diagnosis, Treatment, and Prevention.* New York, JB Lippincott, 1985, pp 111–160.

23. Fackler JC, Nagel JE, Adler WH, et al: Epstein-Barr virus infection in a child with acquired immunodeficiency syndrome. *Am J Dis Child* 1985; 139:1000–1004.

24. Wallace JM, Barbers RG, Oishi JS, et al: Cellular and T-lymphocyte subpopulation profiles in bronchoalveolar lavage fluid from patients with acquired immunodeficiency syndrome and pneumonitis. *Am Rev Respir Dis* 1984; 130:786–790.

25. Lin RY: Severe spirometric defects in systemic lupus erythematosus: A possible role for bronchoalveolar lavage and gallium scanning. *Clin Rheum* 1987; 6:276–281.

26. Crystal RG, Bitterman PB, Rennard SI, et al: Interstitial lung disease of unknown cause. Disorders characterized by chronic inflammation of the lower respiratory tract. *N Engl J Med* 1984; 310:154–166, 235–244.

27. Julsrud PR, Brown LR, Li CY, et al: Pulmonary processes of mature-appearing lymphocytes: Pseudolymphoma, well-differentiated lymphocytic lymphoma, and lymphocytic interstitial pneumonitis. *Radiology* 1978; 127:289–296.

Chapter 38

Thymoma, *Pneumocystis carinii* pneumonia, and AIDS

DANIEL D. BUFF, MD; STEVEN D. GREENBERG, MD; PAULINE LEUNG, MD; FRANK S. PALUMBO, MD

Since the initial descriptions of acquired immunodeficiency syndrome (AIDS), it has become evident that the disorder predisposes patients not only to opportunistic infections, but also to malignancies. Large series have reported a 33–40% incidence of neoplastic disease in patients with AIDS;[1,2] the overwhelming majority of these malignancies are Kaposi sarcoma.[3] An additional 4–10% of patients have non-Hodgkin lymphomas, usually of the

aggressive B-cell type. Case reports of related solid tumors have recently appeared, and although cause and effect have not been proven, the incidence of solid tumors in patients with AIDS may be as high as 5%.[4,5]

We report what appears to be the first case of thymoma in a patient with AIDS. The case is particularly interesting as included in the differential diagnosis is common variable immunodeficiency (Good syndrome), an uncommon immunodeficiency state associated with 5–10% of thymomas.[6]

CASE REPORT

The patient, a 48-year-old man, was in ex-

cellent health until two weeks prior to admission, when fever, anorexia, and a cough productive of yellow sputum developed. His symptoms progressed, and when shortness of breath developed, the patient was referred to a physician. He denied a history of intravenous drug abuse, blood transfusions, or homosexual encounters, but admitted to frequent contacts with prostitutes. He had never been hospitalized before and was not taking any medications.

On physical examination, the patient was noted to be cyanotic, diaphoretic, and in respiratory distress. He was febrile to 104°F, had oral thrush, and, on inspiration, rales were detected in both lung fields. The examination did not reveal adenopathy, organomegaly, or skin lesions.

Routine hematologic tests were signifi-

From the Department of Medicine, Booth Memorial Medical Center, Flushing, NY.

cant for an elevated white blood cell count with a shift to the left, a hemoglobin of 13.8 g/dL, and a normal platelet count. Blood chemistry studies were significant for a total protein of 6.0 g/dL, an albumin of 2.2 mg/dL, a lactate dehydrogenase level of 580 IU/L, and mildly elevated liver enzyme levels. Results of an arterial blood gas test on room air were pH, 7.49; PCO_2, 32 mm Hg; PO_2, 49 mm Hg. A chest film revealed bilateral diffuse interstitial infiltrates and a mediastinal mass approximately 6 cm in diameter.

The patient was admitted to the hospital and was started on trimethoprim/sulfamethoxazole for possible *Pneumocystis* pneumonia. A computed tomographic (CT) scan of the chest revealed a well-defined, homogeneous, noncalcified mass in the anterior mediastinum with no evidence of adenopathy or local invasion (Fig 1). Despite oxygen supplementation and the addition of antituberculous drugs to his regimen, the patient remained febrile, with worsening hypoxia that necessitated intubation.

On the third hospital day, a mediasternotomy was performed with biopsy of the mass and adjacent lung. On gross examination the lesion appeared smooth and tan-colored with an intact capsule. On microscopic analysis, it consisted of spindle-shaped epithelial cells with scattered aggregates of normal-appearing mature lymphocytes (Fig 2). Immunoperoxidase staining showed the spindle cells to be positive for cytokeratin, and well-formed desmosomes were noted between the cells on electron microscopy. The appearance and staining of the mediastinal mass were consistent with spindle cell thymoma, and the intact capsule indicated that the lesion was benign. Silver stains of lung tissue for *Pneumocystis* organisms were positive, while stains for acid-fast bacilli and fungi were negative.

Evaluation of the patient's immune status revealed cutaneous anergy and a strongly

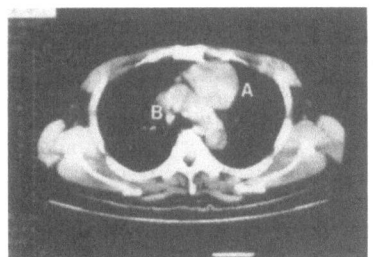

FIGURE 1.   Computed tomographic scan of the chest demonstrating a large mediastinal mass (A) anterior to the great vessels (B).

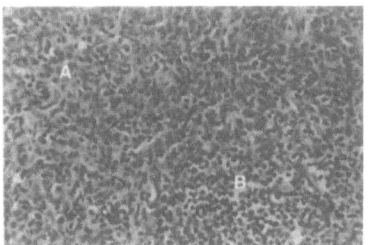

FIGURE 2.   Biopsy specimen from the anterior mediastinal mass. Demonstrated are aggregates of spindle-like epithelial cells (A) and mature lymphocytes (B); hematoxylin-eosin stain, original magnification × 400.

positive human immunodeficiency virus (HIV) titer on ELISA. Gammaglobulin levels were as follows: IgG, 1,090 mg/dL (normal, 750–1,750 mg/dL); IgA, 616 mg/dL (normal, 100–385 mg/dL); IgM, 87.4 mg/dL (normal, 50–250 mg/dL).

Over the next several days, the patient's condition deteriorated, with worsening hypoxia and progressive hypotension. Despite aggressive resuscitation and the administration of pentamidine, the patient died on the seventh day of hospitalization.

DISCUSSION

The documentation of an associated opportunistic infection in a patient with a recognized risk factor and a positive HIV titer are diagnostic of acquired immunodeficiency syndrome. As such, this appears to be the first reported case of thymoma in a patient with AIDS. We do not necessarily propose a cause-and-effect relationship between AIDS and thymoma. As with other case reports involving solid tumors, there is no direct evidence that HIV infection induced or allowed the induction of the patient's tumor. AIDS has become so common that it will now be diagnosed in patients with concomitant but unrelated disorders. However, the predilection of HIV for infecting T lymphocytes and the role of thymus-derived T cells in the immune system may make the development of thymoma and other solid tumors more likely in patients with AIDS.

Although the patient presented had AIDS, included in the differential diagnosis is Good syndrome, a parathymic

immunodeficiency state. Good syndrome is a rather uncommon disorder characterized immunologically by hypogammaglobulinemia (particularly of IgG and IgA), cutaneous anergy, and decreased populations of pre-B, B, and T-helper lymphocytes.[7,8] T-suppressor cell populations appear to be increased, leading to speculation that this is the primary immunologic defect.[8] Clinically, patients are on the average 50 years of age and of either sex.[9] They suffer from recurrent infections involving the respiratory tract, gastrointestinal tract, and skin,[7,8] and *Pneumocystis carinii* pneumonia has been described.[10] On pathologic evaluation, three quarters of thymomas in Good syndrome are of the spindle cell type, and most are benign.[8] The prognosis is poor, as most patients succumb to their infections within several years of diagnosis.[9] In contrast to other parathymic disorders, thymectomy in Good syndrome does not affect the course of the disease; in fact, immunodeficiency can develop many years after removal of a thymoma.[8,10]

REFERENCES

1. Kaplan MH, Susin M, Pahwa SG, et al: Neoplastic complications of HTLV-III infection. Lymphomas and solid tumors. *Am J Med* 1987; 82:389–396.

2. Longo DL, Steis RG, Lane HC, et al: Malignancies in the AIDS patient: Natural history, treatment strategies, and preliminary results. *Ann NY Acad Sci* 1984; 437:421–430.

3. Fauci AS (moderator): Acquired immunodeficiency syndrome: Epidemiologic, clinical, immunologic, and therapeutic considerations. *Ann Intern Med* 1984; 100:92–106.

4. Levine AM: Non-Hodgkin's lymphomas and other malignancies in the acquired immunodeficiency syndrome. *Semin Oncol* 1987; 14:34–39.

5. Groopman JE: Neoplasms in the acquired immune deficiency syndrome: The multidisciplinary approach to treatment. *Semin Onc* 1987; 14:1–6.

6. Rosenow EC 3d, Hurley BT: Disorders of the thymus. A review. *Arch Intern Med* 1984; 144:763–770.

7. Craig JB, Powell BL, Muss HB: Thymoma. *Am Fam Physician* 1984; 29:229–234.

8. Stiehm ER, Fulginiti VA (eds): *Immunologic Disorders in Infants and Children.* Philadelphia, WB Saunders, 1980, pp 321–326.

9. Jeunet FS, Good RA: Thymoma, immunologic deficiencies and hematologic abnormalities. *Birth Defects* 1968; 4:192–203.

10. Velde K te, Huber J, Slikke LB van der: Primary acquired hypogammaglobulinemia, myasthenia, and thymoma. *Ann Intern Med* 1966; 65:554–559.

Chapter 39
Saccharomyces fungemia in a patient with AIDS

Nisha Sethi, MD, William Mandell, MD

Saccharomyces cerevisiae is a yeast that is more commonly known as brewer's yeast. Commercial uses include beer and wine production, health food supplementation, and, more recently, hepatitis B vaccine production by recombinant DNA techniques. Occasionally, *S cerevisiae* has been isolated from clinical specimens and rarely has been a cause of serious infection. Case reports are few, and *S cerevisiae* has frequently been isolated in association with more common pathogenic organisms. We describe a case of *S cerevisiae* septicemia in association with acquired immunodeficiency syndrome (AIDS).

CASE REPORT

A 37-year-old woman with a history of intravenous drug and alcohol abuse sought medical attention in 1985 because of herpes zoster infection and oral candidiasis. The total T4 lymphocyte count was 324/mm^3 with a T4/T8 ratio of 0.73. Antibody against human immunodeficiency virus (HIV) was present. During the following 18 months her renal function deteriorated, with the serum creatinine level ranging from 4 to 6 mg/dL.

One week prior to admission, headache, generalized edema, ascites, pleural effusions, cough, shortness of breath, and fever developed. Examination revealed oral thrush, lymphadenopathy, decreased breath sounds on the right side, hepatomegaly, and anasarca. Serum creatinine and blood urea nitrogen levels were 18.8 mg/dL and 106 mg/dL, respectively. Chest roentgenography showed a right middle lobe infiltrate. Treatment included antibiotics and peritoneal dialysis. During treatment a pericardial effusion developed and the patient's pleural effusions worsened. Pericardial biopsy and pleural fluid stains and cultures were negative.

The patient continued to have temperature elevations. She denied any ophthalmologic complaints and there were no overt signs of infection. Four weeks after admission three sets of blood cultures drawn during a 24-hour period grew *Saccharomyces cerevisiae*. Amphotericin B therapy was begun. Ophthalmologic examination revealed foci of fluffy yellow exudates in the right eye and chorioretinal necrosis of the left eye. Follow-up blood cultures were negative, and the fever subsided. The patient received a total dose of 2,100 mg of amphotericin B. Examination one month after completion of amphotericin B demonstrated disappearance of retinal exudates and chorioretinal scarring at the previous location of necrosis. The patient remained without evidence of saccharomyces infection. However, full-blown AIDS subsequently developed, and she died ten months later.

DISCUSSION

S cerevisiae is generally believed to be nonpathogenic.[1] In experimental studies, subcutaneous inoculation was neither lethal nor invasive for both control and cortisone-treated mice.[2] Although *S cerevisiae* was cultured from some visceral organs six days after challenge in both groups of mice, at 30 days there was no evidence of persistent infection.[2] Colonization and pathogenicity studies have established the safety of *S cerevisiae* as a candidate for a host vector system in recombinant DNA experiments. Colonization could not be established by oral or intravenous inoculation of control or cortisone-treated cynomolgus monkeys.[3]

Saccharomyces is believed to be an occasional, normal commensal in the gastrointestinal tract.[4] It has been isolated from sputum and tracheal aspirates of patients with tuberculosis.[5]

Kiehn et al[6] reviewed 3,340 yeast cultures from cancer patients over a 15-month period and isolated *S cerevisiae* from 19 sputum samples, including one tracheal aspirate and one lung tissue culture. Eng et al[1] described an immunosuppressed patient with dysphagia from whom both *S cerevisiae* and *Candida tropicalis* were isolated from the esophagus. In other patients, the authors[1] isolated *S cerevisiae* from pleural fluid, a kidney, urine, and from a Cowper gland. In many of the reported cases, another pathogenic organism was concomitantly isolated.[1] *S cerevisiae* has also been responsible for postoperative peritoneal infection.[7]

There have been three previous reports of *S cerevisiae* septicemia. The first case report in 1970 described a patient with prosthetic valve endocarditis.[8] The second case involved a 68-year-old man who ingested brewer's yeast in large quantities. The patient recovered without treatment when he stopped ingesting brewer's yeast.[9] The third case of *S cerevisiae* septicemia was in a burn patient on hyperalimentation.[10] In two of the aforementioned cases, fundoscopic examination was reported as normal.

The patient described in this report may have been predisposed to disseminated fungal infection secondary to underlying HIV infection and end-stage renal disease. Invasive fungal infections have previously been described in patients with HIV infection. Dissemination has occurred with *Candida albicans*, *Histoplasma capsulatum*,[11,12] *Coccidioides immitis*,[13] and *Cryptococcus neoformans*.[14,15] In addition, fungal septicemia has been reported in patients receiving peritoneal dialysis.[16] Contrary to the clinical experience with AIDS patients, in whom disseminated fungal infections are difficult to eradicate, this patient showed apparent cure after completing a regimen of 2,100 mg of amphotericin B.

The source of *S cerevisiae* fungemia in this patient is not clear. Dialysate fluid, pleural fluid, pericardial fluid, and sputum failed to grow the organism. Urine and stool were not sent for culture. The lack of a recognizable source is similar to that in cases of salmonellosis[17] or cryptococcosis[15] in patients with AIDS.

From the Department of Medicine, Harlem Hospital Center, College of Physicians and Surgeons, Columbia University, New York.

We conclude that although *Saccharomyces cerevisiae* is a rare pathogen, it may cause serious invasive infection, especially in patients at risk. When isolated from the bloodstream, *S cerevisiae* cannot be dismissed as a nonpathogen and should now be added to the list of opportunistic pathogens that infect patients with AIDS.

REFERENCES

1. Eng RH, Drehmel R, Smith SM, et al: *Saccharomyces cerevisiae* infections in man. *Sabouraudia* 1984; 22:403–407.
2. Holzschu DL, Chandler FW, Ajello L, et al: Evaluation of industrial yeasts for pathogenicity. *Sabouraudia* 1979; 17:71–78.
3. Maejimak K, Shimoda K, Morita C, et al: Colonization and pathogenicity of *Saccharomyces cerevisiae*, MC 16, in mice and cynomolgus monkeys after oral and intravenous administration. *Jpn J Med Sci Biol* 1980; 33:271–276.
4. Rippon JW: *Miscellaneous Yeast Infections in Medical Mycology*, ed 12. Philadelphia, WB Saunders, 1982, pp 559–564.
5. Greer AE, Gemoets HN: The coexistence of pathogenic fungi in certain chronic pulmonary diseases, with especial reference to pulmonary tuberculosis. *Dis Chest* 1943:212–240.
6. Kiehn TE, Edwards FF, Armstrong D: The prevalence of yeasts in clinical specimens from cancer patients. *Am J Clin Pathol* 1980; 73:518–521.
7. Dougherty SH, Simmons RL: Postoperative peritonitis caused by *Saccharomyces cerevisiae* [letter]. *Arch Surg* 1982; 117:248.
8. Stein PD, Folkens AT, Hruska KA: Saccharomyces fungemia. *Chest* 1970; 58:174–175.
9. Jensen DP, Smith DL: Fever of unknown origin secondary to brewer's yeast ingestion. *Arch Intern Med* 1976; 136:332–333.
10. Eschete ML, West BC: *Saccharomyces cerevisiae* septicemia. *Arch Intern Med* 1980; 140:1539.
11. Wheat LJ, Slama TG, Zeckel ML: Histoplasmosis in the acquired immune deficiency syndrome. *Am J Med* 1985; 78:203–210.
12. Mandell W, Goldberg DM, Neu HC: Histoplasmosis in patients with the acquired immune deficiency syndrome. *Am J Med* 1986; 81:974–978.
13. Bonnimann DA, Adam RD, Galgiani JN, et al: Coccidioidomycosis in the acquired immune deficiency syndrome. *Ann Intern Med* 1987; 106:372–379.
14. Zuger A, Loui E, Holzman RS, et al: Cryptococcal disease in patients with the acquired immunodeficiency syndrome. Diagnostic features and outcome of treatment. *Ann Intern Med* 1986; 104:234–240.
15. Kovacs JA, Kovacs AA, Polis M, et al: Cryptococcosis in the acquired immunodeficiency syndrome. *Ann Intern Med* 1985; 103:533–538.
16. Eisenberg ES, Leviton I, Soeiro R: Fungal peritonitis in patients receiving peritoneal dialysis: Experience with 11 patients and review of the literature. *Rev Infect Dis* 1986; 8:309–321.
17. Jacobs JL, Gold JW, Murray HW, et al: Salmonella infections in patients with the acquired immunodeficiency syndrome. *Ann Intern Med* 1985; 102:186–188.

Chapter 40

Candida pneumonia secondary to an acquired tracheoesophageal fistula in a patient with AIDS

ARI KLAPHOLZ, MD; LARRY WASSER, MD; SIDNEY STEIN, MD; WILFREDO TALAVERA, MD

Fungal pneumonias represent approximately 5% of all pulmonary infections occurring in patients with acquired immunodeficiency syndrome (AIDS).[1] The most commonly observed cause of fungal pneumonia is *Cryptococcus neoformans*, followed by *Histoplasma capsulatum* or *Coccidioides immitis*, depending on the geographic location.[2] Despite the prevalence of oral thrush and esophageal candidiasis in patients with AIDS, pneumonia caused by *Candida albicans* is extremely uncommon. The following case report represents, to our knowledge, the first description of a candidal pneumonia secondary to aspiration through a tracheoesophageal fistula in a patient with AIDS.

CASE REPORT

A 36-year-old man with a history of intravenous drug abuse was admitted to Beth Israel Medical Center complaining of a three-week history of severe retrosternal chest pain, weight loss, shortness of breath, and a cough productive of white sputum. The diagnosis of AIDS had been made ten months prior to admission, when the patient was found to have esophageal candidiasis on upper endoscopy. He was initially treated with intravenous amphotericin B and then maintained on ketoconazole, which he took sporadically. Although significant weight loss had occurred, he denied any recent fevers, chills, or night sweats.

Physical examination on admission revealed a cachectic male in no apparent distress. The blood pressure was 100/70 mm Hg, the pulse was 80/min, the respiratory rate was 20/min, and he was afebrile. Examination of the head and neck was unremarkable, and no oral thrush was evident. Moist rales were heard at the base of the left lung posteriorly. The rest of the examination was unrevealing with the exception of a tender, erythematous rectal mucosa with a palpable fissure. A test for occult blood in the stool was negative.

Laboratory evaluation was significant for a white blood cell count of 1,100/mm^3, with a differential of 40% polymorphonuclear leukocytes, 10% band forms, 10% lymphocytes, and 40% monocytes. The hematocrit was 20.3%. Serum chemistry analysis revealed a protein content of 8.2 g/dL; albumin of 2.8 g/dL; alkaline phosphatase of 318 IU/L; and lactate dehydrogenase of 329 IU/L. A chest film revealed an elevated right hemidiaphragm, a left lower lobe retrocardiac infiltrate, and air along the left paratracheal border (Fig 1). There was no evidence of hilar or mediastinal adenopathy, and the heart size was normal. Tests of sputum were negative on Gram stain and culture, and no acid-fast bacilli were seen on smear.

The patient was initially treated with mycostatin oral suppositories and viscous lidocaine for his complaints of retrosternal pain, which was presumably due to the candidal esophagitis. On the sixth hospital day, his rectal temperature spiked to 104°. Physical examination revealed persistent rales at the base of the left lung. After blood and sputum cultures were drawn, he was started on intravenous clindamycin, 600 mg every six

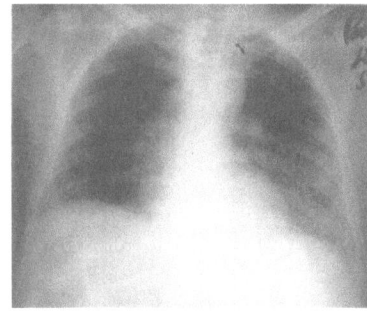

FIGURE 1. Anteroposterior chest film showing a left lower lobe infiltrate and air along the left paratracheal border (arrow).

From the Division of Pulmonary Medicine, Beth Israel Medical Center, New York, NY.

hours, and tobramycin, 80 mg every eight hours. His temperature continued to spike for the next 48 hours despite antibiotic therapy. Arterial blood gas studies revealed a pH of 7.46; PCO_2, 27 mm Hg; PaO_2, 56 mm Hg, and a saturation of 91.2%. Repeat chest film showed worsening of the left lower lobe infiltrate. The antibiotics were changed to intravenous trimethoprim/sulfamethoxazole, 960 mg every six hours, and erythromycin, 750 mg every six hours. On the tenth hospital day, the patient underwent a flexible fiberoptic bronchoscopy. A small opening with irregular borders was noted on the left posterolateral aspect of the trachea, and methylene blue swallowed by the patient was observed to egress from this orifice. Candidal mucous plaques were noted along the left main stem and lower lobe bronchus. Transbronchial biopsies from the left lower lobe revealed pseudohyphae and fungal spores invading the pulmonary parenchyma. The specimens were consistent with *Candida* species. Special stains for acid-fast bacilli were negative. Subsequently the patient was started on antifungal therapy with intravenous amphotericin B, 20 mg/day intravenously. Despite excellent initial improvement, his overall clinical status continued to deteriorate, the dyspnea worsened, and he died on the 23rd hospital day.

DISCUSSION

The most common fungus isolated from respiratory secretions of patients with AIDS is *Candida albicans*, usually representing oropharyngeal colonization.[1] Even with the increased frequency of esophageal candidiasis in AIDS,

candidal pneumonia has rarely been reported, except when secondary to hematogenous dissemination as a preterminal event. Marchevsky et al[3] reviewed the pathology of 70 patients with AIDS and pulmonary involvement. Specimens included transbronchial biopsies and autopsy tissue. Only three cases of invasive candidiasis were found, characterized by the presence of pseudohyphae and spores invading both the bronchial wall and lung parenchyma.

The case reported here is unique in two respects: it identifies a rare case of possible endogenous candidal pneumonia; and the portal of entry, presumably through a tracheoesophageal fistula secondary to longstanding candida esophagitis, has not been previously reported in a patient with AIDS. As with other immunocompromised hosts, the usual portal of entry is via hematogenous spread or aspiration. The first reported case of a tracheoesophageal fistula with an infectious etiology was described by Obrecht et al[5] in a patient with promyelocytic leukemia who was found to have invasive candidiasis and aspergillosis of the esophagus, with fungal organisms protruding from the fistula into the right mainstem bronchus. Sehhat et al[6] also reported a case of esophageal moniliasis, with the formation of an esophagopulmonary fistula and right lung abscess in a 28-year-old

farmer who had no underlying chronic illness.

Although the patient described here initially improved with amphotericin B treatment, it is not certain that his terminal course was due to respiratory failure from a persistent candidal pneumonia with chronic aspiration through a tracheoesophageal fistula. Even in patients with diffuse pulmonary candidiasis secondary to hematogenous spread, the terminal event has usually been bacterial sepsis. However, given the frequency with which candidal esophagitis occurs in the population of AIDS patients, physicians should be cognizant of the potential for development of a tracheoesophageal fistula and fungal aspiration pneumonia.

REFERENCES

1. Talavera W, Mildvan D: Pulmonary infections in the acquired immunodeficiency syndrome. *Semin Respir Infect* 1986; 1:202–211.
2. Armstrong D, Gold JW, Dryjanksi J, et al: Treatment of infections in patients with the acquired immunodeficiency syndrome. *Ann Intern Med* 1985; 103:738–743.
3. Marchevsky A, Rosen MJ, Chrystal G, et al: Pulmonary complications of the acquired immunodeficiency syndrome: A clinicopathologic study of 70 cases. *Hum Pathol* 1985; 16:659–670.
4. Masur H, Rosen PP, Armstrong D: Pulmonary disease caused by *Candida* species. *Am J Med* 1977; 64:914–925.
5. Obrecht WF Jr, Richter JE, Olympio GA, et al: Tracheoesophageal fistula: A serious complication of infectious esophagitis. *Gastroenterology* 1984; 87:1174–1179.
6. Sehhat S, Hazeghi K, Bajoghli M, et al: Oesophageal moniliasis causing fistula formation and lung abscess. *Thorax* 1976; 31:361–364.

Part V
Appendixes

Appendix 1

Ethical issues involved in the growing AIDS crisis*

The Council on Ethical and Judicial Affairs of the American Medical Association recognizes the growing AIDS crisis as a crucial health problem involving the physician's ethical responsibility to his patients and to society. The House of Delegates adopted Report YY (A-87) of the Board of Trustees which provides excellent guidance for a responsible public policy. As stated therein, AIDS patients are entitled to competent medical service with compassion and respect for human dignity and to the safeguard of their confidences within the constraints of the law. Those persons who are afflicted with the disease or who are seropositive have the right to be free from discrimination.

A physician may not ethically refuse to treat a patient whose condition is within the physician's current realm of competence solely because the patient is seropositive. The tradition of the American Medical Association, since its organization in 1847, is that: "when an epidemic prevails, a physician must continue his labors without regard to the risk to his own health." (See Principles of Medical Ethics, 1847, 1903, 1912, 1947, 1955). That tradition must be maintained. A person who is afflicted with AIDS needs competent, compassionate treatment. Neither those who have the disease nor those who have been infected with the virus should be subjected to discrimination based on fear or prejudice, least of all by members of the health care community. Physicians should respond to the best of their abilities in cases of emergency where first aid treatment is essential, and physicians should not abandon patients whose care they have undertaken. (See Section 8.10 of Current Opinions of the Council on Ethical and Judicial Affairs of the American Medical Association, 1986).

Principle VI of the 1980 Principles of Medical Ethics states that "A physician shall in the provision of appropriate patient care, except in emergencies, be free to choose whom to serve, with whom to associate and the environment in which to provide medical services." The Council has always interpreted this Principle as not supporting illegal or invidious discrimination. (See Section 9.11 of Current Opinions, 1986). Thus, it is the view of the Council that Principle VI does not permit categorical discrimination against a patient based solely on his or her seropositivity. A physician who is not able to provide the services required by persons with AIDS should make an appropriate referral to those physicians or facilities that are equipped to provide such services.

At its 1987 Annual Meeting, the House of Delegates adopted Substitute Resolution 18 which asked the Council on Ethical and Judicial Affairs to address "the patient confidentiality and ethical issues raised by known HIV antibody positive patients who refuse to inform their sexual partners or modify their behavior." Physicians have a responsibility to prevent the spread of contagious diseases, as well as an ethical obligation to recognize the rights to privacy and to confidentiality of the AIDS victim. These rights are absolute until they infringe in a material way on the safety of another person or persons. Those who are not infected with the virus are entitled to protection from transmission of the disease. Thus, the societal need for accurate information and public health surveillance must also be respected. As the Board of Trustees stated in Report YY (A-87), "A sound epidemiologic understanding of the potential impact of AIDS on society requires the reporting [on an anonymous or confidential basis to public health authorities] of those who are confirmed as testing positive for the antibody to the AIDS virus."

In those jurisdictions in which the reporting of individuals infected with the AIDS virus to public health authorities is not mandated, a physician who knows that a seropositive patient is endangering a third party faces a dilemma. The physician should attempt to persuade the infected individual to refrain from activities that might result in further transmission of the disease. When rational persuasion fails, authorities should be notified so that they can take appropriate measures to protect third parties. Ordinarily, this action will fulfill the physician's duty to warn third parties; in unusual circumstances when all else fails, a physician may have a common law duty to warn endangered third parties. However, notification of any third party, including public authorities without the consent of the patient may be precluded by statutes in certain states. Therefore, the Council reiterates and strongly endorses Recommendations 16 and 17 of Board Report YY (A-87). They are:

Recommendation 16:

Specific statutes must be drafted which, while protecting to the greatest extent possible the confidentiality of patient information, (a) provide a method for warning unsuspecting sexual partners, (b) protect physicians from liability for failure to warn the unsuspecting third party but, (c) establish clear standards for when a physician should inform the public health authorities, and (d) provide clear guidelines for public health authorities who need to trace the unsuspecting sexual partners of the infected person.

Recommendation 17:

Given the risk of infection being transmitted sexually, and given the dire potential consequences of transmission, serious consideration should be given to sanctions, at least in circumstances where an unsuspecting sexual partner subsequently finds out about a partner's infection and brings a complaint to the attention of authorities. Pre-emptive sanctions are not being endorsed by this recommendation.

The civil rights and liberties of those who are infected with the AIDS virus, as well as those who are not, are entitled to protection. The ethical challenge to the medical profession is to maintain a judicious balance in this regard, including the issue of whether physicians who are HIV-infected must inform their patients or whether they may continue in patient care at all. The Council's new opinion on PHYSICIANS AND INFECTIOUS DISEASES is:

---

* Reproduced from a report of the American Medical Association's Council on Ethical and Judicial Affairs, Report A (I-87). Chicago, American Medical Association, 1987. The Council of the Medical Society of the State of New York has endorsed this report.

A physician who knows that he or she has an infectious disease should not engage in any activity that creates a risk of transmission of the disease to others.

In the context of the AIDS crisis, the application of the Council's opinion depends on the activity in which the physician wishes to engage.

The Council on Ethical and Judicial Affairs reiterates and reaffirms the AMA's strong belief that AIDS victims and those who are seropositive should not be treated unfairly or suffer from discrimination. However, in the special context of the provision of medical care, the Council believes that if a risk of transmission of an infectious disease from a physician to a patient exists, disclosure of that risk to patients is not enough; patients are entitled to expect that their physicians will not increase their exposure to the risk of contracting an infectious disease, even minimally. If no risk exists, disclosure of the physician's medical condition to his or her patients will serve no rational purpose; if a risk does exist, the physician should not engage in the activity. The Council recommends that the afflicted physician disclose his or her condition to colleagues who can assist in the individual assessment of whether the physician's medical condition or the proposed activity poses any risk to patients. There may be an occasion when a patient who is fully informed of the physician's condition and the risks that condition presents may choose to continue his or her care with the seropositive physician. Great care must be exercised to assure that true informed consent is obtained.

In summary, the Council on Ethical and Judicial Affairs believes that:

• A physician may not ethically refuse to treat a patient whose condition is within the physician's current realm of competence solely because the patient is seropositive. Persons who are seropositive should not be subjected to discrimination based on fear or prejudice.

• Physicians are dedicated to providing competent medical service with compassion and respect for human dignity.

• Physicians who are unable to provide the services required by AIDS patients should make referrals to those physicians or facilities equipped to provide such services.

• Physicians are ethically obligated to respect the rights of privacy and of confidentiality of AIDS patients and seropositive individuals.

• Where there is no statute that mandates or prohibits the reporting of seropositive individuals to public health authorities and a physician knows that a seropositive individual is endangering a third party, the physician should: (1) attempt to persuade the infected patient to cease endangering the third party; (2) if persuasion fails, notify authorities; and (3) if the authorities take no action, notify the endangered third party.

• A physician who knows that he or she is seropositive should not engage in any activity that creates a risk of transmission of the disease to others.

• A physician who has AIDS or who is seropositive should consult colleagues as to which activities the physician can pursue without creating a risk to patients.

Appendix 2
Counseling patients about the prevention of AIDS*

The Food and Drug Administration (FDA) is urging that physicians and other health professionals help educate patients about ways to prevent the spread of human immunodeficiency virus (HIV). It should be stressed to patients that because acquired immunodeficiency syndrome (AIDS) is a sexually transmitted disease (STD), sexual abstinence or a mutually monogamous relationship with an uninfected partner is the best insurance against acquiring the disease (except when one partner is an intravenous drug abuser, in which case mutual monogamy offers no protection).

CONDOMS

For sexually active persons, the only instance when condoms are unnecessary for reduction of infection risk is within a long-standing, mutually monogamous relationship in which neither partner uses IV drugs and neither partner is infected with HIV. This applies to any sexual activity where the exchange of semen and/or blood is possible, including vaginal, anal, and oral sex.

Recent studies reported in the press have indicated that natural membrane condoms are not able to contain—and, therefore, are unable to protect against infection from—the HIV virus.

Therefore, FDA allows only latex condoms to be labeled for the prevention of STDs, including AIDS.

Because the diameter of the HIV virus is about 1/25th that of spermatozoa, there was initially some question about whether condoms could contain the virus. Subsequently, however, in vitro tests of latex condoms at the University of California at San Francisco[1] and epidemiologic data[2,3] confirmed that the HIV virus does not pass through an intact latex condom.

To maximize protection against STDs, it is important that condoms be used properly. FDA sent a letter to all US condom manufacturers, importers, and repackagers regarding the labeling of condoms for prevention of STDs. The letter stated that only latex condoms could be labeled for the prevention of STDs, including AIDS. FDA does not allow natural membrane condoms to be so labeled because they have a different permeability than latex and may not lend themselves to the same degree of uniformity. However, regardless of the product's labeling and composition, FDA requested that all condoms contain adequate instructions for use to maximize the degree of protection they afford.

The Agency suggested the following as an acceptable labeling statement for latex condoms:

When used properly, the latex condom may prevent the transmission of many sexually transmitted diseases (STDs) such as syphilis, gonorrhea, chlamydial infections, genital herpes, and AIDS. It cannot eliminate the risk. *For maximum protection, it*

---

* This material is reprinted from the *FDA Drug Bulletin*, September 1987. The Council of the Medical Society of the State of New York has approved the content of this publication on the recommendation of the society's Committee on Preventive Medicine.

is important to follow the accompanying instructions. Failure to do so may result in loss of protection. During intimate contact, lesions and various body fluids can transmit STDs. Therefore, the condom should be applied before any such contact.

In its letter to manufacturers, FDA provided the following example as an acceptable set of instructions:

- Use a condom every time you have sexual intercourse or other acts between partners which involve contact with the penis.
- Put the condom on after the penis is erect and prior to intimate contact, because lesions, pre-ejaculate secretions, semen, vaginal secretions, saliva, urine, and feces can contain sexually transmitted disease (STD) organisms.
- Place the condom on the head of the penis and unroll or pull it all the way to the base.
- Leave an empty space at the end of the condom to collect the semen. Remove any air remaining in the tip of the condom by gently pressing the air out towards the base of the penis.
- If a lubricant is desired, use water-based lubricants such as ———. *Do not use oil-based lubricants,* such as those made with petroleum jelly, mineral oil, vegetable oil, or cold cream, as these may damage the condom.
- After ejaculation, carefully withdraw the penis while it is still erect. Hold onto the rim of the condom as you withdraw so that the condom does not slip off.
- Store condoms in a cool, dark, dry place.
- If the rubber material is sticky or brittle, discolored, or obviously damaged, do not use it.
- Do not reuse condoms.

INFORMATIONAL MATERIALS

Government and private agencies have developed a number of informational materials that health professionals may want to have on hand to help answer patients' questions.

Up to 50 free copies of the following materials, produced jointly by the US Public Health Service (PHS) and the American Red Cross, can be obtained from AIDS, Suite 700, 1555 Wilson Blvd, Rosslyn, VA 22209:

- Poster featuring Patti LaBelle with Toll-free AIDS hot line number.
- Leaflets:

  AIDS, Sex and You

  Facts About AIDS and Drug Abuse

  AIDS and Your Job—Are There Risks?

  Gay and Bisexual Men and AIDS

AIDS and Children—Information for Parents of School Age Children

AIDS and Children—Information for Teachers and School Officials

Caring for the AIDS Patient at Home

If your Test for Antibody to the AIDS Virus is Positive. . .

In addition, PHS has developed the following materials:

- Surgeon General's Report on AIDS (October 1986) from AIDS, PO Box 14252, Washington, DC 20004 (up to 50 free copies)
- Facts About AIDS from AIDS, Suite 700, 1555 Wilson Blvd, Rosslyn, VA 22209 (up to 50 free copies)

Up to 25 free copies of the following scriptographic booklets are available from the Office of Public Inquiries, CDC, Bldg 1, Room B-63, 1600 Clifton Rd, Atlanta, GA 30333:

- What Everyone Should Know About AIDS (also available in Spanish)
- Why You Should Be Informed About AIDS (for health care workers)
- What Gay and Bisexual Men Should Know About AIDS
- AIDS and Shooting Drugs

The following videotapes may be purchased for $55 each from the National Audiovisual Center, 8700 Edgeworth Dr, Capitol Heights, MD 20743-3701; Attn: Customer Service. They may also be borrowed free from Modern Talking Picture Service, 5000 Park St North, St Petersburg, FL 33709; Attn: Film Scheduling:

- AIDS: Fears and Facts (for the general public)
- What If the Patient Has AIDS? (for health care workers)
- AIDS and Your Job (for policemen, firemen, and other emergency personnel)

Practitioners may want to inform patients of the number of the AIDS toll-free national hot line: (1-800) 342-AIDS, and may want to check with the local health department regarding local hot lines.

REFERENCES

1. Conant M, et al: Condoms prevent transmission of AIDS-associated retrovirus [letter]. *JAMA* 1986; 255:1706.

2. Fischl MA, et al: Evaluation of heterosexual partners, children, and household contacts of adults with AIDS. *JAMA* 1987; 257:640-644.

3. Mann J, et al: Condom use and HIV infection among prostitutes in Zaire [letter]. *N Engl J Med* 1987; 316:345.

Appendix 3
Guidelines for effective school health education to prevent the spread of AIDS*

INTRODUCTION

Since the first cases of acquired immunodeficiency syndrome (AIDS) were reported in the United States in 1981, the human immunodeficiency virus (HIV) that causes AIDS and other HIV-related diseases has precipitated an epidemic unprecedented in modern history. Because the virus is transmitted almost exclusively by behavior that individuals can modify, educational programs to influence relevant behavior can be effective in preventing the spread of HIV.[1-5]

The guidelines below have been developed to help school personnel and others plan, implement, and evaluate educational efforts to prevent unnecessary morbidity and mortality associated with AIDS and other HIV-related illnesses. The guidelines incorporate principles for AIDS education that were developed by the President's Domestic Policy Council and approved by the President in 1987 (see Appendix I).

The guidelines provide information that should be considered by persons who are responsible for planning and implementing appropriate and effective strategies to teach young people about how to avoid HIV infection. The guidelines should not be construed as rules, but rather as a source of guidance. Although they specifically were developed to help school personnel, personnel from other organizations should consider these guidelines in planning and carrying out effective education about AIDS for youth who do not attend school and who may be at high risk of becoming infected. As they deliberate about the need for and content of AIDS education, educators, parents, and other concerned members of the community should consider the prevalence of behavior that increases the risk of HIV infection among young people in their communities. Information about the nature of the AIDS epidemic, and the extent to which young people engage in behavior that increases the risk of HIV infection, is presented in Appendix II.

Information contained in this document was developed by CDC in consultation with individuals appointed to represent the following organizations:

American Academy of Pediatrics
American Association of School Administrators
American Public Health Association
American School Health Association
Association for the Advancement of Health Education
Association of State and Territorial Health Officers
Council of Chief State School Officers
National Congress of Parents and Teachers

National Council of Churches
National Education Association
National School Boards Association
Society of State Directors of Health, Physical Education, Recreation and Dance
US Department of Education
US Food and Drug Administration
US Office of Disease Prevention and Health Promotion

Consultants included a director of health education for a state department of education, a director of curriculum and instruction for a local education department, a health education teacher, a director of school health programs for a local school district, a director of a state health department, a deputy director of a local health department, and an expert in child and adolescent development.

PLANNING AND IMPLEMENTING EFFECTIVE SCHOOL HEALTH EDUCATION ABOUT AIDS

The Nation's public and private schools have the capacity and responsibility to help assure that young people understand the nature of the AIDS epidemic and the specific actions they can take to prevent HIV infection, especially during their adolescence and young adulthood. The specific scope and content of AIDS education in schools should be locally determined and should be consistent with parental and community values.

Because AIDS is a fatal disease and because educating young people about becoming infected through sexual contact can be controversial, school systems should obtain broad community participation to ensure that school health education policies and programs to prevent the spread of AIDS are locally determined and are consistent with community values.

The development of school district policies on AIDS education can be an important first step in developing an AIDS education program. In each community, representatives of the school board, parents, school administrators and faculty, school health services, local medical societies, the local health department, students, minority groups, religious organizations, and other relevant organizations can be involved in developing policies for school health education to prevent the spread of AIDS. The process of policy development can enable these representatives to resolve various perspectives and opinions, to establish a commitment for implementing and maintaining AIDS education programs, and to establish standards for AIDS education program activities and materials. Many communities already have school health councils that include representatives from the aforementioned groups. Such councils facilitate the development of a broad base of community expertise and input, and they enhance the coordination of various activities within the comprehensive school health program.[6]

---

* These guidelines were developed by the United States Public Health Service Centers for Disease Control and are reprinted from *Morbidity and Mortality Weekly Reports* 1988; 37(S-2):1–14. The Council of the Medical Society of the State of New York (MSSNY) has adopted these guidelines as MSSNY policy on the recommendation of the society's Committee on Preventive Medicine.

AIDS education programs should be developed to address the needs and the developmental levels of students and of school-age youth who do not attend school, and to address specific needs of minorities, persons for whom English is not the primary language, and persons with visual or hearing impairments or other learning disabilities. Plans for addressing students' questions or concerns about AIDS at the early elementary grades, as well as for providing effective school health education about AIDS at each grade from late elementary/middle school through junior high/senior high school, including educational materials to be used, should be reviewed by representatives of the school board, appropriate school administrators, teachers, and parents before being implemented.

Education about AIDS may be most appropriate and effective when carried out within a more comprehensive school health education program that establishes a foundation for understanding the relationships between personal behavior and health.[7-9] For example, education about AIDS may be more effective when students at appropriate ages are more knowledgeable about sexually transmitted diseases, drug abuse, and community health. It may also have greater impact when they have opportunities to develop such qualities as decision-making and communication skills, resistance to persuasion, and a sense of self-efficacy and self-esteem. However, education about AIDS should be provided as rapidly as possible, even if it is taught initially as a separate subject.

State departments of education and health should work together to help local departments of education and health throughout the state collaboratively accomplish effective school health education about AIDS. Although all schools in a state should provide effective education about AIDS, priority should be given to areas with the highest reported incidence of AIDS cases.

PREPARATION OF EDUCATION PERSONNEL

A team of representatives including the local school board, parent-teachers associations, school administrators, school physicians, school nurses, teachers, educational support personnel, school counselors, and other relevant school personnel should receive general training about a) the nature of the AIDS epidemic and means of controlling its spread, b) the role of the school in providing education to prevent transmission of HIV, c) methods and materials to accomplish effective programs of school health education about AIDS, and d) school policies for students and staff who may be infected. In addition, a team of school personnel responsible for teaching about AIDS should receive more specific training about AIDS education. All school personnel, especially those who teach about AIDS, periodically should receive continuing education about AIDS to assure that they have the most current information about means of controlling the epidemic, including up-to-date information about the most effective health education interventions available. State and local departments of education and health, as well as colleges of education, should assure that such in-service training is made available to all schools in the state as soon as possible and that continuing in-service and pre-service training is subsequently provided. The local school board should assure that release time is provided to enable school personnel to receive such in-service training.

PROGRAMS TAUGHT BY QUALIFIED TEACHERS

In the elementary grades, students generally have one regular classroom teacher. In these grades, education about AIDS should be provided by the regular classroom teacher because that person ideally should be trained and experienced in child development, age-appropriate teaching methods, child health, and elementary health education methods and materials. In ad-

dition, the elementary teacher usually is sensitive to normal variations in child development and aptitudes within a class. In the secondary grades, students generally have a different teacher for each subject. In these grades, the secondary school health education teacher preferably should provide education about AIDS, because a qualified health education teacher will have training and experience in adolescent development, age-appropriate teaching methods, adolescent health, and secondary school health education methods and materials (including methods and materials for teaching about such topics as human sexuality, communicable diseases, and drug abuse). In secondary schools that do not have a qualified health education teacher, faculty with similar training and good rapport with students should be trained specifically to provide effective AIDS education.

PURPOSE OF EFFECTIVE EDUCATION ABOUT AIDS

The principal purpose of education about AIDS is to prevent HIV infection. The content of AIDS education should be developed with the active involvement of parents and should address the broad range of behavior exhibited by young people. Educational programs should assure that young people acquire the knowledge and skills they will need to adopt and maintain types of behavior that virtually eliminate their risk of becoming infected.

School systems should make programs available that will enable and encourage young people who *have not* engaged in sexual intercourse and who *have not* used illicit drugs to continue to—

- Abstain from sexual intercourse until they are ready to establish a mutually monogamous relationship within the context of marriage;
- Refrain from using or injecting illicit drugs.

For young people who *have* engaged in sexual intercourse or who *have* injected illicit drugs, school programs should enable and encourage them to—

- Stop engaging in sexual intercourse until they are ready to establish a mutually monogamous relationship within the context of marriage;
- Stop using or injecting illicit drugs.

Despite all efforts, some young people may remain unwilling to adopt behavior that would virtually eliminate their risk of becoming infected. Therefore, school systems, in consultation with parents and health officials, should provide AIDS education programs that address preventive types of behavior that should be practiced by persons with an increased risk of acquiring HIV infection. These include:

- Avoiding sexual intercourse with anyone who is known to be infected, who is at risk of being infected, or whose HIV infection status is not known;
- Using a latex condom with spermicide if they engage in sexual intercourse;
- Seeking treatment if addicted to illicit drugs;
- Not sharing needles or other injection equipment;
- Seeking HIV counseling and testing if HIV infection is suspected.

State and local education and health agencies should work together to assess the prevalence of these types of risk behavior, and their determinants, over time.

CONTENT

Although information about the biology of the AIDS virus, the signs and symptoms of AIDS, and the social and economic costs of the epidemic might be of interest, such information is not the essential knowledge that students must acquire in order to prevent becoming infected with HIV. Similarly, a single film, lecture, or school assembly about AIDS will not be sufficient to assure that students develop the complex understanding and skills they will need to avoid becoming infected.

Schools should assure that students receive at least the essential information about AIDS, as summarized in sequence in the following pages, for each of three grade-level ranges. The exact grades at which students receive this essential information should be determined locally, in accord with community and parental values, and thus may vary from community to community. Because essential information for students at higher grades requires an understanding of information essential for students at lower grades, secondary school personnel will need to assure that students understand basic concepts before teaching more advanced information. Schools simultaneously should assure that students have opportunities to learn about emotional and social factors that influence types of behavior associated with HIV transmission.

Early Elementary School. Education about AIDS for students in early elementary grades principally should be designed to allay excessive fears of the epidemic and of becoming infected.

AIDS is a disease that is causing some adults to get very sick, but it does not commonly affect children.

AIDS is very hard to get. You cannot get it just by being near or touching someone who has it.

Scientists all over the world are working hard to find a way to stop people from getting AIDS and to cure those who have it.

Late Elementary/Middle School. Education about AIDS for students in late elementary/middle school grades should be designed with consideration for the following information.

Viruses are living organisms too small to be seen by the unaided eye.

Viruses can be transmitted from an infected person to an uninfected person through various means.

Some viruses cause disease among people.

Persons who are infected with some viruses that cause disease may not have any signs or symptoms of disease.

AIDS (an abbreviation for acquired immunodeficiency syndrome) is caused by a virus that weakens the ability of infected individuals to fight off disease.

People who have AIDS often develop a rare type of severe pneumonia, a cancer called Kaposi's sarcoma, and certain other diseases that healthy people normally do not get.

About 1 to 1.5 million of the total population of approximately 240 million Americans currently are infected with the AIDS virus and consequently are capable of infecting others.

People who are infected with the AIDS virus live in every state in the United States and in most other countries of the world. Infected people live in cities as well as in suburbs, small towns, and rural areas. Although most infected people are adults, teenagers can also become infected. Females as well as males are infected. People of every race are infected, including whites, blacks, Hispanics, Native Americans, and Asian/Pacific Islanders.

The AIDS virus can be transmitted by sexual contact with an infected person; by using needles and other injection equipment that an infected person has used; and from an infected mother to her infant before or during birth.

A small number of doctors, nurses, and other medical personnel have been infected when they were directly exposed to infected blood.

It sometimes takes several years after becoming infected with the AIDS virus before symptoms of the disease appear. Thus, people who are infected with the virus can infect other people—even though the people who transmit the infection do not feel or look sick.

Most infected people who develop symptoms of AIDS only live about 2 years after their symptoms are diagnosed.

The AIDS virus cannot be caught by touching someone who is infected, by being in the same room with an infected person, or by donating blood.

Junior High/Senior High School. Education about AIDS for students in junior high/senior high school grades should be developed and presented taking into consideration the following information.

The virus that causes AIDS, and other health problems, is called human immunodeficiency virus, or HIV.

The risk of becoming infected with HIV can be virtually eliminated by not engaging in sexual activities and by not using illegal intravenous drugs.

Sexual transmission of HIV is not a threat to those uninfected individuals who engage in mutually monogamous sexual relations.

HIV may be transmitted in any of the following ways: a) by sexual contact with an infected person (penis/vagina, penis/rectum, mouth/vagina, mouth/penis, mouth/rectum); b) by using needles or other injection equipment that an infected person has used; c) from an infected mother to her infant before or during birth.

A small number of doctors, nurses, and other medical personnel have been infected when they were directly exposed to infected blood.

The following are at increased risk of having the virus that causes AIDS and consequently of being infectious: a) persons with clinical or laboratory evidence of infection; b) males who have had sexual intercourse with other males; c) persons who have injected illegal drugs; d) persons who have had numerous sexual partners, including male or female prostitutes; e) persons who received blood clotting products before 1985; f) sex partners of infected persons or persons at increased risk; and g) infants born to infected mothers.

The risk of becoming infected is increased by having a sexual partner who is at increased risk of having contracted the AIDS virus (as identified previously), practicing sexual behavior that results in the exchange of body fluids (ie, semen, vaginal secretions, blood), and using unsterile needles or paraphernalia to inject drugs.

Although no transmission from deep, open-mouth (ie, "French") kissing has been documented, such kissing theoretically could transmit HIV from an infected to an uninfected person through direct exposure of mucous membranes to infected blood or saliva.

In the past, medical use of blood, such as transfusing blood and treating hemophiliacs with blood clotting products, has caused some people to become infected with HIV. However, since 1985 all donated blood has been tested to determine whether it is infected with HIV; moreover, all blood clotting products have been made from screened plasma and have been heated to destroy any HIV that might remain in the concentrate. Thus, the risk of becoming infected with HIV from blood transfusions and from blood clotting products is virtually eliminated. Cases of HIV infection caused by these medical uses of blood will continue to be diagnosed, however, among people who were infected by these means before 1985. Persons who continue to engage in sexual intercourse with persons who are at increased risk or whose infection status is unknown should use a latex condom (not natural membrane) to reduce the likelihood of becoming infected. The latex condom must be applied properly and used from start to finish for every sexual act. Although a latex condom does not provide 100% protection—because it is possible for the condom to leak, break, or slip off—it provides the best protection for people who do not maintain a mutually monogamous relationship with an uninfected partner. Additional protection may be obtained by using spermicides that seem active against HIV and other sexually transmitted organisms in conjunction with condoms.

Behavior that prevents exposure to HIV also may prevent unintended pregnancies and exposure to the organisms that cause Chlamydia *infection, gonorrhea, herpes, human papillomavirus, and syphilis.*

Persons who believe they may be infected with the AIDS virus should take precautions not to infect others and to seek counseling and antibody testing to determine whether they are infected. If persons are not infected, counseling and testing can relieve unnecessary anxiety and reinforce the need to adopt or continue practices that reduce the risk of infection. If persons are infected, they should: a) take precautions to protect sexual partners from becoming infected; b) advise previous and current sexual or drug-use partners to receive counseling and testing; c) take precautions against becoming pregnant; and d) seek medical care and counseling about other medical problems that may result from a weakened immunologic system.

More detailed information about AIDS, including information about how to obtain counseling and testing for HIV, can be obtained by telephoning the AIDS National Hotline (toll free) at 800-342-2437; the Sexually Transmitted Diseases National Hotline (toll free) at 800-227-8922; or the appropriate state or local health department (the telephone number of which can be obtained by calling the local information operator).

CURRICULUM TIME AND RESOURCES

Schools should allocate sufficient personnel time and resources to assure that policies and programs are developed and implemented with appropriate community involvement, curricula are well-planned and sequential, teachers are well-trained, and up-to-date teaching methods and materials about AIDS are available. In addition, it is crucial that sufficient classroom time be provided at *each* grade level to assure that students acquire essential knowledge appropriate for that grade level, and have time to ask questions and discuss issues raised by the information presented.

PROGRAM ASSESSMENT

The criteria recommended in the foregoing "Guidelines for Effective School Health Education to Prevent the Spread of AIDS" are summarized in the following nine assessment criteria. Local school boards and administrators can assess the extent to which their programs are consistent with these guidelines by determining the extent to which their programs meet each point shown below. Personnel in state departments of education and health also can use these criteria to monitor the extent to which schools in the state are providing effective health education about AIDS.

1. To what extent are parents, teachers, students, and appropriate community representatives involved in developing, implementing, and assessing AIDS education policies and programs?

2. To what extent is the program included as an important part of a more comprehensive school health education program?

3. To what extent is the program taught by regular classroom teachers in elementary grades and by qualified health education teachers or other similarly trained personnel in secondary grades?

4. To what extent is the program designed to help students acquire essential knowledge to prevent HIV infection at each appropriate grade?

5. To what extent does the program describe the benefits of abstinence for young people and mutually monogamous relationships within the context of marriage for adults?

6. To what extent is the program designed to help teenage students avoid specific types of behavior that increase the risk of becoming infected with HIV?

7. To what extent is adequate training about AIDS provided for school administrators, teachers, nurses, and counselors—especially those who teach about AIDS?

8. To what extent are sufficient program development time, classroom time, and educational materials provided for education about AIDS?

9. To what extent are the processes and outcomes of AIDS education being monitored and periodically assessed?

REFERENCES

1. US Public Health Service: Coolfont report: A PHS plan for prevention and control of AIDS and the AIDS virus. *Public Health Rep* 1986; 101:341.
2. Institute of Medicine, National Academy of Sciences: Confronting AIDS: Directions for public health, health care, and research. Washington, DC, National Academy Press, 1986.
3. US Department of Health and Human Services, Public Health Service: Surgeon General's report on acquired immune deficiency syndrome. Washington, DC, US Department of Health and Human Services, 1986.
4. US Public Health Service: AIDS: Information/education plan to prevent and control AIDS in the United States, March 1987. Washington, DC, US Department of Health and Human Services, 1987.
5. US Department of Education: AIDS and the education of our children, a guide for parents and teachers. Washington, DC, US Department of Education, 1987.
6. Kolbe LJ, Iverson DC: Integrating school and community efforts to promote health: Strategies, policies, and methods. *Int J Health Educ* 1983; 2:40–47.
7. Noak M: Recommendations for school health education. Denver, Education Commission of the States, 1982.
8. Comprehensive school health education as defined by the national professional school health education organizations. *J Sch Health* 1984; 54:312–315.
9. Allensworth D, Kolbe L (eds): The comprehensive school health program: Exploring an expanded concept. *J Sch Health* 1987; 57:402–76.

APPENDIX I
The President's Domestic Policy Council's Principles for AIDS Education

The following principles were proposed by the Domestic Policy Council and approved by the President in 1987:

Despite intensive research efforts, prevention is the only effective AIDS control strategy at present. Thus, there should be an aggressive Federal effort in AIDS education.

The scope and content of the school portion of this AIDS education effort should be locally determined and should be consistent with parental values.

The Federal role should focus on developing and conveying accurate health information on AIDS to the educators and others, not mandating a specific school curriculum on this subject, and trusting the American people to use this information in a manner appropriate to their community's needs.

Any health information developed by the Federal Government that will be used for education should encourage responsible sexual behavior—based on fidelity, commitment, and maturity, placing sexuality within the context of marriage.

Any health information provided by the Federal Government that might be used in schools should teach that children should not engage in sex and should be used with the consent and involvement of parents.

APPENDIX II
The Extent of AIDS and Indicators of Adolescent Risk

Since the first cases of acquired immunodeficiency syndrome (AIDS) were reported in the United States in 1981, the human immunodeficiency virus (HIV) that causes AIDS and other HIV-related diseases has precipitated an epidemic unprecedented in modern history. Although in 1985, fewer than 60% of AIDS cases in the United States were reported among persons residing outside New York City and San Francisco, by 1991 more than 80% of the cases will be reported from other localities.[1]

It has been estimated that from 1 to 1.5 million persons in the United States are infected with HIV,[1] and, because there is no cure, infected persons are potentially capable of infecting others indefinitely. It has been predicted that 20%–30% of individuals currently infected will develop AIDS by the end of 1991.[1] Fifty percent of those diagnosed as having AIDS have not survived for more than about 1.5 years beyond diagnosis, and only about 12% have survived for more than 3 years.[2]

By the end of 1987, about 50,000 persons in the United States had been diagnosed as having AIDS, and about 28,000 had died from the disease.[2] Blacks and Hispanics, who make up about 12% and 6% of the US population, respectively, disproportionately have contracted 25% and 14% of all reported AIDS cases.[3] It has been estimated that during 1991, 74,000 cases of AIDS will be diagnosed, and 54,000 persons will die from the disease. By the end of that year, the total number of deaths caused by AIDS will be about 179,000.[1] In addition, health care and supportive services for the 145,000 persons projected to be living with AIDS in that year will cost our Nation an estimated $8–$10 billion in 1991 alone.[1] The World Health Organization projects that by 1991, 50–100 million persons may be infected worldwide.[4] The magnitude and seriousness of this epidemic requires a systematic and concerted response from almost every institution in our society.

A vaccine to prevent transmission of the virus is not expected to be developed before the next decade, and its use would not affect the number of persons already infected by that time. A safe and effective antiviral agent to treat those infected is not expected to be available for general use within the next several years. The Centers for Disease Control,[5] the National Academy of Sciences,[6] the Surgeon General of the United States,[7] and the US Department of Education[8] have noted that in the absence of a vaccine or therapy, educating individuals about actions they can take to protect themselves from becoming infected is the most effective means available for controlling the epidemic. Because the virus is transmitted almost exclusively as a result of behavior individuals can modify (eg, by having sexual contact with an infected person or by sharing intravenous drug paraphernalia with an infected person), educational programs designed to influence relevant types of behavior can be effective in controlling the epidemic.

A significant number of teenagers engage in behavior that increases their risk of becoming infected with HIV. The percent-age of metropolitan teenage girls who had ever had sexual intercourse increased from 30%–45% between 1971 and 1982. The average age at first intercourse for females remained at approximately 16.2 years between 1971 and 1979.[9] The average proportion of never-married teenagers who have ever had intercourse increases with age from 14 through 19 years. In 1982, the percentage of never-married girls who reported having engaged in sexual intercourse was as follows: approximately 6% among 14-year-olds,[10] 18% among 15-year-olds, 29% among 16-year-olds, 40% among 17-year-olds, 54% among 18-year-olds, and 66% among 19-year-olds.[11] Among never-married boys living in metropolitan areas, the percentage who reported having engaged in sexual intercourse was as follows: 24% among 14-year-olds, 35% among 15-year-olds, 45% among 16-year-olds, 56% among 17-year-olds, 66% among 18-year-olds, and 78% among 19-year-olds.[9,12] Rates of sexual experience (eg, percentage having had intercourse) are higher for black teenagers than for white teenagers at every age and for both sexes.[11,12]

Male homosexual intercourse is an important risk factor for HIV infection. In one survey conducted in 1973, 5% of 13- to 15-year-old boys and 17% of 16- to 19-year-old boys reported having had at least one homosexual experience. Of those who reported having had such an experience, most (56%) indicated that the first homosexual experience had occurred when they were 11 or 12 years old. Two percent reported that they currently engaged in homosexual activity.[13]

Another indicator of high-risk behavior among teenagers is the number of cases of sexually transmitted diseases they contract. Approximately 2.5 million teenagers are affected with a sexually transmitted disease each year.[14]

Some teenagers also are at risk of becoming infected with HIV through illicit intravenous drug use. Findings from a national survey conducted in 1986 of nearly 130 high schools indicated that although overall illicit drug use seems to be declining slowly among high school seniors, about 1% of seniors reported having used heroin and 13% reported having used cocaine within the previous year.[15] The number of seniors who injected each of these drugs is not known.

Only 1% of all the persons diagnosed as having AIDS have been under age 20;[2] most persons in this group had been infected by transfusion or perinatal transmission. However, about 21% of all the persons diagnosed as having AIDS have been 20–29 years of age. Given the long incubation period between HIV infection and symptoms that lead to AIDS diagnosis (3 to 5 years or more), some fraction of those in the 20- to 29-year-age group diagnosed as having AIDS were probably infected while they were still teenagers.

Among military recruits screened in the period October 1985–December 1986, the HIV seroprevalence rate for persons 17–20 years of age (0.6/1,000) was about half the rate for recruits in all age groups (1.5/1,000).[16] These data have led some to conclude that teenagers and young adults have an appreciable risk of infection and that the risk may be relatively constant and cumulative.[17]

Reducing the risk of HIV infection among teenagers is important not only for their well-being but also for the children they might produce. The birth rate for U.S. teenagers is among the highest in the developed world;[18] in 1984, this group accounted for more than 1 million pregnancies. During that year the rate of pregnancy among sexually active teenage girls 15–19 years of age was 233/1,000 girls.[19]

Although teenagers are at risk of becoming infected with and transmitting the AIDS virus as they become sexually active, studies have shown that they do not believe they are likely to become infected.[20,21] Indeed, a random sample of 860 teenagers (ages 16–19) in Massachusetts revealed that, although 70% reported they were sexually active (having sexual intercourse or other sexual contact), only 15% of this group reported changing their sexual behavior because of concern about contracting AIDS. Only 20% of those who changed their behavior selected effective methods such as abstinence or use of condoms.[20] Most teenagers indicated that they want more information about AIDS.[20,21]

Most adult Americans recognize the early age at which youth need to be advised about how to protect themselves from becoming infected with HIV and recognize that the schools can play an important role in providing such education. When asked in a November 1986 nationwide poll whether children should be taught about AIDS in school, 83% of Americans agreed, 10% disagreed, and 7% were not sure.[22] According to information gathered by the United States Conference of Mayors in December of 1986, 40 of the Nation's 73 largest school districts were providing education about AIDS, and 24 more were planning such education.[23] Of the districts that offered AIDS education, 63% provided it in 7th grade, 60% provided it in 9th grade, and 90% provided it in 10th grade. Ninety-eight percent provided medical facts about AIDS, 78% mentioned abstinence as a means of avoiding infection, and 70% addressed the issues of avoiding high-risk sexual activities, selecting sexual partners, and using condoms. Data collected by the National Association of State Boards of Education in the summer of 1987 indicated that a) 15 states had mandated comprehensive school health education; eight had mandated AIDS education; b) 12 had legislation pending on AIDS education, and six had state board of education actions pending; c) 17 had developed curricula for AIDS education, and seven more were developing such materials; and d) 40 had developed policies on admitting students with AIDS to school.[24]

The Nation's system of public and private schools has a strategic role to play in assuring that young people understand the nature of the epidemic they face and the specific actions they can take to protect themselves from becoming infected—especially during their adolescence and young adulthood. In 1984, 98% of 14- and 15-year-olds, 92% of 16- and 17-year-olds, and 50% of 18- and 19-year-olds were in school.[25] In that same year, about 615,000 14- to 17-year-olds and 1.1 million 18- to 19-year-olds were not enrolled in school and had not completed high school.[26]

REFERENCES

1. US Public Health Service: Coolfont report: A PHS plan for prevention and control of AIDS and the AIDS virus. *Public Health Rep* 1986; 101:341.

2. CDC: Acquired immunodeficiency syndrome (AIDS) weekly surveillance report—United States. Cases reported to CDC. December 28, 1987.

3. CDC: Acquired immunodeficiency syndrome (AIDS) among blacks and Hispanics—United States. *MMWR* 1986; 35:655-8, 663-6.

4. World Health Organization: Special program on AIDS: strategies and structure projected needs. Geneva, World Health Organization, 1987.

5. CDC: Results of a Gallup Poll on acquired immunodeficiency syndrome—New York City, United States. *MMWR* 1985; 34:513-4.

6. Institute of Medicine, National Academy of Sciences: Confronting AIDS: Directions for public health, health care, and research. Washington, DC, National Academy Press, 1986.

7. US Department of Health and Human Services, Public Health Service: Surgeon General's report on acquired immune deficiency syndrome. Washington, DC, US Department of Health and Human Services, 1986.

8. US Department of Education: AIDS and the education of our children, a guide for parents and teachers. Washington, DC, US Department of Education, 1987.

9. Zelnick M, Kantner JF: Sexual activity, contraceptive use, and pregnancy among metropolitan-area teenagers: 1971-1979. *Fam Plann Perspect* 1980; 12:230-7.

10. Hofferth SL, Kahn J, Baldwin W: Premarital sexual activity among United States teenage women over the past three decades. *Fam Plann Perspect* 1987; 19:46-53.

11. Pratt WF, Mosher WD, Bachrach CA, et al: Understanding US fertility: Findings from the National Survey of Family Growth, cycle III. *Popul Bull* 1984; 39:1-42.

12. Teenage pregnancy: The problem that hasn't gone away. Tables and References. New York, The Alan Guttmacher Institute, June 1981.

13. Sorensen RC: Adolescent sexuality in contemporary America. New York, World Publishing, 1973.

14. Divison of Sexually Transmitted Diseases, Annual Report, FY 1986. Center for Prevention Services, Centers for Disease Control, US Public Health Service, 1987.

15. Johnston LD, Bachman JG, O'Malley PM: Drug use among American high school students, college, and other young adults: National trends through 1986. Rockville, Md, National Institute on Drug Abuse, 1987.

16. CDC: Trends in human immunodeficiency virus infection among civilian applicants for military service—United States, October 1985-December 1986. *MMWR* 1987; 36:273-6.

17. Burke DS, Brundage JF, Herbold JR, et al: Human immunodeficiency virus infections among civilian applicants for United States military service, October 1985 to March 1986. *N Engl J Med* 1987; 317:131-6.

18. Jones EF, Forrest JD, Goldman N, et al: Teenage pregnancy in developed countries: determinants and policy implications. *Fam Plann Perspect* 1985; 17:53-63.

19. National Research Council. Risking the future: Adolescent sexuality, pregnancy, and childbearing (vol 1). Washington, DC, National Academy Press, 1987.

20. Strunin L, Hingson R: Acquired immunodeficiency syndrome and adolescents: Knowledge, beliefs, attitudes, and behaviors. *Pediatrics* 1987; 79:825-8.

21. DiClemente RJ, Zorn J, Temoshok L: Adolescents and AIDS: A survey of knowledge, attitudes, and beliefs about AIDS in San Francisco. *Am J Public Health* 1986; 76:1443-5.

22. Yankelovich Clancy Shulman: Memorandum to all data users from Hal Quinley about Time/Yankelovich Clancy Shulman Poll findings on sex education, November 17, 1986. New York City, Yankelovich Clancy Shulman, 1986.

23. United States Conference of Mayors: Local school districts active in AIDS education. *AIDS Information Exchange* 1987; 4:1-10.

24. Cashman J: Personal communication on September 8, 1987, about the National Association of State Boards of Education survey of state AIDS-related policies and legislation. Washington, DC, National Association of State Boards of Education.

25. US Department of Commerce, Bureau of the Census: Statistical abstract of the United States, 105th ed. Washington, DC, US Department of Commerce, 1985.

26. US Department of Commerce, Bureau of the Census: School enrollment—Social and economic characteristics of students: October 1984. Current Population Reports. Washington, DC, US Department of Commerce, 1985 (Series P-20, No. 404).

Appendix 4

Public Health Service guidelines for counseling and antibody testing to prevent HIV infection and AIDS*

These guidelines are the outgrowth of the 1986 recommendations published in the *MMWR*;[1] the report on the February 24–25, 1987, Conference on Counseling and Testing;[2] and a series of meetings with representatives from the Association of State and Territorial Health Officials, the Association of State and Territorial Public Health Laboratory Directors, the Council of State and Territorial Epidemiologists, the National Association of County Health Officials, the United States Conference of Local Health Officers, and the National Association of State Alcohol and Drug Abuse Directors.

Human immunodeficiency virus (HIV), the causative agent of acquired immunodeficiency syndrome (AIDS) and related clinical manifestations, has been shown to be spread by sexual contact; by parenteral exposure to blood (most often through intravenous [IV] drug abuse) and, rarely, by other exposures to blood; and from an infected woman to her fetus or infant.

Persons exposed to HIV usually develop detectable levels of antibody against the virus within 6–12 weeks of infection. The presence of antibody indicates current infection, though many infected persons may have minimal or no clinical evidence of disease for years. Counseling and testing persons who are infected or at risk for acquiring HIV infection is an important component of prevention strategy.[1] Most of the estimated 1.0 to 1.5 million infected persons in the United States are unaware that they are infected with HIV. The primary public health purposes of counseling and testing are to help uninfected individuals initiate and sustain behavioral changes that reduce their risk of becoming infected and to assist infected individuals in avoiding infecting others.

Along with the potential personal, medical, and public health benefits of testing for HIV antibody, public health agencies must be concerned about actions that will discourage the use of counseling and testing facilities, most notably the unauthorized disclosure of personal information and the possibility of inappropriate discrimination.

Priorities for public health counseling and testing should be based upon providing ready access to persons who are most likely to be infected or who practice high-risk behaviors, thereby helping to reduce further spread of infection. There are other considerations for determining testing priorities, including the likely effectiveness of preventing the spread of infection among persons who would not otherwise realize that they are at risk. Knowledge of the prevalence of HIV infection in different populations is useful in determining the most efficient and effective locations providing such services. For example, programs that offer counseling and testing to homosexual men, IV-drug abusers, persons with hemophilia, sexual and/or needle-sharing partners of these persons, and patients of sexually transmitted dis-

ease clinics may be most effective since persons in these groups are at high risk for infection. After counseling and testing are effectively implemented in settings of high and moderate prevalence, consideration should be given to establishing programs in settings of lower prevalence.

INTERPRETATION OF HIV-ANTIBODY TEST RESULTS

A test for HIV antibody is considered positive when a sequence of tests, starting with a repeatedly reactive enzyme immunoassay (EIA) and including an additional, more specific assay, such as a Western blot, are consistently reactive.

The *sensitivity* of the currently licensed EIA tests is 99% or greater when performed under optimal laboratory conditions. Given this performance, the probability of a false-negative test result is remote, except during the first weeks after infection, before antibody is detectable.

The *specificity* of the currently licensed EIA tests is approximately 99% when repeatedly reactive tests are considered. Repeat testing of specimens initially reactive by EIA is required to reduce the likelihood of false-positive test results due to laboratory error. To further increase the specificity of the testing process, laboratories must use a supplemental test—most often the Western blot test—to validate repeatedly reactive EIA results. The sensitivity of the licensed Western blot test is comparable to that of the EIA, and it is highly specific when strict criteria are used for interpretation. Under ideal circumstances, the probability that a testing sequence will be falsely positive in a population with a low rate of infection ranges from less than 1 in 100,000 (Minnesota Department of Health, unpublished data) to an estimated 5 in 100,000.[3,4] Laboratories using different Western blot reagents or other tests or using less stringent interpretive criteria may experience higher rates of false-positive results.

Laboratories should carefully guard against human errors, which are likely to be the most common source of false-positive test results. All laboratories should anticipate the need for assuring quality performance of tests for HIV antibody by training personnel, establishing quality controls, and participating in performance evaluation systems. Health department laboratories should facilitate the quality assurance of the performance of laboratories in their jurisdiction.

GUIDELINES FOR COUNSELING AND TESTING FOR HIV ANTIBODY

These guidelines are based on public health considerations for HIV testing, including the principles of counseling before and after testing, confidentiality of personal information, and the understanding that a person may decline to be tested without being denied health care or other services, except where testing is required by law.[5] Counseling before testing may not be practical when screening for HIV antibody is required. This is true for donors of blood, organs, and tissue; prisoners; and immigrants

---

* These guidelines were developed by the United States Public Health Service Centers for Disease Control and are reprinted from *Morbidity and Mortality Weekly Report* 1987; 36:509–514. The Council of the Medical Society of the State of New York (MSSNY) has adopted these guidelines as MSSNY policy on the recommendation of the society's Committee for Preventive Medicine.

for whom testing is a Federal requirement as well as for persons admitted to state correctional institutions in states that require testing. When there is no counseling before testing, persons should be informed that testing for HIV antibody will be performed, that individual results will be kept confidential to the extent permitted by law, and that appropriate counseling will be offered. Individual counseling of those who are either HIV-antibody positive or at continuing risk for HIV infection is critical for reducing further transmission and for ensuring timely medical care.

Specific recommendations follow:

1. *Persons who may have sexually transmitted disease.* All persons seeking treatment for a sexually transmitted disease, in all health-care settings including the offices of private physicians, should be routinely* counseled and tested for HIV antibody.

2. *IV-drug abusers.* All persons seeking treatment for IV-drug abuse or having a history of IV-drug abuse should be routinely counseled and tested for HIV antibody. Medical professionals in all health-care settings, including prison clinics, should seek a history of IV-drug abuse from patients and should be aware of its implications for HIV infection. In addition, state and local health policy makers should address the following issues:

   • Treatment programs for IV-drug abusers should be sufficiently available to allow persons seeking assistance to enter promptly and be encouraged to alter the behavior that places them and others at risk for HIV infection.

   • Outreach programs for IV-drug abusers should be undertaken to increase their knowledge of AIDS and of ways to prevent HIV infection, to encourage them to obtain counseling and testing for HIV antibody, and to persuade them to be treated for substance abuse.

3. *Persons who consider themselves at risk.* All persons who consider themselves at risk for HIV infection should be counseled and offered testing for HIV antibody.

4. *Women of childbearing age.* All women of childbearing age with identifiable risks for HIV infection should be routinely counseled and tested for HIV antibody, regardless of the health-care setting. Each encounter between a health-care provider and a woman at risk and/or her sexual partners is an opportunity to reach them with information and education about AIDS and prevention of HIV infection. Women are at risk for HIV infection if they:

   • Have used IV drugs.

   • Have engaged in prostitution.

   • Have had sexual partners who are infected or are at risk for infection because they are bisexual or are IV-drug abusers or hemophiliacs.

   • Are living in communities or were born in countries where there is a known or suspected high prevalence of infection among women.

   • Received a transfusion before blood was being screened for HIV antibody but after HIV infection occurred in the United States (e.g., between 1978 and 1985).

Educating and testing these women before they become pregnant allows them to avoid pregnancy and subsequent intrauterine perinatal infection of their infants (30%-50% of the infants born to HIV-infected women will also be infected).

All pregnant women at risk for HIV infection should be routinely counseled and tested for HIV antibody. Identifying

---

* "Routine counseling and testing" is defined as a policy to provide these services to all clients after informing them that testing will be done. Except where testing is required by law, individuals have the right to decline to be tested without being denied health care or other services.

pregnant women with HIV infection as early in pregnancy as possible is important for ensuring appropriate medical care for these women; for planning medical care for their infants; and for providing counseling on family planning, future pregnancies, and the risk of sexual transmission of HIV to others.

All women who seek family planning services and who are at risk for HIV infection should be routinely counseled about AIDS and HIV infection and tested for HIV antibody. Decisions about the need for counseling and testing programs in a community should be based on the best available estimates of the prevalence of HIV infection and the demographic variables of infection.

5. *Persons planning marriage.* All persons considering marriage should be given information about AIDS, HIV infection, and the availability of counseling and testing for HIV antibody. Decisions about instituting routine or mandatory premarital testing for HIV antibody should take into account the prevalence of HIV infection in the area and/or population group as well as other factors and should be based upon the likely cost-effectiveness of such testing in preventing further spread of infection. Premarital testing in an area with a prevalence of HIV infection as low as 0.1% may be justified if reaching an infected person through testing can prevent subsequent transmission to the spouse or prevent pregnancy in a woman who is infected.

6. *Persons undergoing medical evaluation or treatment.* Testing for HIV antibody is a useful diagnostic tool for evaluating patients with selected clinical signs and symptoms such as generalized lymphadenopathy; unexplained dementia; chronic, unexplained fever or diarrhea; unexplained weight loss; or diseases such as tuberculosis as well as sexually transmitted diseases, generalized herpes, and chronic candidiasis.

Since persons infected with both HIV and the tubercle bacillus are at high risk for severe clinical tuberculosis, all patients with tuberculosis should be routinely counseled and tested for HIV antibody.[6] Guidelines for managing patients with both HIV and tuberculous infection have been published.[7]

The risk of HIV infection from transfusions of blood or blood components from 1978-1985 was greatest for persons receiving large numbers of units of blood collected from areas with high incidences of AIDS. Persons who have this increased risk should be counseled about the potential risk of HIV infection and should be offered antibody testing.[8]

7. *Persons admitted to hospitals.* Hospitals, in conjunction with state and local health departments, should periodically determine the prevalence of HIV infections in the age groups at highest risk for infection. Consideration should be given to routine testing in those age groups deemed to have a high prevalence of HIV infection.

8. *Persons in correctional systems.* Correctional systems should study the best means of implementing programs for counseling inmates about HIV infection and for testing them for such infection at admission and discharge from the system. In particular, they should examine the usefulness of these programs in preventing further transmission of HIV infection and the impact of the testing programs on both the inmates and the correctional system.[9] Federal prisons have been instructed to test all prisoners when they enter and leave the prison system.

9. *Prostitutes.* Male and female prostitutes should be counseled and tested and made aware of the risks of HIV infection to themselves and others. Particularly prostitutes who are HIV-antibody positive should be instructed to discontinue the practice of prostitution. Local or state jurisdictions should adopt procedures to assure that these instructions are followed.

PARTNER NOTIFICATION/CONTACT TRACING

Sexual partners and those who share needles with HIV-infected persons are at risk for HIV infection and should be routinely counseled and tested for HIV antibody. Persons who are HIV-antibody positive should be instructed in how to notify their partners and to refer them for counseling and testing. If they are unwilling to notify their partners or if it cannot be assured that their partners will seek counseling, physicians or health department personnel should use confidential procedures to assure that the partners are notified.

CONFIDENTIALITY AND ANTIDISCRIMINATION CONSIDERATIONS

The ability of health departments, hospitals, and other health-care providers and institutions to assure confidentiality of patient information and the public's confidence in that ability are crucial to efforts to increase the number of persons being counseled and tested for HIV infection. Moreover, to assure broad participation in the counseling and testing programs, it is of equal or greater importance that the public perceive that persons found to be positive will not be subject to inappropriate discrimination.

Every reasonable effort should be made to improve confidentiality of test results. The confidentiality of related records can be improved by a careful review of actual record-keeping practices and by assessing the degree to which these records can be protected under applicable state laws. State laws should be examined and strengthened when found necessary. Because of the wide scope of "need-to-know" situations, because of the possibility of inappropriate disclosures, and because of established authorization procedures for releasing records, it is recognized that there is no perfect solution to confidentiality problems in all situations. Whether disclosures of HIV-testing information are deliberate, inadvertent, or simply unavoidable, public health policy needs to carefully consider ways to reduce the harmful impact of such disclosures.

Public health prevention policy to reduce the transmission of HIV infection can be furthered by an expanded program of counseling and testing for HIV antibody, but the extent to which these programs are successful depends on the level of participation. Persons are more likely to participate in counseling and testing programs if they believe that they will not experience negative consequences in areas such as employment, school admission, housing, and medical services should they test positive. There is no known medical reason to avoid an infected person in these and ordinary social situations since the cumulative evidence is strong that HIV infection is not spread through casual contact. It is essential to the success of counseling and testing programs that persons who are tested for HIV are not subjected to inappropriate discrimination.

REFERENCES

1. CDC: Additional recommendations to reduce sexual and drug abuse-related transmission of human T-lymphotropic virus type III/lymphadenopathy-associated virus. *MMWR* 1986; 35:152-5.
2. CDC: Recommended additional guidelines for HIV antibody counseling and testing in the prevention of HIV infection and AIDS. Atlanta, Georgia, US Department of Health and Human Services, Public Health Service, 1987.
3. Burke DS, Brandt BL, Redfield RR, et al: Diagnosis of human immunodeficiency virus infection by immunoassay using a molecularly cloned and expressed virus envelope polypeptide. *Ann Intern Med* 1987; 106:671-6.
4. Meyer KB, Pauker SG: Screening for HIV: Can we afford the false positive rate? *N Engl J Med* 1987; 317:238-41.
5. Bayer R, Levine C, Wolf SM: HIV antibody screening: an ethical framework for evaluating proposed programs. *JAMA* 1986; 256:1768-74.
6. CDC: Tuberculosis provisional data—United States, 1986. *MMWR* 1987; 36:254-5.
7. CDC: Diagnosis and management of mycobacterial infection and disease in persons with human T-lymphotropic virus type III/lymphadenopathy-associated virus infection. *MMWR* 1986; 35:448-52.
8. CDC: Human immunodeficiency virus infection in transfusion recipients and their family members. *MMWR* 1987; 36:137-40.
9. Hammett TM: AIDS in correctional facilities: issues and options. 2nd ed. Washington, DC, US Department of Justice, National Institute of Justice, 1987.

Appendix 5
Immunizations for children with HIV infections*

Addressing theoretical concerns that vaccination with live, attenuated vaccine viruses may produce serious adverse events in symptomatic HIV-infected children, and that antigenic stimulation might lead to a deterioration of clinical status of HIV-infected children,[1,2] the Immunization Practices Advisory Committee (ACIP) has established recommendations for immunizations of HIV-infected children in the United States.

The complete recommendations were published in the *MMWR* of Sept 26, 1986.[3] The following is a summary of the recommendations for oral polio vaccine (OPV), inactivated polio vaccine (IPV), and vaccines for measles, mumps, and rubella (MMR), bacille Calmette-Guérin (BCG), diphtheria, pertussis, and tetanus (DPT), haemophilus influenzae type B (Hib), influenza, and pneumococcus.

CHILDREN WITH SYMPTOMATIC HIV INFECTIONS

- *OPV, MMR, BCG* and other live vaccines should not be given to children and young adults who are immunosuppressed as a manifestation of HIV infection. These persons should receive IPV and should be excused for medical reasons from regulations requiring measles, rubella, and/or mumps immunization.

- *DPT, IPV, Hib*: The potential benefits of immunization outweigh the theoretical concerns that stimulation of the immune system by immunization with inactivated vaccines might cause deterioration in immune function. Such effects have not been noted thus far among children with AIDS or other immunosuppressed individuals. Immunization with DTP, IPV, and Hib vaccines is recommended, although immunization may be less effective than in immunocompetent children.

- *Flu, pneumococcal vaccines*: As with other conditions producing immunosuppression, annual immunization with inactivated influenza vaccine is recommended for children over 6 months of age, and one-time administration of pneumococcal vaccine is recommended for children over 2 years of age.

- *Immune globulins*: As with other immunosuppressed patients, children with clinical manifestations of HIV infection may be at increased risk of having serious complications of infectious diseases such as measles and varicella and therefore, following significant exposure to these diseases, should receive passive immunization with immune globulin or varicella-zoster immune globulin, respectively.

CHILDREN WITH PREVIOUSLY DIAGNOSED ASYMPTOMATIC HIV INFECTION

- *MMR*: Pending further data, it is recommended that these children be vaccinated with MMR and followed for possible adverse reactions and for the occurrence of vaccine-preventable diseases, since immunization may be less effective than for other children.

- *OPV*: Available data suggest that OPV can be administered without adverse consequences to HIV-infected children who do not have overt clinical manifestations of immunosuppression. However, because family members may be immunocompromised due to HIV infection, it may be prudent to use IPV routinely to immunize these children.

- *DTP, Hib*: Immunization with DTP and Hib vaccines in accordance with ACIP recommendations is recommended.

CHILDREN RESIDING IN THE HOUSEHOLD OF A PATIENT WITH AIDS

- *OPV*: Children living with others known to be immunocompromised due to AIDS or other HIV infections should not receive OPV because they would be likely to excrete vaccine viruses that would be communicable to their immunosuppressed family members.

- *MMR*: MMR may be given to such a child because extensive experience has shown that live, attenuated MMR vaccine viruses are not transmitted from vaccinated individuals to others.

REFERENCES

1. ACIP: General recommendations on immunization. *MMWR* 1983; 32:1–8, 13–17.
2. Zagury D, et al: Long-term cultures of HTLV-III-infected T-cells: a model of cytopathology of T-cell depletion in AIDS. *Science* 1986; 231:850–853.
3. ACIP: Immunization of children infected with Human T-Lymphotropic Virus Type III/Lymphadenopathy-Associated Virus. *MMWR* 1986; 35:595–598, 603–606.

---

* This material is reprinted from the *FDA Drug Bulletin*, September 1987. The Council of the Medical Society of the State of New York (MSSNY) has approved the content of this publication on the recommendation of the society's Committee on Preventive Medicine.

Appendix 6
Immunization of children infected with human immunodeficiency virus—supplementary ACIP statement*

The Immunization Practices Advisory Committee (ACIP) recently reviewed data both on the risks and benefits of immunizing children infected with human immunodeficiency virus (HIV)[1] and on severe and fatal measles in HIV-infected children in the United States.[2] Since this review, the committee has revised its previous recommendations for measles vaccination and for mumps and rubella vaccination.

Previously published ACIP statements on immunizing HIV-infected children have recommended vaccinating children with asymptomatic HIV infection, but not those with symptomatic HIV infection.[3] After considering reports of severe measles in symptomatic HIV-infected children, and in the absence of reports of serious or unusual adverse effects of measles, mumps, and rubella (MMR) vaccination in limited studies of symptomatic patients,[4,5] the committee feels that administration of MMR vaccine should be considered for all HIV-infected children, regardless of symptoms. This approach is consistent with the World Health Organization's recommendation for measles vaccination.[6]

If the decision to vaccinate is made, symptomatic HIV-infected children should receive MMR vaccine at 15 months, the age currently recommended for vaccination of children without HIV infection and for those with asymptomatic HIV infection. When there is an increased risk of exposure to measles, such as during an outbreak, these children should receive vaccine at younger ages. At such times, infants six to 11 months of age should receive monovalent measles vaccine and should be revaccinated with MMR at 12 months of age or older. Children 12–14 months of age should receive MMR and do not need revaccination.[7]

The use of high-dose intravenous immune globulin (IGIV) (approximately 5 gm% protein) administered at regular intervals is being studied to determine whether it will prevent a variety of infections in HIV-infected children. It should be recognized that MMR vaccine may be ineffective if administered to a child who has received IGIV during the preceding three months.

Immune globulin (IG) (16.5 gm% protein) can be used to prevent or modify measles infection in HIV-infected children if administered within six days of exposure. IG is indicated for measles-susceptible[†] household contacts of children with asymptomatic HIV infection, particularly for those under one year of age and for measles-susceptible pregnant women. The recommended dose is 0.25 mL/kg intramuscularly (maximum dose, 15 mL).[7]

In contrast, exposed symptomatic HIV-infected patients should receive IG prophylaxis regardless of vaccination status. The standard postexposure measles prophylaxis regimen for such patients is 0.5 mL/kg of IG intramuscularly (maximum dose, 15 mL).[7] This regimen corresponds to a dose of protein of approximately 82.5 mg/kg (maximum dose, 2,475 mg). Intra-

muscular IG may not be necessary if a patient with HIV infection is receiving 100–400 mg/kg IGIV at regular intervals and received the last dose within three weeks of exposure to measles. Based on the amount of protein that can be administered, high-dose IGIV may be as effective as IG given intramuscularly. However, no data exist on the efficacy of IGIV administered postexposure in preventing measles.

Although postexposure administration of globulins to symptomatic HIV-infected patients is recommended regardless of measles vaccine status, vaccination prior to exposure is desirable. Measles exposures are often unrecognized, and postexposure prophylaxis is not always possible.

While recommendations for MMR vaccine have changed, those for other vaccines have not.[3] A summary of the current ACIP recommendations for HIV-infected persons follows (Table I). These recommendations apply to adolescents and adults with HIV infection as well as to HIV-infected children.

TABLE I. Recommendations for Routine Immunization of HIV-Infected Children—United States, 1988*

| Vaccine | HIV Infection | |
	Known Asymptomatic	Symptomatic
DTP[†]	yes	yes
OPV[§]	no	no
IPV[¶]	yes	yes
MMR**	yes	yes[††]
HbCV[§§]	yes	yes
Pneumococcal	no	yes
Influenza	no	yes

* See accompanying text and previous ACIP statement[3] for details.
† DTP = Diphtheria and tetanus toxoids and pertussis vaccine.
§ OPV = Oral, attenuated poliovirus vaccine; contains poliovirus types 1, 2, and 3.
¶ IPV = Inactivated poliovirus vaccine; contains poliovirus types 1, 2, and 3.
** MMR = Live measles, mumps, and rubella viruses in a combined vaccine.
†† Should be considered.
§§ HbCV = *Haemophilus influenzae* type b conjugate vaccine.

REFERENCES

1. Von Reyn CF, Clements CJ, Mann JM: Human immunodeficiency virus infection and routine childhood immunisation. *Lancet* 1987; 2:669–672.
2. Centers for Disease Control: Measles in HIV-infected children—United States. *MMWR* 1988; 37:183–186.
3. Immunization Practices Advisory Committee: Immunization of children infected with human T-lymphotropic virus type III/lymphadenopathy-associated virus. *MMWR* 1986; 35:595–598, 603–606.
4. McLaughlin P, Thomas PA, Onorato I, et al: Use of live virus vaccines in HIV-infected children: A retrospective survey. *Pediatrics* (in press).
5. Krasinski K, Borkowsky W, Krugman S: Antibody following measles immunization in children infected with human T-cell lymphotropic virus-type III/lymphadenopathy associated virus (HTLV-III/LAV) [Abstract], In *Program and Abstracts of the International Conference on Acquired Immunodeficiency Syndrome.* Paris, France, June 23–25, 1986.
6. Global Advisory Group, World Health Organization: Expanded programme on immunization. *Wkly Epidem Rec* 1987; 62:5–9.
7. Immunization Practices Advisory Committee: Measles prevention. *MMWR* 1987; 36:409–418, 423–425.

* These guidelines are reprinted from *Morbidity and Mortality Weekly Reports* 1988; 37:181–183. The prior Immunization Practices Advisory Committee recommendations for immunization of HIV-infected children were published in the May 1988 issue of the *Journal*.
† Persons who are unvaccinated or do not have laboratory evidence or physician documentation of previous measles disease.[7]

Index